OXFORD MEDICAL PUBLICATIONS

**Preventive medicine
in general practice**

OXFORD GENERAL PRACTICE SERIES

Editorial Board
G. H. FOWLER, J. A. M. GRAY,
J. C. HASLER, A.-L. KINMOUTH,
D. C. MORRELL

1. Paediatric problems in general practice
   M. Modell and R. D. H. Boyd
2. Geriatric problems in general practice
   G. K. Wilcock, J. A. M. Gray, and P. M. M. Pritchard
3. Preventive medicine in general practice
   edited by J. A. M. Gray and G. H. Fowler
4. Women's problems in general practice
   edited by A. McPherson and A. Anderson
5. Locomotor disorders in general practice
   edited by M. I. V. Jayson and R. Million

In preparation
   Management in general practice
   P. M. M. Pritchard, K. B. Low, and M. Whalen
   Chronic disease in general practice
   edited by J. C. Hasler and T. P. C. Schofield
   The consultation: an approach to learning and teaching
   D. A. Pendleton, P. H. L. Tate, P. B. Havelock, and T. P. C. Schofield

Preventive medicine in general practice

Oxford General Practice Series 3

Edited by

MUIR GRAY
Community Physician, Oxfordshire Health Authority

and

GODFREY FOWLER
General Practitioner; Clinical Reader in General Practice, University of Oxford

OXFORD   NEW YORK   TOKYO
OXFORD UNIVERSITY PRESS

Oxford University Press, Walton Street, Oxford OX2 6DP
Oxford New York Toronto
Delhi Bombay Calcutta Madras Karachi
Petaling Jaya Singapore Hong Kong Tokyo
Nairobi Dar es Salaam Cape Town
Melbourne Auckland
and associated companies in
Beirut Berlin Ibadan Nicosia

Oxford is a trade mark of Oxford University Press

© Muir Gray and Godfrey Fowler, 1983

First published 1983
Reprinted 1985, 1986

All rights reserved. No part of this publication may be reproduced, stored in
a retrieval system, or transmitted, in any form or by any means, electronic,
mechanical, photocopying, recording, or otherwise, without the prior
permission of Oxford University Press

This book is sold subject to the condition that it shall not, by way
of trade or otherwise, be lent, re-sold, hired out or otherwise circulated
without the publisher's prior consent in any form of binding or cover
other than that in which it is published and without a similar condition
including this condition being imposed on the subsequent purchaser

British Library Cataloguing in Publication Data
Preventive medicine in general practice.—(Oxford
general practice series; 3).—(Oxford medical
publications)
1. Medicine. Preventive—Great Britain
I. Gray, Muir II. Fowler, Godfrey
362.1'72'0941 RA485
ISBN 0-19-261299-9

Library of Congress Cataloging in Publication Data
Main entry under title:
Preventive medicine in general practice.
(Oxford general practice series; 3)
Bibliography: p.
Includes index.
1. Family medicine. 2. Medicine, Preventive.
I. Gray, J. A. Muir (John Anthony Armstrong Muir)
II. Fowler, Godfrey. III. Series. [DNLM:
1. Preventive medicine. 2. Family practice. W1
OX55 no. 3/WA 108 P94553]
R729.5.G4P734 1983 613 82–18920
ISBN 0-19-261299-9 (pbk.)

Printed and bound in Great Britain by
Biddles Ltd, Guildford and King's Lynn

Foreword

by

John Horder
Formerly President, Royal College of General Practitioners

Prevention is an old and obvious principle but during the last half century those who have advocated it as a way of thinking and acting in medicine have been small, neglected voices. Pharmacology and surgery have brought success after success to the care and cure of established diseases. Their effective use calls for earlier and earlier diagnosis and for case-finding when patients come to the doctor about something else.

But today we find that effective treatment in some parts of medicine has exposed other parts in which a new sort of exploration is needed. Sir George Young, when at the Ministry of Health, described it well: 'If you look at most of the big killer diseases today, they are not caused by Nature, but by our way of life. I am thinking particularly of cancer, heart attack, stroke and road accidents. For these illnesses and injuries medicine has at best cures which are expensive and partly successful, at worst no cure at all. The answer is not cure, but prevention.'

Sir George was pointing to the responsibility of politicians, but what he says applies just as much to doctors, since success in prevention depends on influencing both public opinion and the beliefs and behaviour of individuals.

Doctors as a group have set an outstanding example in this country, demonstrating how one single change in behaviour can achieve a dramatic reduction in their own chances of early death and premature disability.

Yet each general practitioner's list of patients includes 40 per cent who still smoke cigarettes. The great majority claim that they want to stop. How can we understand their individual beliefs and difficulties, help them towards the same sense of responsibility for their own futures, convince them it can be done? Does our relationship with them give us any special opportunities? Would this be as valuable a use of limited time as the way in which we use it now?

The campaign against cigarettes promises the most significant gains, even if we each achieve only 25 long-term successes each year. What are the other worthwhile targets? Can the health visitors and nurses share the tasks? Who will organize? What limited experiments will provide the figures, graphs, and histograms that will reveal success and add another form of satisfaction to the traditional one of seeing an individual recover from an illness?

These are the sort of questions which the writers of this book attack.

This book is the product of two editors who practise what they preach – a community physician trained to think of populations and a general practitioner trained to think of individuals. It gives practical advice whenever the evidence is beyond dispute; where this is not yet so, the issues are discussed. I see it above all as a challenge to general practitioners to make experiments and explorations at an advancing boundary of their work. What a chance for relating the community physician not only to the practitioner but to every member of the primary care team in a wide choice of important common tasks!

Preface

This book is aimed primarily at general practitioners – established principals and trainees. We have tried to provide useful information for those who see the potential contribution of the general practitioner in the face of the epidemic of behaviourally determined disease which characterizes developed societies in the final decades of the twentieth century. It reviews the evidence for preventive policies, makes recommendations for actions, and provides guidelines for achievement. Although directed mainly at general practitioners it should also interest many others, notably the health visitor, hitherto perhaps the only health professional with an acknowledged educational role, district nurse, the practice nurse, health education officer, and the community physician.

But the general practitioner remains the key to preventive medicine. In helping patients to stop smoking it has been suggested on the basis of good research work that the general practitioners – if they tried – could be as effective as ten thousand anti-smoking clinics. One million consultations a day offers immense scope for the type of preventive medicine which is required in the twentieth century.

Oxford   M.G.
April 1982   G.F.

Acknowledgements

Many colleagues have contributed to the preparation of this book. In particular we should like to mention Paddy McCarthy, Gills McKay, Theo Schofield, John Howie, Elizabeth Fanshawe, and Sarah Lomas who made valuable comments on sections of the text. Rosemary Lees and Maggie Dennis deserve a special vote of thanks for coping with the typing and collation of the references as pleasantly, helpfully, and efficiently as they cope with all the problems that we set them.

Contents

List of contributors   xi

Part I: Principles of prevention

1. The scope of preventive medicine
   Muir Gray and Godfrey Fowler   3
2. Opportunities for prevention in general practice
   Godfrey Fowler and Muir Gray   20
3. Record systems in preventive medicine
   Alastair Tulloch   33
4. Patient education in general practice
   Simon Smail   56
5. Obstacles to prevention
   Muir Gray   70
6. The politics of prevention – the scope for individual action
   Michael Daube and Muir Gray   86
7. Screening
   Godfrey Fowler   94
8. Resources for prevention
   Godfrey Fowler, Muir Gray, Max Blythe, and Elaine Fullard   117

Part II: Practising prevention

9. Smoking
   Godfrey Fowler   133
10. Diet
    Jim Mann   149
11. Exercise
    Archie Young   160
12. Alcohol
    Peter Anderson   180
13. Mental illness
    Gordon Lennox   208
14. Accident prevention
    Muir Gray   229
15. Prevention of disability and handicap
    Muir Gray   243

x   *Contents*

16. Prevention in old age
    Muir Gray   257
17. The future of preventive medicine in general practice
    Godfrey Fowler and Muir Gray   275
Index   285

Contributors

Peter Anderson
Formerly General Practitioner, Oxford. Trainee in Community Medicine.

Max Blythe
Formerly Director, Oxfordshire Health Education Unit,
Principal, Davies, Long and Dick Sixth Form College, London, W2.

Michael Daube
Senior Lecturer, Department of Community Medicine, University of Edinburgh.

Godfrey Fowler
General Practitioner, Oxford, and Clinical Reader in General Practice,
University of Oxford.

Elaine Fullard
Formerly Health Visitor, Oxford.
Project Director, Oxford Heart Attack and Stroke Prevention Project.

Muir Gray
Community Physician, Oxfordshire Health Authority.

Gordon Lennox
General Practitioner, Didcot, and Tutor in General Practice,
University of Oxford.

Sue Lousley
Chief Dietician, Radcliffe Infirmary, Oxford.

Jim Mann
University Lecturer in Social and Community Medicine, University of Oxford.

Simon Smail
General Practitioner, Cardiff, and Senior Lecturer in General Practice,
Welsh National School of Medicine.

Alistair Tulloch
General Practitioner, Bicester, and Research Assistant, Unit of Clinical Epidemiology,
University of Oxford.

Archie Young
Clinical Lecturer and Honorary Consultant Physician, Nuffield Departments of
Orthopaedic Surgery and Clinical Medicine, University of Oxford.

Part I

Principles of prevention

1 The scope of preventive medicine

Muir Gray and Godfrey Fowler

The expectations of life of men and women probably increased by no more than a small amount from prehistoric times until the middle of the nineteenth century. There were periods when the expectation of life must have decreased, during the Black Death for example, and other times when it increased more rapidly than the average, but the general trend has been a very slow increase in average life span.

The reasons for the improvement before the nineteenth century are not clear but it was certainly not due to the development of effective cures and it can therefore be concluded that the reason that the expectation of life increased was because certain causes of death were prevented. However, it seems likely that the prevention of disease was not the result of any conscious attempt at prevention, although there were many of them. Some, such as the forty-day quarantine, a term derived from the Italian *quaranta* meaning forty, were based on the scientific theories of the day; some were magical; some were religious; and some represented an amalgam of scientific, magical, and religious ideas about disease which is not surprising because science, magic, and religion were all intimately related to one another. A few of these measures may have had some effect, for example the Jewish proscription of pork may have prevented trichinosis, but it is probable that their effectiveness owed as much to chance as to scientific reasoning, that is to say the reasons that the pig was selected as being unclean was not because it harboured *Trichinella* but for some other reason. Almost all these measures were completely ineffective and some were actually harmful (Cipolla 1962).

There are many aspects of the decline in mortality during this epoch which have not been explained, for example the reasons why leprosy and plague vanished from Europe are not understood. However, it is now generally agreed that one important reason for the decline in mortality in the period before 1850 was that food supplies became more plentiful and more stable. There were lean years of course; for example there were epidemics of typhus in 1718, 1728, and 1741, each following a bad harvest, and another great epidemic in 1846–8 following the Irish Potato Famine, but improvements in agriculture and the growth of trade improved and stabilized food supplies. The policies which achieved these improvements and all other related politices such as the development of powerful armies and navies to guard trade routes and the aquisition of colonies can therefore be classified as policies which prevented disease, although that was not their objective at that time (McNeill 1976).

THE GREAT LEAP FORWARD

Our data are much more dependable for the latter half of the nineteenth century, because registration of births and deaths was introduced in 1838, and during this period there was a dramatic reduction in mortality (Fig. 1.1).

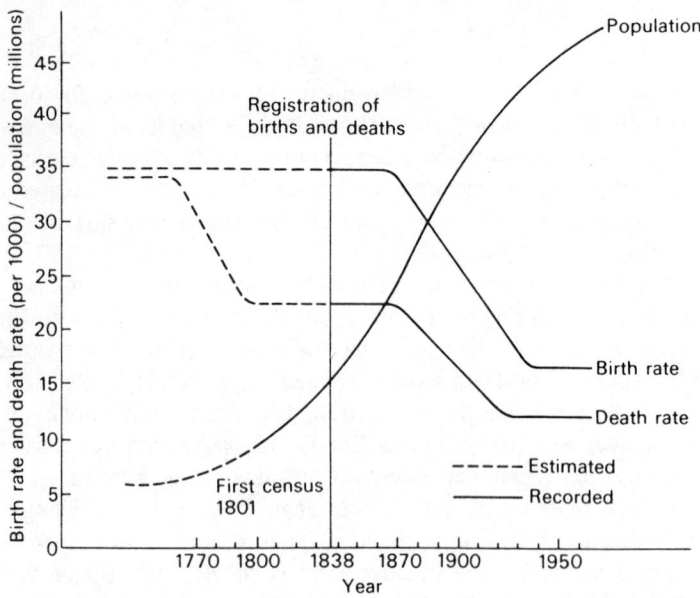

Fig. 1.1. Population, birth rate, and death rate: England and Wales. (From McKeown and Lowe (1974).)

Thomas McKeown has argued that a decline in tuberculosis mortality was responsible for nearly one half of the total drop; a decrease in typhus and typhoid mortality for about one fifth; a decrease in scarlet fever deaths for another fifth; a decrease in those from cholera, dysentry, and diarrhoea for one tenth; and a decline in smallpox deaths for one twentieth. Only in the case of smallpox was a preventive measure which focused on the individual important; for the rest of these diseases the decrease can be attributed to environmental changes which affected the whole community, namely the provision of pure water, the disposal of sewage, the provision of better housing and a further improvement in nutrition (McKeown 1979). However, these were only the tools of prevention. The real reason why the incidence of these diseases declined was that there were a number of social changes which made the necessary legislation for environmental improvement acceptable to the majority. One change was the growth of scientific knowledge in the nineteenth century, although it must be emphasized that the bacterial transmission of disease was not clearly understood until some decades after the most important laws had been passed, but there were many other relevant trends in nineteenth century society. Philanthropy and paternalism became more important philosophies, the latter fostered to some degree by the need to have a healthy work force. Secondly, poor people became more articulate and rich people became very afraid of some of the diseases, particularly of cholera which spread from the insalubrious conditions of the nineteenth-century city. Finally, Britain became wealthy enough to implement the changes which Parliament deemed necessary.

Prevention in the nineteenth century required Government action, legislation, and this legislation improved the quality of life of the majority of the people who enjoyed clean safe water, better working conditions, freedom from offensive smells, and other 'nuisances'. That is not to say there was no opposition to preventive medicine in the nineteenth century. On the contrary, there was vociferous and vehement opposition both to vaccination and to environmental improvement, not so much because of the measures involved, which were in themselves generally welcomed, but because they were imposed by law and because they increased the power of central government (Gray 1979).

In developed countries in the twentieth century the causes of death and disease and therefore the scope for preventive medicine are different.

THE SCOPE FOR PREVENTION TODAY

In a paper published in 1975 Sir Douglas Black and J. D. Pole, a health economist, set out the burden on services that different diseases caused (Black and Pole 1975). They chose five separate indices of burden and tried to assess how much of a burden each of the common types of disease created for society. Their analysis can be criticized for it does not include obesity, diabetes, or alcohol misuse as causes of burden, neither does it include disability (see p. 241) as a category of burden though there is scope for prevention of all these major problems. Nevertheless it provides a very useful summary of the burden of different diseases and a basis for considering the scope for prevention (Table 1.1).

Prevention of mortality

The prevention of cardiovascular disease

The scope for prevention of death from ischaemic heart disease and other forms of cardiovascular disease appears to be considerable. The most dramatic evidence of this for people working in the United Kingdom is offered by a comparison of its mortality rates with the mortality rates in America and Australia (Fig. 1.2).

It has been estimated that if the rates in the United Kingdom had declined as quickly as in America there would be a decline of 25 000 deaths every year and the secular changes in mortality in many other countries show how much scope there is for prevention and how much prevention has already occurred (Fig. 1.3).

6 The scope of preventive medicine

Table 1.1. *Rank order of categories of disease, according to five types of burden.*

For each list, a double line is drawn below the conditions which cause 50 per cent of the total burden. Under each list is given the percentage of total burden accounted for by the conditions listed; and the percentage of total burden due to causes other than classifiable disease, described as 'unaccounted burden'.

	Percentage of total burden
1. *Inpatient days*	
Mental illness	31.31
Mental handicap	15.19
Cerebrovascular disease	4.86
Malignant neoplasma	4.18
Digestive disorders	3.80
Child-birth	3.69
Accidents and suicide	3.44
Peripheral vascular disease	2.43
Neurological disorders	2.14
Ischaemic heart disease	2.11
Other cardiac diseases	2.06
Cumulative burden of ranked categories	75.21
'Unaccounted burden.	6.31
2. *Outpatient referrals*	
Neurological disorders	9.82
Accidents and suicide	7.84
Bone and joint disease (other than arthritis)	6.87
Digestive disorders	6.72
Skin diseases	5.90
Urogenital disease	5.50
Mental disorders	3.96
Arthritis and rheumatism	3.72
Peripheral vascular disease	3.70
Respiratory infections	3.70
Bronchitis and asthma	3.63
Cumulative burden of ranked categories	61.36
'Unaccounted burden'	17.32
3. *GP consultations*	
Respiratory infections	16.03
Mental disorders	7.73
Bronchitis and asthma	5.07
Skin diseases	4.84
Accidents and suicide	4.63
Digestive disorders	4.05
Arthritis and rheumatism	3.99
'Other heart disease'	3.06
'Other bone and joint disease'	2.79
Ischaemic heart disease	2.63
Ear diseases	2.60
Hypertension	2.48
Neoplasms	2.40
Peripheral vascular disease	2.25
Neurological disorders	2.00
Cumulative burden of ranked categories	66.55
'Unaccounted burden'	15.94

4.	Days of sickness benefits	
	Bronchitis and asthma	11.46
	Mental disease	9.55
	Accidents and suicide	8.81
	Arthritis and rheumatism	7.22
	Respiratory infections	7.17
	Ischaemic heart disease	5.73
	Digestive disorders	5.73
	Neurological disorders	5.16
	'Other bone and joint disease'	3.64
	Other respiratory disease	2.82
	Hypertension	2.56
	Peripheral vascular disease	2.36
	Cumulative burden of ranked categories	72.21
	'Unaccounted burden'	10.27
5.	Mortality (loss of life expectancy)	
	Ischaemic heart disease	21.51
	Neoplasms	20.63
	Cerebrovascular disease	10.68
	'Other cardiovascular disease'	8.74
	Respiratory infections	7.11
	Accidents and suicide	6.51
	Bronchitis and asthma	4.10
	Peripheral vascular disease	3.39
	Congenital anomalies	3.17
	Digestive disorders	2.48
	'Other respiratory disease'	1.54
	Neurological disorders	1.41
	Hypertension	1.30
	Rheumatic heart disease	1.27
	Cumulative burden of ranked categories	93.84
	'Unaccounted burden'	5.54

From Black and Pole (1975).

The reason why ischaemic heart disease is declining more in some countries than in others is not fully understood. From the epidemiological evidence available a number of risk factors have been identified which are known to be risk factors for ischaemic heart disease (Table 1.2).

The same factors are associated with atherosclerosis in other parts of the body, although cigarette smoking is relatively more important in comparison with other risk factors in the development of this disease.

The prevention of stroke

The scope for the prevention of stroke also seems to be considerable. The decline in America has been dramatic but there has been an even greater decline in other countries (Fig. 1.4).

The Working Party on the Prevention of Arterial Disease set up by the Royal College of General Practitioners concluded that 'about half of all strokes and a

8   The scope of preventive medicine

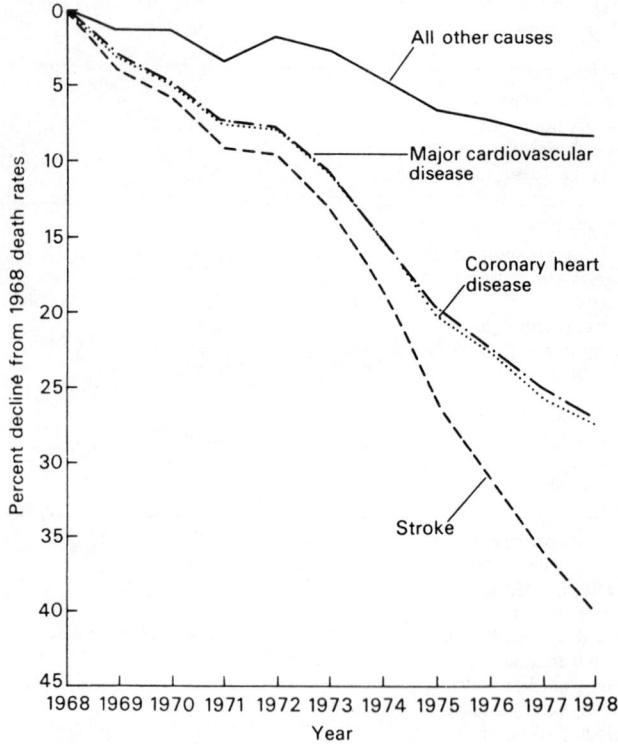

Fig. 1.2. Trends in cardiovascular disease and all other causes of mortality: decline by age-adjusted death rates, ages 35–74, 1968–1978, United States. (US Department of Health and Human Services 1981.)

quarter of all deaths from coronary heart disease in people under 70 are probably preventable by the application of existing knowledge' (RCGP 1981) and the main means of prevention of stroke is the detection and control of high blood pressure (see p. 99). The Americans have been successful – we have not.

The prevention of cancer

Four types of cancer are responsible for more than half of all cancer deaths – cancers of the lung, breast, large intestine, and stomach – and there is good evidence that these cancers are largely preventable.

The evidence is firstly that the onset rates of lung cancer and stomach cancer have changed dramatically in almost all developed countries – in many countries lung cancer rates have doubled and stomach cancer rates have halved every 20 to 30 years.

Secondly, for all four types of cancer there are great differences in the incidence recorded in different countries.

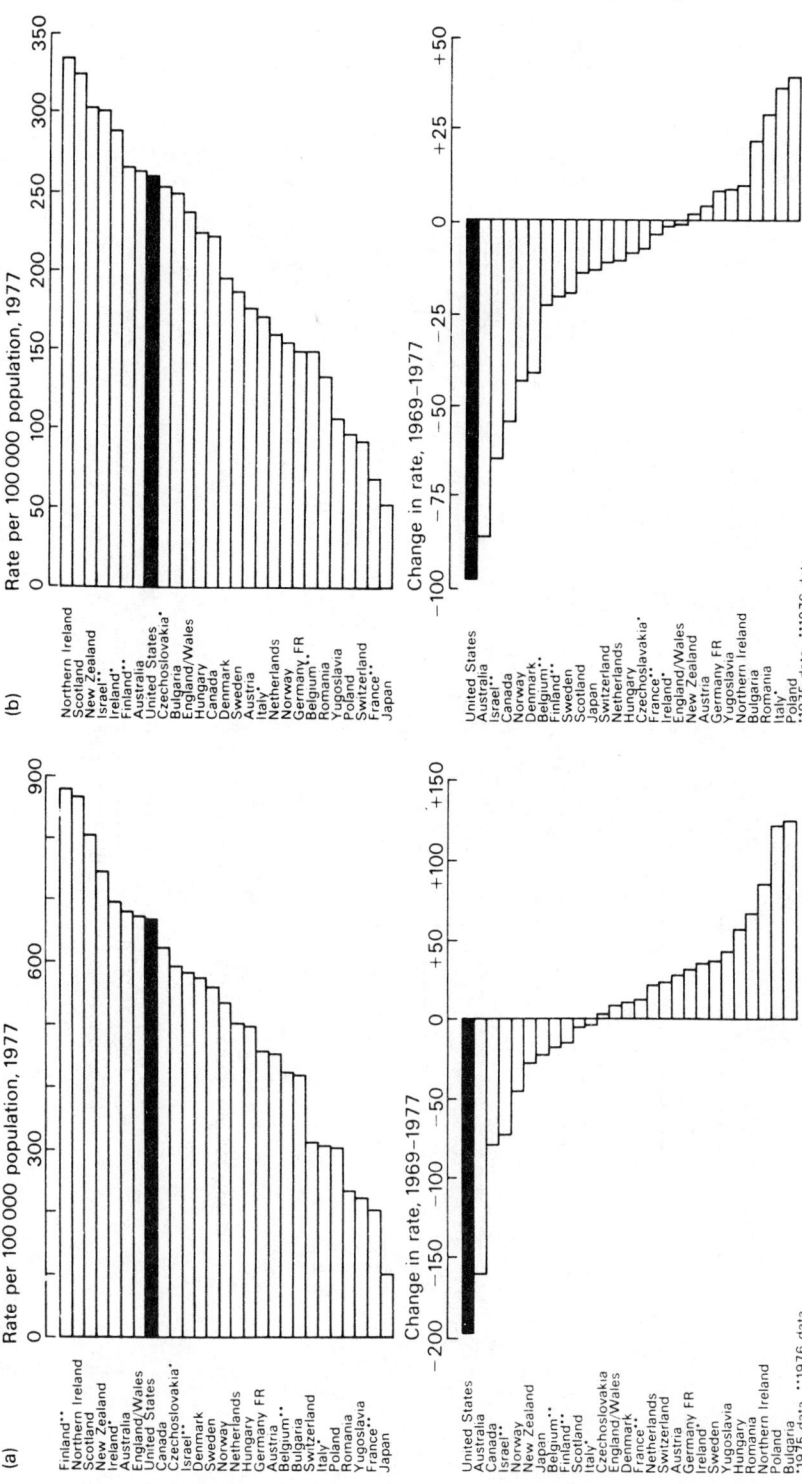

Fig. 1.3. (a) Death rate for coronary heart disease by country. (a) Men 35–74 years of age. (b) Women 35–74 years of age. (From National Heart, Lung and Blood Institute (1981).).

10 *The scope of preventive medicine*

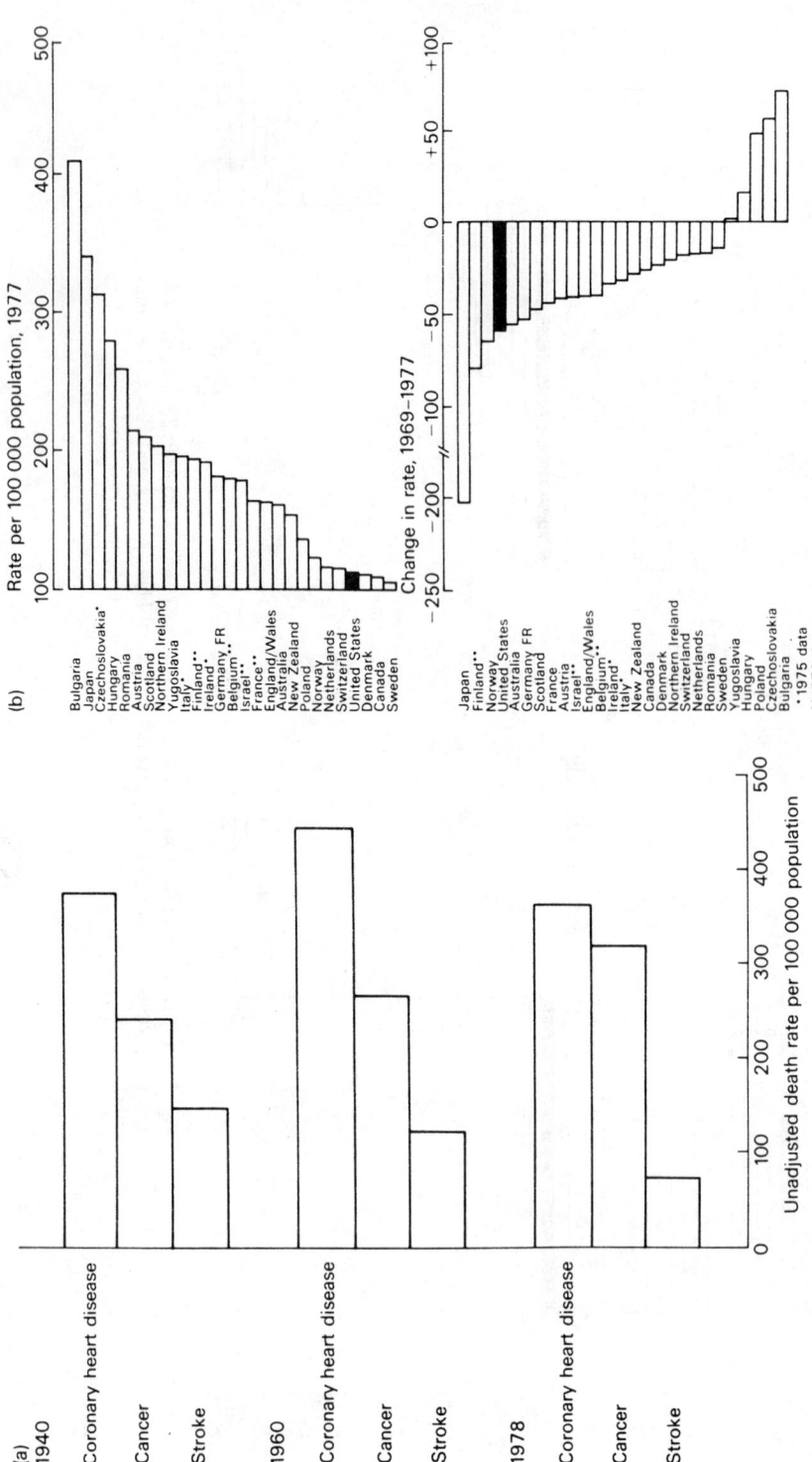

Fig. 1.4. (a) Mortality rates for three leading causes of death; ages 35–74; United States; 1940, 1960, 1978. (b) Death rates for cerebrovascular disease by country; men 35–74 years of age. (From National Heart, Lung and Blood Institute (1981).)

Table 1.2. *Risk factors for coronary heart disease*

	Characteristic	Effect on the risk of coronary heart disease
Principal risk factors	Smoking (cigarettes)	The greater the amount smoked currently, the greater the risk
	Blood pressure	The higher the pressure the greater the risk
	Blood cholesterol	The greater the concentration the greater the risk
	Diabetes	People with diabetes have a higher risk
	Family history	The longer parents live, the less the risk for their children
	Obesity	Being overweight *may* increase the risk (unproven)
	Stress	Stress *may* increase the risk (unproven)
	Personality	Some types *may* be more prone than others (unproven)
	Physical activity	The less exercise customarily taken, the greater *may* be the risk (unproven)
	Hardness of tap water	The softer the tap water the greater *may* be the risk (unproven)

Note: In most cases of coronary heart disease it is likely that more than one factor is present. Only the first three characteristics given below have been shown to operate as risk factors independently of others. A combination of factors is likely to increase the risk.
From Department of Health and Social Security (1981). *Avoiding heart attacks*. DHSS, London.

Thirdly, where it has been possible to study the incidence of cancer in migrants it has been shown that they develop cancer at rates more similar to the rates that prevail in the population they join than the rates which prevail in the genetically related population they have left.

On such evidence Sir Richard Doll and Richard Peto have calculated that about 90 per cent of lung cancer and 80 to 90 per cent of large intestine and breast cancer might be avoidable in Britain and America (Doll and Peto 1982).

Unfortunately it is not yet known how cancer of the breast, large intestine, and stomach can be prevented. Some very interesting correlations have been found, for example the correlation between meat consumption and colon cancer, and fat consumption and breast cancer but the evidence is not so firm that we can embark on a programme to reduce fat and meat consumption (Fig 1.5).

For lung cancer the causal agent is known with confidence – cigarette smoking. At present tobacco is the principal known cause of cancer. However, as Sir Richard Doll and Richard Peto have argued in their excellent review of *The causes of cancer* (Doll and Peto 1982) dietary factors may prove to be as important as tobacco when all the causes of cancer have been identified (Table 1.3).

12 The scope of preventive medicine

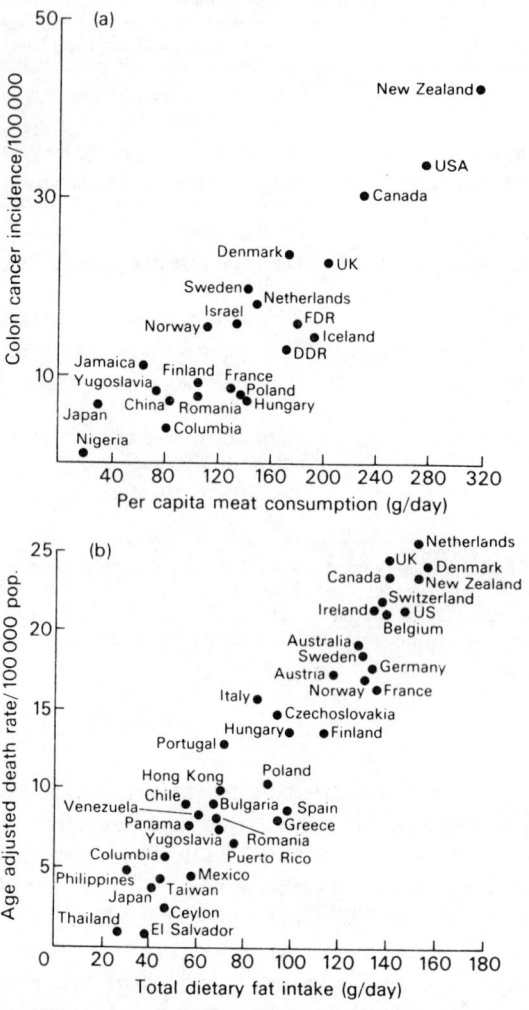

Fig. 1.5. (a) Relationship between meat consumption in various countries and the risk in those countries of developing cancer of the colon. (b) Relationship between fat consumption in various countries and the risk in those countries of death from breast cancer. 'In these graphs, each point represents one country (and the cancer rates per 100 000 women relate to women of similar age, and so are not materially affected by the greater risks of premature death from other causes in poor countries). The (generally prosperous) countries where meat or fat consumption is highest are those where women of a given age are at greatest risk of developing cancer of the colon or breast. But, although the explanation of this remains obscure, this is *not* strong evidence that either fat or meat are important causes of these cancers, merely strong evidence that these cancers have causes' (Peto 1981).

Table 1.3. *Developing and current knowledge of causes*

Future perfect

Estimate of the proportions of cancer deaths that will be found to be attributable to various factors †

	Percent of all US cancer deaths	
	Best estimate	Range of acceptable estimate
Tobacco	30	25–40
Alcohol	3	2–4
Diet	35	10–70
Food additives	<1	−5*–2
Sexual behaviour	1	1
Yet-to-be-discovered hormonal analogues of reproductive factors	−6	−112–0
Occupation	4	2–8
Pollution	2	1–5
Industrial products	<1	<1–2
Medicines and medical procedures	1	0.5–3
Geophysical factors (mostly natural background radiation and sunlight)	3	2–4
Infective processes	10?	1–?
Unknown	?†	?
Total	200% or more †	

*The net effects of food additives may be protective, e.g. against stomach cancer.

† Since one cancer may have two or more causes, the grand total in such a table will probably when more knowledge is available, greatly exceed 200 per cent. (It is merely a coincidence that the suggested figures in the present table happen to add up to nearly 100 per cent.)

Present imperfect

Reliably established (as of 1981), practicable* ways of avoiding the onset of life-threatening cancer

	Percent of all US cancer deaths known to be thus avoidable
Avoidance of tobacco smoke	30%
Avoidance of alcoholic drinks or mouthwashes	3%
Avoidance of obesity	2%
Regular cervical screening and genital hygiene	1%
Avoidance of inessential medical use of hormones or radiology	<1%
Avoidance of unusual exposure to sunlight	<1%
Avoidance of current levels of exposure to currently known effects of carcinogens (for which there is good epidemiological evidence of human hazard) in	
(i) occupational context	<1%
(ii) food, water or urban air	<1%

*Excluding ways such as prophylactic prostatectomy, mastectomy, hysterectomy, oophorectomy, artificial menopause or pregnancy (Peto 1981).

The scope of preventive medicine

Prevention of respiratory infections, bronchitis, and asthma

The general practitioner is also in the best position to prevent these causes of death, which are together responsible for over 11 per cent of loss of life expectancy, by influenza immunization, helping people who want to stop smoking, because cigarette smoking is now the major cause of bronchitis, and by the effective treatment and continuing surveillance of all patients with asthma.

The prevention of accidents and suicide

The general practitioner has an important part to play in the prevention of deaths from these causes (see pp. 227 and 223).

Prevention of morbidity

The first important point to emphasize is that although many people criticize preventive medicine because they believe that it simply postpones mortality and increases the numbers of disabled elderly 'geriatric' people, this is not the case. The effect of preventive medicine, and of clinical medicine, is not to increase the biological life span, which appears to lie somewhere between 75 and 80, but to increase life expectancy. That is to say that a higher proportion of people survive to die of 'senescent' deaths, to use a demographer's term describing deaths from normal aging, and fewer people die of 'anticipated' or premature deaths as a result of disease. The terminal peak in 'the curve of deaths', as it is called in the actuarial literature, becomes taller and more symmetrical with the same number dying before the peak as after it. This is illustrated in Fig. 1.5 which shows the actual curve of deaths, and the two constituent curves of premature or anticipated deaths and senescent deaths.

Demographers are now in agreement that the proportion of deaths due to the cumulative effects of normal aging is steadily increasing in all developed

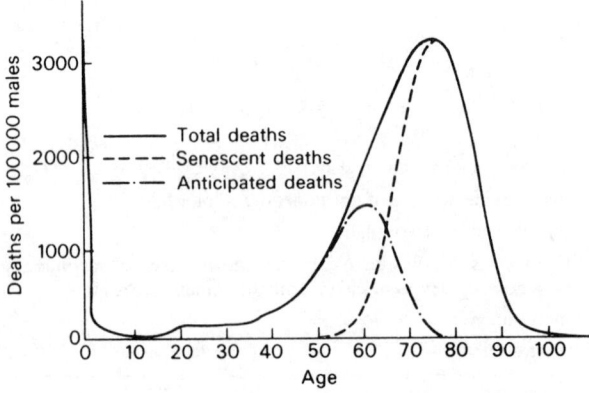

Fig. 1.6. Curve of deaths; England; males. (From Benjamin and Overton (1980).)

The scope for prevention today   15

Table 1.4. *Senescent deaths as a proportion of total. England and Wales*

Life Tables	Period of deaths	Males Peak age	Senescent deaths % of total	Females Peak age	Senescent deaths % of total
ELT 1	1841	72.0	39.9	73.5	41.0
ELT 8	1910–12	73.5	51.5	76.0	55.3
ELT 11	1950–52	75.7	69.4	80.3	70.3
ELT 12	1960–62	74.8	74.5	80.6	72.3
ELT 13	1970–72	74.4	84.1	82.6	72.9

From Benjamin and Overton (1980).

countries, with an increase in life expectancy but no significant increase in life span (Table 1.4).

This trend can be expressed diagrammatically either as a change in the shape of the curve of deaths which shows a taller, narrower, more symmetrical peak, nearer to four score years than to three score and ten (Fig. 1.7).

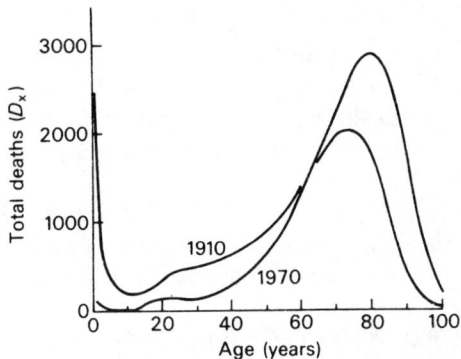

Fig. 1.7. Total deaths per year against age; United States; 1910 and 1970. There is an increase in early deaths with a corresponding increase in late deaths in 1970 as compared with 1910. (From Fries and Crapo (1981).)

Alternatively it can be shown on the survival curve, which plots the percentage of each cohort surviving at each age. Its effect on the survival curve has been called the 'rectangularization' of the survival curve (Fig. 1.8).

However, preventive medicine does not simply prevent premature deaths due to disease; by preventing the diseases themselves it also prevents disability. Thus the effect is not to postpone the onset of disability but to shorten the period of terminal disability and dependency: Sir Richard Doll once said that his wish

16   *The scope of preventive medicine*

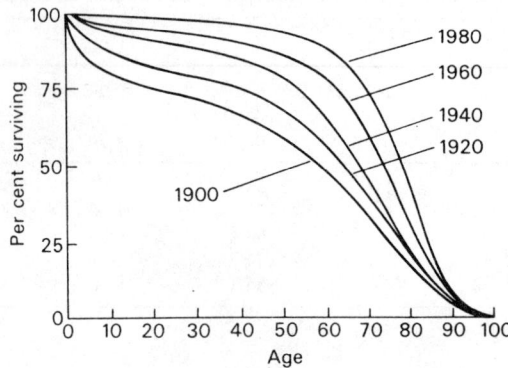

Fig. 1.8. Human survival curves for 1900, 1920, 1940, 1960, and 1980. The curves converge at the same maximum age, thereby demonstrating that the maximum age of survival has been fixed over this period of observation. (From Fries and Crapo (1981).)

was to 'die young as late as possible' and it seems that this is the effect of preventive medicine. The investment of energy and resources in prevention will therefore not increase the burden of disability – the opposite is true and the trends which have taken place and which will continue may be summarized in the following list of hypotheses.

The span of life is fixed although life expectancy is increased.

The age at which disability develops has increased and will continue to increase.

The duration of disability and dependence will therefore decrease.

The good news for policy makers, doctors, and consumers is therefore that modern medicine prevents more disability than it creates.

Prevention of disorders that use in-patient facilities

Three conditions are responsible for the occupation of more than half of all hospital beds – mental illness, mental handicap, and cerebrovascular disease.

The principal causes of hospitalization for mental illness are schizophrenia and Alzheimer's disease. Neither of these are preventable but hospitalization is preventable by the provision of appropriate support for the sufferer and his family (see p. 263).

The exact proportion of cases of mental handicap that is preventable depends on the significance of sex-linked mental retardation, a topic still under debate, but with our present knowledge there is scope for prevention; but as we are not discussing prevention in pregnancy and childhood in this book we will not consider this subject in detail. However, the cigarette smoking, alcohol misuse, and rubella are three causes of mental handicap that the general practitioner can prevent before the woman becomes pregnant (see pp. 133, 178).

The fact that many strokes are preventable has been discussed in the context of the prevention of premature mortality but the prevention of the morbidity due to stroke, and the demands made on health and personal social services are also of vital importance, not only because of the prevention of grief and suffering but also because of the prevention of unnecessary use of health service resources which are thus freed to meet other needs.

Prevention of disorders for which people consult general practitioners

Some of the disorders for which people consult general practitioners are preventable, for example influenza. However, in recent years more attention has been paid to the prevention of consultation for 'trivial' conditions that do not need medical attention by the 'modification of help seeking behaviour', that is by educating patients about the way in which they use their general practitioner's time (see p. 56). However, this approach is not without its drawbacks, not only because it may alienate patients whose views of triviality and seriousness often differ from the views of the medical profession (Hannay 1979) but also because it reduces the opportunities for opportunistic health education or for prevention by case finding. These do not, however, seem to be major problems.

Prevention of disorders referred to out-patient departments

As with other types of burden discussed, there is scope for both the prevention of the diseases which are referred and for the prevention of 'unnecessary' referrals, that is the referral of problems that could be managed by primary care services if they had adequate resources, for example a community physiotherapy service, or open access to resources that are necessarily sited in a large hospital, for example laboratory services. A priority for the development of primary care is therefore to examine the factors that influence referral to out-patients and to try to invest the resources in primary care that would reduce the number of referrals of conditions that could be effectively managed by the general practitioner.

It would be unwise, however, to assume that closer examination of out-patient referrals would necessarily lead to significant savings in hospital services because there are many people with problems who should be referred and the development of anticipatory care would discover an unmet need for hospital referral.

Prevention of disorders causing sickness absence from work

Although general practitioners cannot do much to prevent occupational diseases unless they are employed, part time, in industry they have an influence on sickness absence but it is important to distinguish between the disorders that cause short-term absence and those which cause long-term absence when considering their contribution. Long-term sickness absence is usually caused by a chronic disabling disease although social factors are always of relevance, whereas short-term sickness absence is primarily a social phenomenon although the people who are off sick for a few days usually have an acute self-limiting disease.

A Department of Health and Social Security survey found that the diseases that caused it were the diseases that are the common cause of disabilities (Fig 1.9).

The length of time a person stays off work is affected by the nature of his contribution. In the Department of Health and Social Security survey it was found that those who were in physically demanding jobs had to stay off longer than those who were in light office jobs. Those who were off sick from less

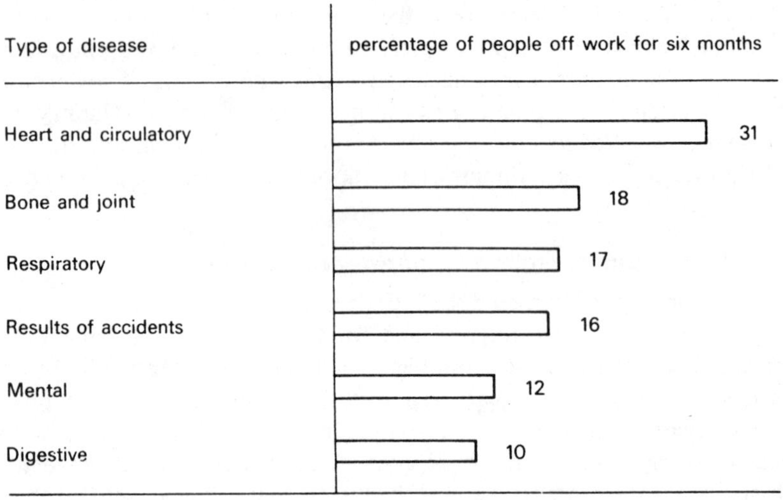

Type of disease	percentage of people off work for six months
Heart and circulatory	31
Bone and joint	18
Respiratory	17
Results of accidents	16
Mental	12
Digestive	10

Fig. 1.9. Principal causes of long-term sickness absence 1973/74. (From Martin and Morgan (1975).)

skilled jobs were less frequently covered by sick pay and they more frequently lost their jobs as a result of their sickness absence. The consequence of this was that they sometimes not only became unemployed but also, because the causes of long-term sickness absence occur in middle age and often have permanent effects, virtually unemployable. The research workers were emphatic in their conclusion that 'it does not seem from our results that lack of motivation to return to work in itself causes sickness to be prolonged. The long-term sick seemed to want to return to work but the practical problems many faced frequently made their return extremely difficult'.

Because of the difficulty that disabled people have in returning to work or finding new work the most effective contribution the general practitioner can make to the prevention of long-term sickness absence is to prevent the causal disease in the first place, and the principal means of doing this is to try to prevent stroke, heart disease, and bronchitis, for the main causes of long-term sickness absence are social, not occupational.

The prevention of short-term sickness absence is more a matter for the management and Unions, especially the former, than it is for the medical profession. This is not to suggest that all short-term sickness absence is due solely to social and psychological factors. Most people who are off sick for a few days are suffering from a disease but the decisions a person who has a disease makes about whether or not he should stay off work and how long he stays off are influenced by social and psychological factors, which are therefore the major preventable causes of short-term sickness absence.

REFERENCES

Benjamin, B. and Overton, E. (1981). Prospects for mortality decline in England and Wales. *Population Trends* 22–8.

Black, D. A. K. and Pole, J. D. (1975). Priorities in biomedical research. *Br. J. prevent. soc. Med.* **29**, 222–7.

Cipolla, C. M. (1962). *The economic history of world population.* Penguin, London.

Doll, R. and Peto, R. (1982). *The causes of cancer.* Oxford University Press.

Fries, J. F. and Crapo, L. M. (1981). *Vitality and aging: implications of the rectangular curve.* Freeman, San Francisco.

Gray, J. A. M. (1979). *Man against disease,* pp. 12–23. Oxford University Press.

Hannay, D. R. (1979). *The symptom iceberg: a study of community health.* Routledge and Kegan Paul, London.

McNeill, W. H. (1976). *Plagues and people.* Penguin, London.

Martin, J. and Morgan, M. (1975). *Prolonged sickness absence and the return to work.* HMSO, London.

Peto, R. (1981). Why cancer? The causes of cancer in developed countries. *The Times Health Supplement* 6 November, pp. 12–14.

Royal College of General Practitioners (1981). *The prevention of arterial disease.* RCGP, London.

2 Opportunities for prevention in general practice

Godfrey Fowler and Muir Gray

Without becoming enmeshed in a web of semantics it is appropriate to define some of the terms that are used in this book.

PRIMARY, SECONDARY, AND TERTIARY PREVENTION

Primary prevention

This is the removal of the causes of disease. In the context of the present-day prevalence of behaviourally determined disease, avoidance of cigarette smoking is the example par excellence of primary prevention. It is the ideal level of prevention – removal of the cause – but one which largely requires doctors to adopt an educational rather than a diagnostic/therapeutic role. Given the word 'doctor' is derived from the Latin *docere*, to teach, the adoption of this role should be feasible but medical education places little emphasis on it.

Secondary prevention

This is the early detection of disease at a stage before this is manifest as symptoms or disordered function and when action may halt or even reverse the disease process. Detection of hypertension is one such example. Elevation of blood pressure is a *risk factor* strongly associated with cardiovascular disease, particularly stroke. It is asymptomatic – except when the damage has been done. Its discovery depends on the use of a sphygmomanometer, an examination taking approximately one minute (Buchan and Richardson 1973).

There is one use of this term that may cause confusion and that is the term 'secondary prevention' in the context of coronary heart disease because many people use the term to mean the prevention of a recurrence of angina or infarction in someone who has symptomatic and clinical evidence of coronary atherosclerosis.

Secondary prevention is usually associated with the term '*screening*'. Broadly, screening is the application of sorting procedures – history, examination; or investigations – to populations: it is doctor initiated; it is usually episodic; and its intention is to identify in an apparently healthy population those who have disease or who are at special risk of disease (see p. 94). In fact for some people screening and secondary prevention are synonymous but a new means of secondary prevention has received prominence in recent years – case finding.

Case finding is also doctor initiated, but the initiative is limited to the 'opportunistic' approach, that is to the incidental detection of disease or risk factors in the patient who is consulting about an unrelated problem. Case finding contrasts with the more aggressive pursuit of the uncomplaining individual, usually regarded as one of the hallmarks of screening, and a case-finding approach incorporates secondary prevention into daily practice rather than having it as a separate activity.

To the general practitioner who is faced with a heavy workload, seeing 50, 60, or even more patients a day in an industrial area, the case-finding approach may seem unattainable and it is important to recognize that many general practitioners still face such heavy demands that it is difficult to remember all the risk factors that could be detected at every consultation and for many practices therefore a combination of case finding and screening is appropriate. For example, a doctor may try to achieve a recent blood pressure recording on every person who consults but work with his practice manager to set up a screening service for women at risk of cervical cancer.

Tertiary prevention

This is the management of established disease. The 'prevention' is the avoidance or limitation of disability or handicap. Conventional medical treatment necessarily incorporates this function, but seduction by the glamour and excitement of emergency and acute medicine has ensured relegation of tertiary prevention to a background role. The opportunities for better tertiary prevention by, for example, careful long-term supervision of diabetics or asthmatics are primarily available in general practice because of the part that the general practitioner plays in the provision of a comprehensive health service. Preventive and curative medicine are not mutually exclusive alternatives, although they often have to compete for the same scarce resources. They simply attack at different points in its natural history and although the service offered to the individual patient differs the general approach is, or to be more accurate should be, the same. This approach has been called anticipatory care.

Anticipatory care

This approach to medicine is, as the name implies, one in which an attempt is made to anticipate and preclude problems and it is relevant to primary, secondary, and tertiary prevention (Royal College of General Practitioners 1981). However, anticipatory care requires not only a thoughtful approach to each consultation, for example one which uses the opportunity of a consultation for influenza to discuss smoking cessation, it also requires a systematic approach to the whole community for which the general practitioner is responsible, namely all the patients on his list. This in turn requires a record system that allows all those who are at risk in some way or who have some particular disease, such as diabetes, to be identified easily and accurately, and the transition of general practice from a branch of medicine dominated by the demands of the patient to one in which both demands and hidden needs are tackled – this is the changing nature of general practice (Tudor Hart 1981).

THE CHANGING NATURE OF GENERAL PRACTICE

The traditional view of the doctor, particularly the general practitioner, sitting in his shop waiting for sick patients to present themselves, is changing. No longer is it enough for him to require the provision of symptoms before offering appropriate remedy or advice. To do so may be to miss the opportunity to influence what happens. The chronic bronchitis of the lifelong smoker and the hemiplegia of the undiagnosed hypertensive leave little scope for medical intervention. How much more beneficial might effective anti-smoking advice or detection and treatment of hypertension have been if implemented a decade or two earlier.

The adequacy of a symptom-management approach to medical care is being questioned and there is increasing acknowledgement that the major opportunities for doctors, particularly at the primary care level, to influence the health of their patients lie in the field of prevention. This implies a major philosophical change from the passive role of 'shopkeeper' to the active one of 'teacher'.

What is it about general practice that makes it such a promising medium for preventive medicine? There are many reasons why primary care provides the ideal framework for prevention or 'anticipatory care'. This is especially true of National Health Service general practice in Great Britain with its characteristics of accessibility, availibility, comprehensiveness, continuing responsibility, and long-term doctor/patient relationships. Furthermore, the identification of a defined population as a practice enhances the opportunities to influence the health of a finite number of people.

One of the essential features of the general practitioner is that he is the first medical professional to whom the ill patient turns. This is not to deny the importance of self-care (a vital aspect of prevention) and of non-professional sources of advice about health and illness. Health and illness. What do these terms mean?

The WHO definition of health as 'a state of complete physical, mental, and social wellbeing' is utopian.

Only a very small proportion of people would admit to enjoying this. A more realistic view of health is of a state of dynamic equilibrium between the individual and his environment. Ill-health is then a disturbance of this equilibrium and has two components – illness and disease. Illness is the experience of ill-health by the individual. Disease is ill-health which could be ascribed to demonstrable pathology. An individual may feel ill, i.e. have symptoms, without any pathological lesion or defect being evident. For example, most patients with headache. Conversely, particularly in the early stages of disease, patients may

Circle **A** comprises a given population

Circle **B** defines those who are ill, i.e. have symptoms

Circle **C** defines those who have disease, i.e. demonstrable pathology

x = those who are ill but have no demonstrable pathology

y = those who have disease but are asymptomatic

z = those who are ill and have disease

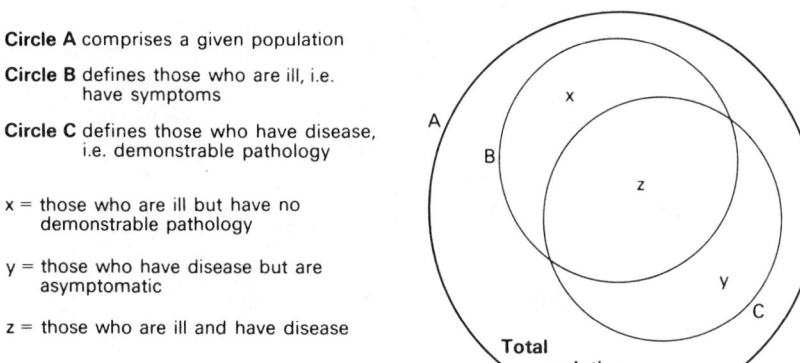

Fig. 2.1. The relationship between disease and illness.

be asymptomatic and do not feel ill. Examination or investigation may, however, demonstrate abnormality. In some cases, for example hypertension, this asymptomatic phase of disease may be prolonged and screening may have particular relevance. The relevance between illness and disease is illustrated in Fig. 2.1.

Conventionally it is those with symptoms who concern doctors, but this excludes a substantial number with asymptomatic disease, for example the 40-year-old man with undiagnosed hypertension, or his wife with undetected breast cancer. But of course not all patients with symptoms consult doctors either. Indeed, studies have shown that only a small proportion of symptoms lead to medical consultations (Morrell and Wale 1976). The decision to seek medical help is a complex one and the probability of symptoms leading to a medical consultation is influenced by numerous factors and especially the anxiety which a given symptom generates in the patient.

The concept of the iceberg or morbidity (Last 1963) illustrated in Fig. 2.2 is helpful in understanding the limited involvement of doctors in the management of illness. It acknowledges that much illness is 'below the surface' in the sense that it does not reach the medical care system. It illustrates furthermore that there are various levels of care. The first of these is self-care. The vast amount of minor illness is managed by individuals without reference to any other source of help. Self-care may include the use of medication and about one-third of expenditure on drugs in Britain is on self-medication; in a two-week period about half of all adults will have taken some over-the-counter medicine (Dunnell and Cartwright 1972). Supplementary to self-care, advice may be sought from a variety of non-professional sources, such as family and friends, and when buying over-the-counter medicines from local chemists.

Opportunities for prevention in general practice

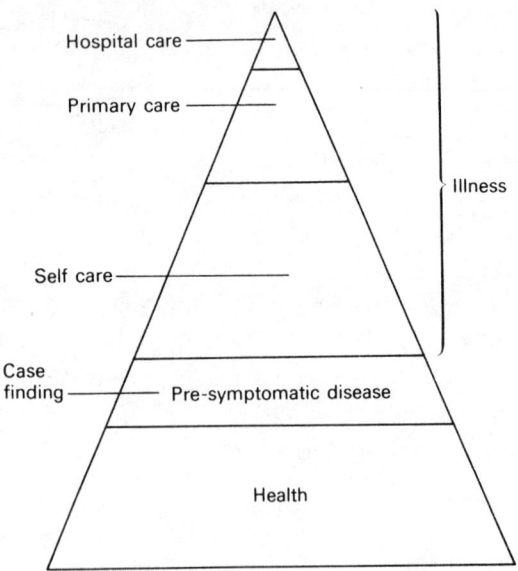

Fig. 2.2. The iceberg of morbidity.

The next stage, the seeking of professional advice, is as mentioned complex. Many factors influence it, including personal, social, and cultural characteristics as well as the nature of the symptoms and their perceived seriousness. The expectations that patients have of doctors and their previous experience of medical services are also important. In Britain the professional advice first sought will usually be that of a general practitioner. But elsewhere it may be that of a nurse or specialist.

Of the problems about which patients do consult doctors, more than 90 per cent are dealt with entirely at a primary care level, without reference to any other agency. The tip of the iceberg representing hospital and specialist secondary care is a minute proportion – about 1 per cent – of the total morbidity of the population at any given time. General practice is therefore in a key position. It has a vital role as the portal of entry to the medical care system. As a link between self-care and professional medical care it profoundly influences the overall level of care and the use of resources. Moreover, not only does it defend the expensive, technologically based hospital care system from extravagant and inappropriate usage, but it also protects certain patients from unnecessary and even harmful investigations and treatment.

Important amongst the characteristics of general practice are availability and accessibility. While many of the problems presented to him do not require his immediate availability, the crisis intervention role of the GP is a highly valued one. There is some evidence that this feature is less prominent than it was. The tendency to group practices and the growth of out-of-hours rotas, while ensuring the continued availability of a doctor, may undermine the benefits derived from the special knowledge of the patient which is the preserve of the personal doctor. Likewise the congregation of doctors into health centres and group practices, the establishment of rigid appointment systems, and the growth of less personal 'practice teams' may impair the accessibility of the doctor.

As the point of first contact with the medical care system, general practice must provide a wide-ranging comprehensive service to the patient. The variety of problems which may be brought to the general practitioner is infinite. Many of these problems will be ill-defined and in elucidating them he will be greatly assisted by his close relationship with, and special knowledge of, the patient. Often such occasions will provide opportunity for health education and preventive medicine, rather than a therapeutic approach and in this context the personal relationship may have particular value in enhancing the influence of such advice.

The continuity of care which the general practitioner provides has many valuable implications. It provides the basis for the development of the doctor-patient relationship which is such a vital element of general practice, and for the acquisition of that knowledge of the patient – personal, social, and medical – which is essential to proper management of his or her problems. The continuing nature of medical contact in general practice allows the doctor to learn about the natural history of disease and about the influence of the patient's response to illness.

The job of the general practitioner

These characteristics for general practice are reflected in the job description of the general practitioner, approved by the European Working Party on General Practice: 'The general practitioner is a licensed medical graduate who gives personal, primary, and continuing care to individuals, families, and the practice population, irrespective of age, sex, and illness. It is the synthesis of these functions which is unique. He will attend his patients in his consulting room, in their homes, and sometimes in a clinic or hospital. His aim is to make early diagnoses. He will include and integrate physical, psychological, and social factors in his considerations about health and illness. This will be expressed in the care of his patients. He will make an initial decision about every problem which is presented to him as a doctor. He will undertake the continuing management of his patients with chronic, recurrent, or terminal illness. Prolonged contact means that he can use repeated opportunities to gather information at a pace appropriate to each patient and build up a relationship of trust which he can use professionally. He will practice in co-operation with other colleagues, medical and non-medical. He will know how and when to intervene through treatment, prevention, and education, to promote the health of his patients and their families. He will recognize that he also has a professional responsibility to the community.'

Organization of general practice

The organization of general practice in Britain has undergone big changes since the inception of the National Health Service. Wheras in the early years almost half of the general practitioners practised single-handed and less than a fifth in partnerships of three or more, the situation is now reversed. Only one in six doctors works solo; two-thirds are in practices of at least three doctors. Over the last decade there has been a steady increase in the number of general practitioners to the present figure of about 26 000 so that average list sizes have fallen from 2500 to about 2300. Like all averages these figures hide variations from a few hundred on islands and in remote rural areas to three or four thousand in some industrial areas. As indicated by Tudor Hart's 'Inverse Care Law' (Hart 1971) the availability of medical services is generally inversely related to need. The great majority of doctors practise from adapted premises and in spite of an increase in the number of health centres over the last decade, only about one in six doctors works from a health centre. In addition, the general practitioner has begun to work more closely with other professionals.

The development of the team approach

The development of teams began in the mid-sixties with the attachment of health visitors to certain practices and was subsequently extended to include nurses, midwives, social workers, and others. The majority of practices now have 'primary care teams' but the extent to which these have developed is very variable. In addition to attached Health Authority staff some practices now employ their own team members, especially nurses for treatment room duties. Other professionals who have in some instances been incorporated into such teams include occupational therapists, physiotherapists, dieticians, and clinical psychologists.

Inevitably views about this development are polarized. On the one hand are those who recognize that doctors do not have a monopoly of primary care skills and that other health care professionals not only have their own contribution to make to the care of the patients in the community but that primary care generally would be enhanced by the greater delegation and co-operation in the team approach. However, others claim the sharing of care between several professionals results in fragmentation of medical services but from the viewpoint of preventive medicine there are strong arguments in support of primary care teams. Not only may the performance of routine procedures such as dressings and injections by others free the doctor to spend more time on prevention, but preventive medical procedures themselves may be carried out equally well by others – particularly practice nurses. Immunizations are already accepted as an appropriate nursing function. Monitoring hypertensive patients is another preventive activity which can be performed by suitably trained nurses.

The health visitor is no newcomer to prevention. This is, and always has been, her primary role. She is a health educator. To many health visitors, who have struggled to convince general practitioner colleagues, the signs of awakening interest in preventive medicine in general practice must be a welcome relief (see p. 277).

Undoubtedly the problems of working in multidisciplinary teams have been underestimated (Pritchard 1981) but they are now being appreciated and tackled (Department of Health and Social Security 1981).

THE CHANGING PATTERN OF CONSULTATION

Like list sizes, consultation rates vary widely. The average patient consults his doctor between three and four times a year. But there are variations from less than two to more than six consultations per patient each year. The average general practitioner will therefore experience rather less than 10 000 doctor–patient contacts a year, an average of 30 or 40 a day. The great majority of these contacts are surgery consultation and home visiting rates are now only about a third of what they were in the early days of the National Health Service. This means that only about one in ten of doctor–patient contacts take place in the patient's home. Although, as previously stated, long-term care is an important feature of general practice and about two-thirds of patients keep the same doctor for at least five years, there is nevertheless about a 10 per cent annual turnover in the average practice, usually because patients move.

About two-thirds of patients consult at least once a year and more than 90 per cent at least once every five years. These facts have important implications for preventive care. They mean that the great majority of patients provide opportunities at regular intervals when not only may a 'case finding' approach to preventive care be pursued, but also for health education at a time when they may be expected to be particularly receptive to advice. About half of consultations are initiated by the patient presenting with a new symptom. The others are 'continuing' in the sense that they are concerned with the management of longstanding problems and are often at the specific request of the doctor. The young and the old have the highest consulting rates and at all ages except in infancy females consult more than males.

Reasons for consultation

The view once prevailed that general practice is a sort of 'watered down' form of hospital medicine. This view is no longer tenable. The content of general practice in terms of morbidity pattern is remarkably similar in developed countries and is very different from that of hospital 'secondary' care.

About two-thirds of illness seen in general practice is minor, that is to say transient, self-limiting, and without sequelae. There may, however, be important social and psychological components. Of the remaining third, most is chronic illness in the sense that there is some permanent impairment of normal function. This category of illness accounts for a substantial amount of general practice workload and provides the potential for minimizing disability and handicap by careful surveillance and optimum management (tertiary prevention). Only about 10 per cent of illness seen in general practice consists of acute major illness, most of which may be managed at a primary care level, so some will require the expertise, nursing, and technical resources of hospital care, and this group includes life-threatening illnesses. Table 2.1 lists the minor illnesses seen in an average British general practice in a year.

Although 'minor' these conditions are not insignificant or trivial. They are the illnesses most commonly occurring in the population. They cause disproportionate anxiety to the patients and their economic importance as the cause of sick absence from work is considerable. Such illness is not seen in hospital. Experience of its management is confined to general practice. Table 2.2 shows the pattern of acute major illness in the average practice.

These are the conditions most commonly seen in hospital, but comparatively rarely in primary care. A major task of the general practitioner is to remain alert to their possibility and to manage them competently when they arise. Table 2.3 indicates the amount of chronic illness in the typical practice.

These conditions cause varying degrees of disability and handicap. Many are a source of frequent consultation and may require regular and sustained supervision. Such supervision may be shared with a hospital clinic, but there is increasing recognition that this may be unnecessary or even undesirable and that the proper place for surveillance is in primary care, particularly as they are so frequently complicated by social problems (Table 2.4).

The process of consultation

The most crucial feature of medical care, especially of general practice, is the consultation. In the words of Sir James Spence, 'The essential unit of medical practice is the occasion when, in the intimacy of the consulting room or sickroom, a person who is ill or believes himself to be ill, seeks the advice of a doctor whom he trusts. This is a consultation and all else in medicine derives from it.'

The average length of a consultation in general practice in Britain is about six minutes, but it may vary from half a minute to half an hour. Within this time a number of tasks need to be pursued. First of these will be the establishment or reinforcement of a relationship which will facilitate effective communication. Then comes the elucidation of the reasons for the patient's attendance and their formulation in physical, psychological, and social terms. The patient's own ideas about aetiology and effects need also to be elicited, especially the sources of anxiety about the illness and the expectations that the patient has of the doctor. Following assessment and the formulation of solutions, the patient's involvement in the plans for management of the problems may help to ensure his understanding and encourage his willingness to comply. This is particularly

Table 2.1. *Minor illness (of short duration and minimal disability). An average general practice of 2500 persons per annum in the United Kingdom*

	Persons consulting
Upper respiratory infections	500
Common gastro-intestinal 'infections and dyspepsias'	250
Skin disorders	225
Emotional disorders	200
Acute otitis media	50
Wax in external meatus	50
'Acute back' syndrome	50
Migraine	30
Hay fever	25
Acute urinary infections	50

From Royal College of General Practitioners (1970). *Present state and future needs of general practice,* 2nd edn. RCGP, London.

Table 2.2. *Acute major illness (life-threatening). An average general practice of 2500 persons per annum in the United Kingdom*

	Persons consulting
Pheumonia and acute bronchitis	50
Acute myocardial infarction	7
Acute appendicitis	5
All new cancers	
Lung	1–2 per year
Breast	1 per year
Large bowel	2 every 3 years
Stomach	1 every 2 years
Bladder	1 every 3 years
Cervix	1 every 3 years
Pancreas	1 every 4 years
Ovary	1 every 5 years
Oesophagus	1 every 7 years
Brain	1 every 10 years
Uternine body	1 every 12 years
Lymphadenoma	1 every 15 years
Thyroid	1 every 20 years
	Persons consulting
Severe depression	12
Suicide	1 every 4 years
Attempted suicide	2 every year
Acute glaucoma	1
Acute strokes	5
Killed in road accident	1 every 3 years

From Royal College of General Practitioners (1970). *Present state and future needs of general practice,* 2nd edn. RCGP, London.

Table 2.3. Chronic illnesses. An average general practice of 2500 persons per annum in the United Kingdom

	Persons consulting
Chronic rheumatism	100
Rheumatoid arthritis	10
Chronic mental illness	55
Severe subnormality	5
Educationally subnormal	3*
Vulnerable adults	40
Child guidance	4*
Chronic bronchitis	50
Anaemia	40
Pernicious anaemia	2
Hypertension	25
Asthma	25
Peptic ulcer	25
Strokes	15
Epilepsy	10
Diabetes	10
Parkinsonism	3
Multiple sclerosis	2
Pulmonary tuberculosis	2
Chronic pyelonephritis	1

*Persons attending school or clinic.
From Royal College of General Practitioners (1970). *Present state and future needs of general practice*, 2nd edn. RCGP, London.

Table 2.4. Social pathology. An average general practice of 2500 persons per annum in the United Kingdom

	Persons
Poverty-receiving supplementary social security benefits	100
Aged over 75	100
Lonely – living alone	50
Broken homes (children under 15 living with only one parent)	60
Illegitimate births	4
Problem families	5–10
Divorce	1–2
Adult committed to prison	1
Juvenile delinquents	4
Chronic alcoholics – known	5
probable	25
Male homosexuals	50
Deaf (requiring hearing aids)	25
Blind (registered)	5
Severe physical disability – registered	6

From Royal College of General Practitioners (1970). *Present state and future needs of general practice*, 2nd edn. RCGP, London.

important in view of the evidence that less than half the information communicated to patients is remembered shortly after the consultation is over. Throughout the general practice consultation a prime consideration is the establishment of and maintenance of a good relationship with the patient, acknowledging that this relationship is a key factor in enhancing the therapeutic potential of the doctor and the willingness of the patient to accept his advice.

The conventional concept of the consultation tends to be limited to the diagnosis and management of symptoms presented by the patient and of any pre-existing disease which he may have. But to these must be added the potential consultations provide for health education and preventive medicine. Objectives which derive from this potential have been identified as 'the modification of help-seeking behaviour' and 'opportunistic health promotion' (Fig. 2.3). The former implies health education aimed at influencing the patient's future behaviour when ill, and is especially concerned with encouraging self-care for minor ailments (Morrell *et al.* 1980). Opportunistic health promotion refers to the scope in the consultation for preventive medicine, both the promotion of health and the early detection of disease.

A	B
Management of presenting problems	Modification of help-seeking behaviour
C	D
Management of continuing problems	Opportunistic health promotion

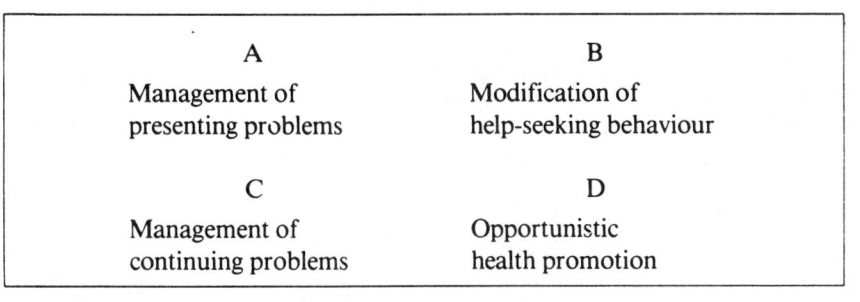

Fig. 2.3. The potential in each primary care consultation – an *aide-mémoire* (Stott and Davis 1979).

Health education is not traditionally a function of the medical consultation. But increasing awareness of the contribution of faulty lifestyles and behaviour to present day illness, requires that greater attention be paid to the opportunities offered in many consultations for the identification of relevant aspects of these in any individual. The vulnerability of the sick patient makes it likely that he will be more receptive to advice. The potent influence of the doctor's role and the effectiveness of the one-to-one transaction are further powerful potentiating factors. So the combination of these provides a unique educational opportunity. But the realization of the potential this provides naturally depends on the willingness and ability of the patient to comply. Such compliance requires that not only is the patient better informed but that his greater knowledge leads to a behaviour change (Sackett and Haynes 1976). This issue is discussed in detail in Chapter 4.

REFERENCES

Buchan, I. C. and Richardson, I. M. (1973). *Time study of consultations in General Practice.* Scottish Home and Health Department, Edinburgh.

Department of Health and Social Security (1981). *The Primary Health Care Team.* Report of a Joint Working Group of the Standing Medical Advisory Committee and the Standing Nursing and Midwifery Advisory Committee. HMSO, London.

Dunnell, K. and Cartwright, A. (1972). *Medicine takers, prescribers and hoarders.* Routledge and Kegan Paul, London.

Hart, J. T. (1971). The inverse care law. *Lancet* i, 405.

—— (1981). A new kind of doctor. *J. R. Soc. Med.* 871–83.

Last, J. M. (1963). The clinical iceberg. *Lancet* ii, 28–31.

Morrell, D. C., Avery, A. J., and Watkins, C. J. (1980). Management of minor illness. *Br. med. J.* i, 769.

—— and Wale, J. (1976). Symptoms perceived and recorded by patients. *J. R. Coll. gen. Pract.* 26, 398.

Pritchard, P. M. (1981). *Manual of primary health care: its nature and organization,* pp. 47–67. Oxford University Press.

Royal College of General Practitioners (1981). *Health and prevention in primary care:* Report from General Practice No. 18. RCGP, London.

Sacket, D. L. and Haynes, R. B. (1976). *Compliance in therapeutic regimens.* Johns Hopkins University Press.

Stott, N. C. H. and Davis, R. H. (1979). The exceptional potential in each primary care consultation. *J. R. Coll. gen. Practrs* 29, 201.

3 Record systems in preventive medicine

Alistair Tulloch

Order and simplification are the first steps towards the mastery of a subject – the real enemy is the unknown.
                                            Thomas Mann *The Magic Mountain*

No professional activity can be properly planned, organized, administered, maintained, and reviewed without complete records of all the relevant facts. Yet many doctors, including some with otherwise impeccable standards, tend to ignore this elementary consideration, probably because they do not fully appreciate the potential contribution of records to medical care. Good records are a *sine qua non* in prophylaxis and the lack of such records and a means of processing them has slowed the trend towards preventive medicine by general practitioners. This change has been further hobbled by the fact that medical education has been dominated hitherto by clinicians who have taught students that the only 'real' medicine is clinical care. The implication of this is that epidemiology is interesting academic work but peripheral to 'real' medicine. Such teachers have also tended to value records only insofar as they underpinned clinical care and few of them have recognized the role of records as a dynamic tool. Even today the contribution of epidemiology to patient care is underestimated but more doctors now recognize that facts are the tools of prevention. Medical records are likewise the building bricks of epidemiology which is itself the key to high standards of preventive medicine, but they need to be recorded with care, marshalled, integrated, deployed, and processed in such a fashion as to express their message clearly.

FAULTS OF THE CONVENTIONAL RECORDS SYSTEM

The present system of medical records taught in medical schools has much to commend it but it does also have certain limitations both of design and use.

First there is a lack of emphasis on the importance of assembling *all* the facts likely to influence health status. In particular social, occupational, and environmental data are often poorly recorded although they may be of fundamental value in certain groups, e.g. the elderly and the disabled. Even in medical school I seem to recall the 'social history' rarely embraced much more than 'Smokes a packet of cigarettes per day and is occasional social drinker'.

Firm and unreliable data are mixed freely and not infrequently are indistinguishable from each other. Urinary infection may be diagnosed when the only sympton is dysuria. In many instances no MSU is sent off and the patient may really have had, for example, vaginitis.

The classification of disease used is too inflexible especially for the vague syndromes so often found in general practice and there is an over-emphasis on the importance of making an early diagnosis. Thus when the patient has been fully investigated the doctor feels guilty if he cannot make at least a provisional diagnosis. The result is that some Procrustan diagnoses are made which do not fit the facts.

Little attempt is made to highlight important records in progress notes which are, as a result, a relatively poor source of reference.

Objectives of care are virtually never recorded although they may occasionally be important, e.g. the target blood pressure one is seeking to achieve in hypertension.

Important findings which cannot be explained on investigation, e.g. unexplained hypochromic anaemia, tend to be conveniently forgotten. They should be highlighted for future reference when their significance may become clear.

Rarely does one find a conventional record file with an index and when present it virtually never records paramedical data.

Finally the file supplied for use in general practice is obsolete. It is not a true file in the modern sense but merely a record envelope which encourages 'ragbag' rather than chronological filing and is not the correct size to take most modern reports (many now of international size A4) received by family doctors, unfolded. Reference to reports is thus discouraged as they have to be withdrawn, unfolded, refolded, and inserted in the file each time. Also space is not really adequate when, for example, a full psychiatric history is being taken which may cover several pages.

As a result of all these problems the current record system is inadequate, incomplete, a poor source of reference, does not express its message clearly and is difficult to retrieve and process.

In the course of a study (unpublished) done for an MD thesis, the contents of 400 records reaching the practice were reviewed and the following findings made:

– One hundred and ten items of information on medical disorders (excluding data on oral contraception and obstetrics) useful or vital to health were not recorded in the files including past history of asthma, thyrotoxicosis, severe depression, open-heart surgery, rheumatic fever, duodenal ulcer, renal failure, Caesarian section, hysterectomy, and ankylosing spondylitis.

– Only 5 per cent had any form of indexing, however crude, of the more important contents and none had a complete index.

– Less than half the files had progress cards arranged in chronological order and this figure is almost certainly flattering as doctors were given the benefit of the doubt when only two cards were present.

– There was no highlighting of important data (however basic) in 85 per cent of progress notes.

– None of those patients on long-term therapy had a treatment chart.

– Only 22 per cent of pregnancies had any record, however basic, of all pregnancies and none had a *full* record each.

– Only a third of those patients taking a contraceptive tablet had this fact recorded in their files.

Taking all these factors into account there was certainly more than one piece of information, likely to prove helpful to the doctor in patient care, missing from these files on average.

REQUIREMENTS OF A RECORD SYSTEM FOR PREVENTIVE MEDICINE

1. The record system must overcome the faults listed above and thus meet the following requirements:

(i) There must be complete cover of all the relevant facts including social, functional, economic, environmental, and occupational data.

(ii) Important material must be easily accessible, files should be indexed, important data highlighted, etc. This should also be organized in such a manner as to facilitate planning, administration, and management of the practice, as well as computer input and epidemiology.

(iii) Records should indicate clearly whether diagnoses are firm or equivocal, assessment being recorded at the level of the doctor's understanding of the problem, i.e. where not even a provisional diagnosis is possible it is perfectly respectable to label the condition by the main presenting symptom.

(iv) Records must be properly integrated so that they express their message clearly on the progress of the disorder and response to treatment (e.g. in diabetes or hypertension).

(v) In selected cases objectives of care should be recorded (e.g. target blood pressure in hypertension).

(vi) The record system should employ a flexible nomenclature and taxonomy of disease.

2. Confidentiality of sensitive records must be preserved since there will be better access to all important material.

3. A record system for prophylaxis must be able to identify 'high-risk' cases. It must have a facility built in to prompt the doctor when such cases are due for review and also facilities for recalling them.

4. The system should be as simple as possible, adaptable, capable of being transferred to other practices and should include a formal and fool-proof method of updating.

To my knowledge only one system has been designed to meet these requirements – Problem-oriented Medical Records (POMR) – devised by Lawrence Weed, Professor of Medicine at the University of Vermont. The system has already been described in detail (Weed 1969; Bjorn and Cross 1970; Petrie and McIntyre) but its main elements are as follows:

1. *The data base* – this consists of all the pertinent health-related information, medical, social, economic, occupation, recreational, and environmental. In my Bicester practice this is generated from a health questionnaire (Appendix 3.1) completed when the patient joins the list together with the information in the patient's file when it arrives some time later.

2. *The problem list* (Appendix 3.2) – this consists of the health problems formulated from the data base which are classified as currently active or resolved. A problem, in this context, is defined as a factor which worries the patient or the doctor (or both) because it is a threat to health or there is a reasonable probability that it may become so in the future. Such problems may take the form of diagnoses, abnormal physical findings or investigation results or any social, economic, occupational, recreational, or functional factor affecting health. There is no place here for the guess or provisional diagnosis and problems are recorded at the level of understanding of the recorder.

This health profile makes important information easily available and enables a doctor to assess the current complaint in the context of the past medical and social history with the optimal chance of him making the correct diagnosis. Computerization and record retrieval which are essential to the organization of preventive medicine are also facilitated by these problem lists.

Weed recommends that problems should be numbered and linked to similarly numbered entries in the progress notes but the author does not find this necessary.

3. *Plans* – in the management of patients, especially where long-term care is involved, careful plans for the management of each problem should be made and recorded under the following headings:

   (i) diagnostic;
   (ii) therapeutic;
   (iii) patient education.

The plans for an obese patient of 48 with a family history of diabetes and a blood pressure of 150/105 might be:

   (i) – Haemoglobin, blood film, urea, creatine lipids, triglycerides, blood sugar, CXR, ECG.
   – Target blood pressure 130/90.
   (ii) – Weight reduction (with target weight to be allowed).
   – Propranol 80 mg b.d.
   – Stop smoking.
   – Reduce saturated fats in diet.

   (iii) – Advise patient of the risks of uncontrolled hypertension and of his increased risk of developing diabetes in the future – stress especially the importance of weight reduction and giving up cigarettes – emphasize the need for strict compliance with therapy and regular review.

4. *Structured progress notes* (Appendix 3.3) – these are laid out in a formal structure, which seeks to highlight important data, under the following headings.

― Subjective data (S) ― the patient's complaint and any medical or paramedical data elicited from him.

― Objective data (O) ― physical examination and investigation results.

― Assessment (A) ― interpretation of the above data and any other relevant information at the level of understanding of the recorder ― there may be a case here for the educated guess or provisional diagnosis, *provided it is identified as such.*

― Plans (P) ― these are recorded for diagnostic, therapeutic and patient education purposes once again.

The acronym SOAP is often used to describe this type of structuring of progress notes.

5. *Flow charts* ― chronic disorders are monitored by reviewing a number of clinical criteria and these results are usually scattered throughout the progress notes. Flow charts are simply a means of bringing them together in tabular or graphic form to express their message more clearly and to indicate *at a glance* the progress of the disease and the response to treatment.

Thus by using the hypertension flow chart (Appendix 3.4) the doctor would have easy access to the following facts:

(i) Clear identifying details including social status and date of birth.

(ii) A record of when hypertension was first noted and the manner in which it was diagnosed.

(iii) Important data on previous medical, family, and weight history together with smoking behaviour.

(iv) Current therapy.

(v) Physical findings.

(vi) Assessment of the findings at the level of understanding of the clinician involved.

(vii) Clear objectives of care.

(viii) Graphic presentation of systolic and diastolic blood pressure readings and recording of weight.

(ix) Valuable comments on compliance with review and treatment.

(x) Clear dated recordings of investigations which also remind the doctor when they are due to be re-checked.

(xi) Clear details of past treatment with reported side-effects.

(xii) Recording of when the next appointment is due which helps the doctor to monitor compliance.

Thus the flow chart acts as a check list and a means of collating records so that they give a clear profile of the progress of the disorder.

FILING SYSTEMS

Few subjects in general practice polarize opinion so sharply as this. Both the Family Practitioner Committee record file and the A4 file have their fervent advocates and the pros and cons of the argument are summarized below:

FPC file (7" × 5")	A4 file (12¼" × 9½")
Type – simply a record envelope and not a true modern file which encourages 'rag-bag' rather than chronological, filing	A true modern file which encourages chronological filing
Size – small, easy to carry, and does not clutter the surgery desk – space for records not always adequate – may lead to under-recording but advocates say that it discourages over-elaborate recording. Reports often have to be folded before insertion and unfolded after withdrawal	Larger and therefore clumsier for use in surgery and on calls. Plenty of space for recording but may encourage the prolix

Reports are almost always filed flat |
Thickness – files at six per inch	Files at 3–4 per inch
Source of reference – poor in view of the above factors especially in the case of bulky files	Excellent
Cost to provide, maintain, file, and post – low	More expensive (especially as the doctor may have to provide his own)
Use – rarely found outside general practice	Almost universal in other disciplines and branches of the profession

Advocates of the FPC file further claim that the expense of transferring to A4 files is unjustifiable since computers will make them obsolete. The idea that computers will make hard-copy files obsolete even within the next decade is a triumph of hope over experience. The cost of computers is falling but remains a considerable disincentive as is the organization of records which is a prerequisite to any form of data-processing. Finally the discipline required for the development and maintanance of such a system is far from being universal.

Personally I prefer the A4 system which I have used with complete satisfaction for more than eight years. Few people who have used it return to the FPC file with all its shortcomings. However, it must be acknowledged that A4 files are not a *sine qua non* for the development of a POMR system as has been shown by Tait (1979) and Maycock (1978) although the former has now partly converted to A4 files.

IMPLEMENTATION OF A MODERN SYSTEM

The problems of introducing a modern record system are usually underestimated not least in relation to preventive care. These difficulties need to be clearly defined and understood by anyone embarking on this task.

The initial difficulty lies in persuading doctors of the need for change and motivating them to become involved. Next all members of the care team must agree on the data to be collected and the manner in which it is to be recorded. Since important (and sometimes sensitive) information is more easily accessible, fears about breach of confidentiality must be overcome by careful record design, i.e. sensitive data will be coded or extracted and kept in a special file. The cost of using a modern record system especially if it involves computerization may be considerable. This must be justified although benefits are not always easy to *demonstrate*. Fears about bulkier files leading to increased storage costs need to be appreciated, and can be offset by record culling. Form filling is tedious and must be kept to a minimum while fears of the computer, although often irrational need to be resolved.

It must be appreciated that staff (and especially doctors) are being asked to change the habits of a lifetime and adopt a new record system with strict rules calling for them to be disciplined and obsessional in making entries. Furthermore, the value of this record system has not been fully established by research and likewise there are doctors who regard prophylaxis itself (especially where it involves screening and surveillance) as being of questionable value especially as it can be time-consuming.

Taking all these factors into account it can be no mean task to convince workers that the work involved is justified and the best use is being made of available resources.

USES OF A MODERN RECORD SYSTEM IN PROPHYLAXIS

In 1963, Last drew our attention to the 'clinical iceberg' commenting that a 'considerable amount of undetected disease, some of which is serious and some controllable, might be found fairly easily without adding greatly to the burden of the day's work'. Good records are fundamental to any programme designed to achieve this because they help to identify high-risk groups. This can be illustrated by the screening and surveillance of old people undertaken by the author in his practice in Bicester. High-risk elderly patients are identified from the following check list by doctors, nurses, social workers, relatives, or neighbours:

Socio-economic factors	Medical disorders
(i) Advanced age – 75 years or more	(i) Impaired vision or hearing
(ii) Social isolates who live alone or lack social contact	(ii) Patients with a painful or disabling chronic disease especially involving the musculo-skeltal, circulatory, or nervous system
(iii) Patients with an infirm partner or poor support in the event of other than serious illness	
(iv) Lonely patients (not always socially isolated)	(iii) Disorders of the feet – corns, oedema, ulcers. Anaemia. Breathlessness.
(v) Patients with reduced mobility (especially housebound)	

(vi) The recently bereaved or recently discharged from hospital
(vii) Indigent patients
(viii) Patients unfit for all the activities of daily living – dressing, cooking, feeding, toilet, housework, and shopping
(ix) Old people in unsuitable accommodation
(x) Patients with depression, boredom, lack of purpose, loss of identity, and especially those adapting poorly to their problems

Disturbed bowel or bladder habit.
Emotional or mental disturbance especially depression.
Any disability
(iv) Patients showing withdrawal – perhaps the highest risk of all

These patients are screened using questionnaires (Appendixes 3.5 and 3.6) which record and scale socio-economic, health, and disability problems together with an estimation of the patient's adaptation to them in each case. Records are also kept of the names of relatives, neighbours, or friends ready to provide help in the event of illness.

With all these records available it is possible to work out a programme of care appropriate to each patient, making use of the primary care team, the social worker, physiotherapist, occupational therapist, chiropodist, relatives, neighbours, and voluntary workers with the family doctor acting as a co-ordinator of care. Finally the patient's risk rating is assessed and this helps the doctor plan continuing surveillance, after their initial screening, either at home or in a geriatric clinic.

IDENTIFICATION AND REGISTRATION OF HIGH-RISK PATIENTS

These at risk patients need to be identified and this can be done in two ways:

1. By case finding during a clinical consultation, when reports are received on the patient from hospital or other authorities or on record review.

2. By formally screening a given population with the intention of identifying a specific disease or group of disorders.

Both methods have been used in the identification of cases of diabetes and hypertension in the past. The former method is much more practical and therefore useful but blanket screening of populations has been largely discredited (Nuffield Provincial Hospitals Trust 1968) except for certain conditions such as phenylketonuria.

The files of such patients must then be 'tagged' to facilitate retrieval and the Royal College of General Practitioners has devised a colour code for certain common diseases (Appendix 3.7).

Certain other colour codes are also available to enable the doctor to identify other special groups.

Coloured stickers using this code and overprinted with the name of the disease involved are supplied by a drug firm (Winthrop Ltd.). They are equally suitable for use on the current medical record envelope or the A4 file.

When 'at-risk' patients have been identified it is necessary to enter the name, address, sex, and date of birth of each in a register and two of these are especially useful: (i) the disease or morbidity register; (ii) the handicap register.

Disease or morbidity register

Several such registers already exist such as:

(i) The E Book (Eimerl 1973; Eimerl and Laidlaw 1969) which can act as a disease index or (because frequency of attacks can be recorded) as a morbidity register – to remain effective it needs annual review and updating.

(ii) The F Book designed by Kuennsberg (1964) which gives a profile of family morbidity.

(iii) The W Book (Walford 1963) – this disease index is cumulative and is intended for the registration of 'important' conditions only.

By tagging and the use of ad hoc registers care can be focused on vulnerable patients with special needs by members of the primary care team.

THE USES OF A COMPUTER IN PROPHYLAXIS

The value of the computer in prophylaxis lies in its capacity to store large amounts of data, to provide rapid access to these data, easy analysis, and quick recall. In this way population review and screening can be facilitated so that 'at-risk' patients can be identified to enable attention to be focused on their particular needs.

Thus the computer can provide:

1. A tabulation of any particular group of patients by age and sex.
2. A listing of patients at special risk because of chronic disease, handicap, etc. and this may be provided simply as an alphabetical tabulation or categorized by disease or handicap.
3. A means therefore of planning screening and surveillance programmes for all high-risk groups so that appropriate priorities can be established.
4. Recall facilities to assist the scheduling of clinics.
5. A means of identifying patients defaulting on review.
6. Indirect benefits in prophylaxis by facilitating audit, research, and teaching.
7. Help in integrating the primary care team by providing the above administrative help to receptionists and secretaries and clinical facilities to nurses and health visitors.
8. A prompting facility to remind medical and nursing staff when a special service, e.g. inoculation or cervical smearing is due.

42   Record systems in preventive medicine

9. A problem list or flow chart which will help the doctor planning review of individual cases or groups of patients.

Thus the planning, administration, and practice of prophylaxis can be facilitated.

This chapter has sought to indicate how important records and data processing are to prophylaxis in patient care. Hitherto the profession has been slow to recognize the central role of medical records and epidemiology in preventive medicine. However, attitudes are changing and with the technological advances predicted in the near future, data assembly and manipulation are sure to play a much greater role in years to come in the prevention and management of disease.

Sir William Osler neatly encapsulated the spirit of this chapter in commenting 'If you have the good fortune to command a large clinic remember that one of your chief duties is the tabulation and analysis of the carefully recorded experience' – and that was almost 100 years ago.

REFERENCES

Bjorn, J. C. and Cross, H. D. (1970). *Problem oriented practice*. McGraw Hill, Chicago.

Eimerl, T. S. (1973). The E-Book system for record-keeping in general practice. *Medical Care* 11, Suppl., 138–44.

—— and Laidlaw, A. J. (1969). *Handbook for research in general practice,* 2nd edn. Churchill Livingstone, Edinburgh.

Kuenssberg, E. V. (1964). Recordings of morbidity of families, F Book. *J. R. Coll. Gen. Practrs* 7, 410–22.

Last, J. M. (1963). The clinical iceberg. *Lancet* ii, 28–31.

Maycock, C. (1978). GP records: a simple and inexpensive system. *Br. med. J.* ii, 1510–11.

Nuffield Provincial Hospital Trust (1968). *Screening in medical care.* Oxford University Press, London.

Petrie, J. C. and McIntyre, N. (1979). *The problem orientated medical record. Its use in hospitals, general practice and medical education.* Churchill Livingstone, Edinburgh.

Tait, I. G. (1979). The clinical record in general practice. *Br. med. J.* ii, 683–8.

Walford, P. A. (1963). The practice index. *J. R. Coll. Gen. Practrs* 6, 225–32.

Weed, L. L. (1969). *Medical records, medical education and patient care.* The Press of Case Western Reserve, University of Queensland.

APPENDIX 3.1

APPENDIX 1

HEALTH DATA FORM 2

THIS INFORMATION WILL BE TREATED AS PRIVATE AND CONFIDENTIAL

You have just joined our list and it may be some months before your records reach us. This may of course be important and the absence of these records may impair the service which we wish to give you. It is therefore in the interests of both yourself and your doctor to fill in the questionnaire below for each member of your family. Please use a ballpoint pen. If you have any doubts about any question, just leave it blank and the nurse will help you to fill it in when you see her.

SURNAME ..... OTHER

FORENAMES ..... ABRAHAM N.

ADDRESS ..... BUCKINGHAM MEWS ..... NEWTOWN

NHS No SACC64/6 ... Date of Birth 18.6.28

Please place a tick in appropriate box:

~~Married /-/ Single /-/ Widowed /-/~~
Divorced /✓/   ~~Separated /-/~~

1. Occupation
   1. Present Computer programmer
   2. Previous Clerical officer

   If a housewife / /
   Please give husband's occupation   n/r

   If a child / /   n/r
   Please give father's occupation

2. Smoking
   How long? 40 years
   Current rate? 15 a day
   Intervals off cigarettes? None

3. Have you had any previous illnesses, accidents or operations, not including trivial illnesses, e.g. influenza, colds, sore throats, etc., unless they keep recurring. If so, please enter them below with the year in which they occurred?

Year	Condition	Year	Condition
1932	Scarlet fever	1969	Pneumonia
1946	Rubella	1971	Appendicectomy
1950	Bacillary dysentery (Egypt)		
1961	Road traffic accident (hosp 24 hrs)		Asthma recurring since 1965

4. If any of the illnesses necessitated hospital admission, please state the name of the hospital, whether you had an operation, and what the operation was if you know?

Year	Condition	Hospital	Operation
1961	Head injury -RTA	Hull Infirmary	
1971	Appendicectomy		

5. Treatment at present (tablets, capsules, medicines, etc.) and dosage

1. Ventolin Inhaler   5.
2.   6.
3.   7.
4.   8.

Appendix 3.1 45

6. Are you allergic to anything? YES/NO Please specify ....Septrin........................

7. In the case of a woman:
   i. How many pregnancies have you had? ....n/r............
   ii. Have any them ended in miscarriage, stillbirth, or diffcult delivery, e.g. breech delivery, forceps, or Caesarian section?   YES/NO Please specify ....
   iii. If you are on an oral contraceptive (the "Pill") at the moment, how long have you been taking it. YES/NO ....Brand ....
   iv. If not, have you taken the pill in the past? YES/NO   For how long? ....
   When stopped? ....
   v. Have you had a cervical (cancer) smear? YES/NO
   Date of last smear ....

8. Have you been immunised against:
   i. Diptheria Date.............../NO
   ii. Polio Date ..../NO
   iii. Tetanus Date .1976......../NO
   vii. Any Other Date ..../NO
   iv. Smallpox Date..1952........./NO
   v. Measles Date................/NO
   vi. Whooping Cough Date................/NO

9. Have you had any major handicap or disability e.g. blind, deaf, amputated limb, etc. ?   XXYES/NO Details ....
   ....

10. Is there any history of disease in the family such as diabetes, raised blood pressure, heart disease, or mental disorder? YES/NO Details: ..Mother.&.one.aunt.diabetic
   ....

11. Do you have any major social problems, e.g. unsatisfactory housing, marital problems, disabled child, etc? XYES/NO Details ....
   ....
   ....

12 a. Current Weight ..11.st...6.lbs:.. Height ....5'8"......... Blood Group (if known)
   Group.Not.known.RH..........
   b. Are you taking any medicine at present NOT prescribed by a doctor?   YES/NO Details ....
   ....

PLEASE FILL OUT ONE OF THESE FORMS FOR EACH MEMBER OF THE FAMILY BUT NOTE THAT THIS DOES NOT MEAN YOU ARE REGISTERED WITH THE PRACTICE. REGISTRATION ONLY TAKES PLACE WHEN YOUR SIGNED MEDICAL CARD IS HANDED OVER. IF YOU ARE ON LONG TERM TREATMENT BRING YOUR MEDICAL CONTAINERS OR A TREATMENT CARD (IF YOU HAVE ONE) WHEN YOU COME TO SEE THE DOCTOR.

l systems in preventive medicine

X 3.2

APPENDIX 2

___M LIST   Date:

Full name: A.N. OTHER

Registers
1 — Chronic disease

    a) ordinary — ✓

    b) high risk —

2 — handicap — ✓

3 — other risks —

Address: BUCKINGHAM MEWS

          NEWTOWN

m/~~f~~

d.o.b. 18.6.28

Occupation

Date	Active	Inactive	Code	u/d
1932		Scarlet fever-quite severe attack but no sequelae		
1946		Rubella		
1950		Bacillary dysentery x 2 (while in Egypt on Nat. Service)		
1961		Road traffic accident K.O'd x ½ hr.-kept in hospital 24 hrs. X-rays- NAD		
1969		Pneumonia		
1965	Started having asthmatic attacks			
1971		Appendicectomy		
1974		Pains L.I.F. recurrently for several months Investigation negative		
	REACTION TO SEPTRIN			
1977	Anxiety Depression Marital difficulties			
1978	Wife has left him Depression Confidential entry **			

(** this refers to his wife's discovery that he has had an homosexual relationship -such sensitive details are kept in a locked confidential file and are <u>not</u> entered in the problem list)

APPENDIX 3.3 (a)

APPENDIX 3 (a)

	National Health Service Number	
CLINICAL NOTES	Surname (Block Letters) EINSTEIN	Forenames (Block Letters) ERASMUS
	Address SEBASTOPOL TERRACE BICESTER Oxon.	Occupation Building Labourer — Date of Birth 9.10.1930

Date	*		
1970			
8.2.70	S-	Cough, brick-coloured spit, pain (L) side, worse on coughing. Temp. malaise, headache x 2 days	POMR progress notes as designed by Weed
VC14	O-	T101.2° P.106 R: 36 (with dilated alae) R.S.-Dull (R) base. Bronchial breathing & coarse creps	
	A-	Probable pneumonia	
	P-	Inj.crys.penicillin 500,000 units 6 hourly I.M. Tab.DF118 Sputum to path/w.b.c.	
9.2.70 V.	S- O-	No change Physical findings ISQ	
10.2.70 V.	S- O-	Sl.better. Breathing easier Dullness less marked. Fewer creps. Wbc 17,500	
11.3.70 V	S O-	urther improvement Apyrexial. Dullness clearing Spt.:pneumococci	
	A-	Pneumonia	
	P-	Continue treatment	
14.2.70 V.	O-	Continued progress Dullness almost cleared	
19.2.70	S-	Mobile but weak	
23.2.70 VC7	P-	Chest X-ray	
30.2.70 ACF(Mon)		Cleared	

* This column has been provided for doctors to enter A, V or C at their discretion

FORM FP111 F

48 *Record systems in preventive medicine*

APPENDIX 3.3 (b)

APPENDIX 3 (b)

CLINICAL NOTES

National Health Service Number		
Surname (Block Letters) EINSTEIN	Forenames (Block Letters) ERASMUS	
Address SEBASTOPOL TERRACE BICESTER Oxon	Occupation: Building labourer	Date of Birth 9.10.1930

Date	*		
8.10.70	A-	A-Follicular tonsillitis P-Tabs.penicil.V-IC 250 mg.qds (28)	Author's modification of POMR progress notes for use in general practice
1972 14.4.72	A-	Vague para-umbilical pain recurrently in last 2-3 days-constipated-sick x 2 this morning -no other symptoms-2 previous similar attacks in 1969 P.82 T.99 R.18 Chest NAD Abdo-vague tenderness below umbilicus (no rebound)-no guarding.P.R.NAD A ? P.rest light diet R.review 24 hours	
15.4.72		Cleared	
~~1975~~ 18.9.75		Tired-requesting a tonic-no worry or stress at home or work-insomnia- appetite poor-no localising symptoms. O.E. NAD A endogenous depression P Tabs.amitriptyline 25 mg. x 2 nocte R. 2/52	
2.10.75		improving gradually	

* This column has been provided for doctors to enter A, V or C at their discretion

FORM FP111 F

APPENDIX 3.4

```
                    APPENDIX 4
```

HYPERTENSION FLOW CHART 1	Name LADY MACBETH Address 10 MAIN STREET NEWTOWN.
Presentation Age of onset [Slight toxaemia (1954) in 2nd pregnancy- Age 28 yrs. 140/95 Insurance medical -36 yrs. (1960)	Tel No Newtown 2646 D.O.B. 18.6.26 NHS No ABCD 64/2 Hosp. No.
Previous Medical History Recurrent urinary infection since 1966 (5 attacks)	Family Doctor Dr.J.Bloggs The Health Centre, Newtown. Tel No. Newtown 4428
	Family History Aunt hypertensive Father diabetic Mother grossly overweight
Smoking Habits 20/day x 22 yrs.	
Weight History Overweight since age of 19 yrs.	

Other Pertinent Information
Previous doctor reports default
on review and compliance with
drug therapy.
	Current Therapy
	  June 1971(on joining list)
	  Tabs.methyldopa 250 mg. qds

Occupation Housewife	

Initial Examination   Date 16.6.71

Personality   Plethoric subject. Untidy appearance   Weight 92 kgs.
                                                               Height 5'4"

Physique	Flabby	Fundi L)			
		Fundi R) NAD		Thyroid	
C V S	NAD	Pulses Normal			
J.V.P.		P.R. 82			
A.B.		B.P. 170/105			
R.S.	NAD	Abdomen NAD			
C.N.S.	NAD				

                              Albumin Nil
                              Urine — sugar Nil
Other   ketones Nil

Assessment	**Objectives**
Essential hypertension	1. SBP 140 2. DBP 90 3. Initial weight target -70 kg. 4. Watch for diabetes

REVIEW CRITERIA

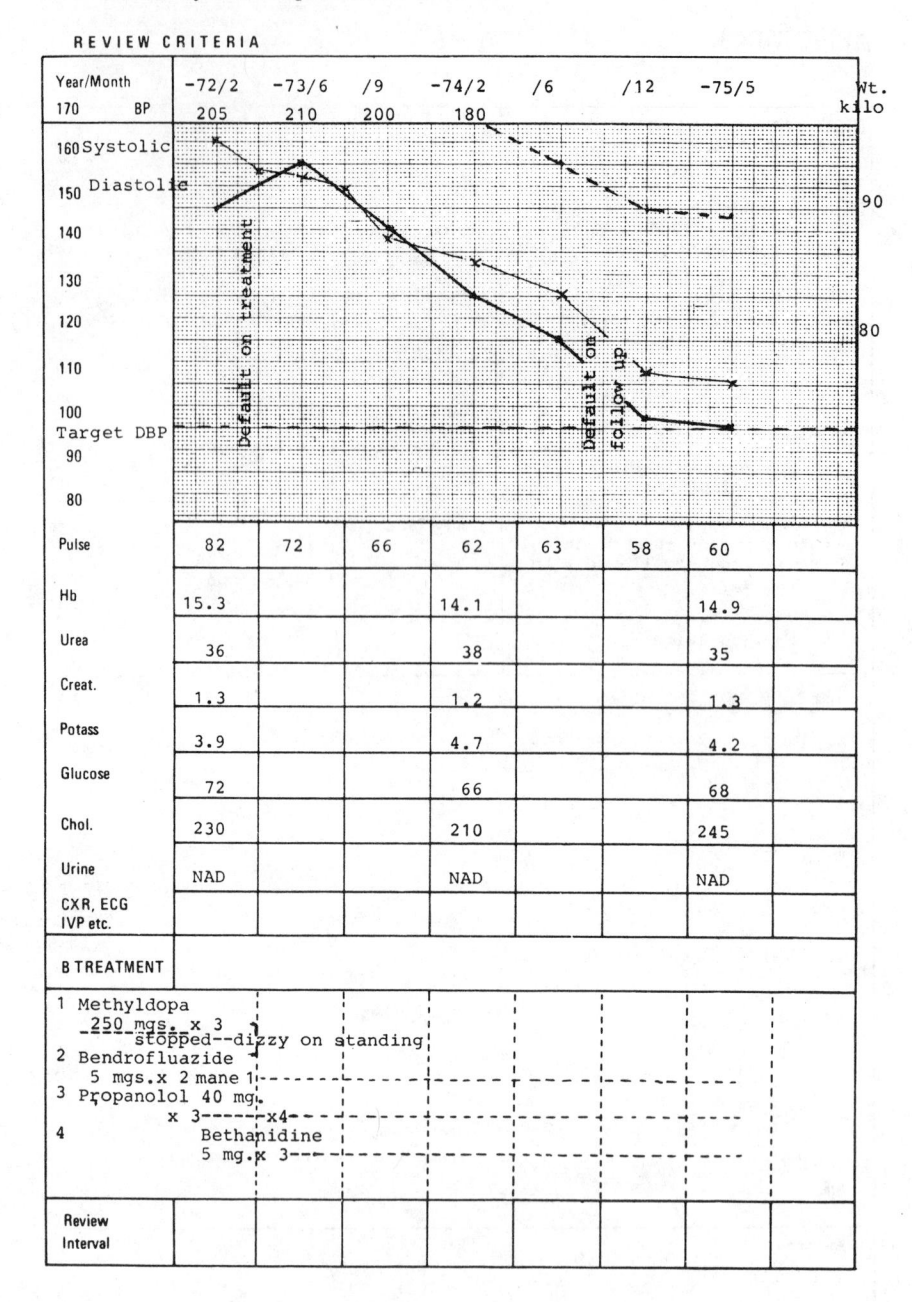

Year/Month	-72/2	-73/6	/9	-74/2	/6	/12	-75/5	Wt. kilo
BP	205	210	200	180				
Pulse	82	72	66	62	63	58	60	
Hb	15.3			14.1			14.9	
Urea	36			38			35	
Creat.	1.3			1.2			1.3	
Potass	3.9			4.7			4.2	
Glucose	72			66			68	
Chol.	230			210			245	
Urine	NAD			NAD			NAD	
CXR, ECG IVP etc.								

B TREATMENT

1 Methyldopa
   250 mgs. x 3
         stopped--dizzy on standing
2 Bendrofluazide
   5 mgs.x 2 mane 1
3 Propanolol 40 mg.
       x 3-----x4
4   Bethanidine
        5 mg.x 3

Review Interval

(Graph shows Systolic and Diastolic BP over time with annotations "Default on treatment", "Default on follow up", and "Target DBP" line at 90)

APPENDIX 3.5

```
                        APPENDIX 5
-------------------------------------|---------------------------------------
CARE OF THE ELDERLY    CHART 1       | Surname    PATIENT
-------------------------------------|
                                     | Forenames  A
                        Date         |
                                     | Address   331 OXFORD ROAD
-------------------------------------|                BICESTER
A.  SOCIO-ECONOMIC PROBLEMS          |
-------------------------------------| D.O.B. 18.6.02   Marital status
1. Day to day support                |                            WIDOW
   i.   Lives with spouse            | Past occupation DOMESTIC SERVANT
   ii.  Lives with children          |---------------------------------------
   iii. Lives with other relations   | 5. Economic Status
   iv.  Lives with friends           |    i.   Satisfactory
  (v.)  Lives alone with periodic    |   (ii.) Borderline
         outside support             |    iii. Inadequate
   vi.  Lives alone without outside  |
                         support     | 6. Recent Bereavement
-------------------------------------|    During the past year patient has
2. Illness support                   |                                 cost
   When confined to bed the patient  |    i.  nobody
   has                               |    ii. a close friend, in-law, or
   i.   full support                 |        relative outside the immediate
   ii.  day-time support only        |        family
  (iii.) uncertain support           |    iii. a parent
   iv.  no support                   |   (iv.) a husband, wife or child
                                     |
-------------------------------------|---------------------------------------
3. Accommodation  A-good B-fair C-poor| 7. Loneliness
   Structural state                  |    The patient feels lonely
   Heating                           |    i.   never
   Running h. & c.                   |   (ii.) occasionally
   Toilet facilities                 |    iii. often
   Lighting                          |    iv.  almost all the time
   Decoration                        |
                                     |---------------------------------------
  - Rating of structure & facilities | 8. Accident risk            Detail
   i.   Excellent                    |    i.   minimal
   ii.  Good                         |    ii.  average
  (iii.) Fair                        |   (iii.) above average
   iv.  Poor                         |
   v.   Unacceptable                 |---------------------------------------
                                     | 9. Other Problems
  - Suitability of accommodation     |   (a) Infirm partner       YES/NO
   i.   Good              Detail     |   (b) Frustration          YES/NO
   ii.  Fair                         |   (c) Boredom              YES/NO
  (iii.) Poor                        |    d) Lack of role/purpose YES/NO
              Steep stairs           |    e)
                                     |
-------------------------------------|---------------------------------------
4. Social contact                    |10. Need for
   Relatives, friends or neighbours  |   (a) meals on wheels
   seen                              |   (b) voluntary support (transport,etc)
   i.   daily                        |   (c) day centre
  (ii.) two- three times a week      |    d) day hospital
   iii. weekly                       |    e)
   iv.  sporadically                 |    f)
   v.   rarely                       |    g)
```

B. **PROBLEMS OF DISABILITY**

---

1. **Mobility**
   i. Fully mobile
   ii. Moderate impairment of mobility
   iii. Marked limitation of mobility (no aid or assistance)
   iv. Mobile only with aid
   v. Mobile only with assistance
      (iii, iv & v usually housebound)
   vi. Bed or chair fast

---

2. **Continence**
   i. Fully continent
   ii. Occasional accident due to restricted mobility or stress incontinence
   iii. Nocturnal incontinence of urine
   iv. Urinary incontinence day and night
   v. Double incontinence

---

3. **Domestic Care**
   Cooking:
   i. Able to prepare all meals
   ii. Able to prepare some food only
   iii. Unable to prepare food/meals at all

   Housework:
   i. Able to do all own housework
   ii. Requires assistance with housework
   iii. Requires full time help

   Shopping:
   i. Able to do all own shopping
   ii. Requires assistance with shopping
   iii. Unable to do any shopping

   Rating:
   i. scores 1 in all indices
   ii. scores 2 on no more than one index
   iii. scores 2 on more than one index
   iv. scores 3 on two or three indices

---

4. **Nutrition**
   i. Adequate
   ii. Borderline
   iii. Unsatisfactory

5. **Self Care**
   Dressing:
   i. Independent
   ii. Requires assistance with shoes and socks only
   iii. Able to assist in dressing
   iv. Unable to assist in dressing

   Feeding:
   i. Independent
   ii. Requires assistance with cutting up food only
   iii. Able to assist in feeding
   iv. Unable to assist in feeding

   Toilet:
   i. Independent day and night
   ii. Requires assistance at night only
   iii. Requires assistance day and night but remains continent
   iv. Incontinent despite assistance

   Rating:
   i. Fully independent - scores 1 in each
   ii. Minor disability - scores 1 in each except dressing, where he may score 2
   iii. Partial independence - scores 2 or 3 on feeding and/or toilet or 3 on dressing
   iv. Dependent - scores 4 on at least one index
   v. Wholly dependent - scores 4 on two or three indices

---

6. **Other Problems**

   Lives 3 miles from surgery - poor bus service on this route - cannot get in to see doctor as often as she feels she needs to do.

APPENDIX 3.6

APPENDIX 6   A.PATIENT 18.6.02

CARE OF THE ELDERLY   CHART 2   Date ....

BASIC HEALTH QUESTIONNAIRE	YES	AMPLIFICATION BY QUESTIONER OR PATIENT
1. Is your sight poorer than last year ?		No
2. Is your hearing poorer than last year ?		No
3. Do you feel more tired than you might expect to be	Yes	
4. Is your concentration poorer than last year ?		No
5. Is memory now poorer than last year— a) for recent events b) for remote events		No
6. Do you get more a) anxious b) depressed than a year ago ?		No
7. Do you have dizzy spells or blackouts		No
8. Is your sleep pattern disturbed	Yes	
9. Do you have pain especially in a) head b) chest c) abdomen d) legs on walking		No
10. Has your weight changed How much		No
11. Do you get breathless much more easily than a year ago ?	Yes	
12. Have you a chronic cough		No
13. Do you have indigestion		No
14. Is your bowel function disturbed		No
15. Do you pass water more often -especially at night		No
16. Can you control urination	Yes	
17. Have you any foot problems		No
18. Do your ankles swell regularly	Yes	- occas
19. Have you been in hospital during the past year		No
20. Can you get about as well as a year ago	Yes	
21 Have you any other problems		No

Health problems
1. Medical disorders

   i) mild congestive heart failure
   ii) osteo-arthritis R hip

2. Socio-economic problems

   i)   poor day to day support
   ii)   uncertain illness support
   iii) unsuitable accommodation
   iv)   economic status : borderline
   v)   recently lost husband (Nov. 1980)
   vi)   above average accident risk
   vii) bored frustrated & occasionally lonely

3. Disabilities

   i) mobility slightly impaired
   ii) needs help with housekeeping & shopping. 3) needs transport surgery.

Adaptation -   good /   fair/   poor

Next of kin

   Mr. R. Higgins,
     2, Edinburgh Close,
        Kidlington.

Relatives/friends prepared to help in crisis

Mr. J. Smith : 329, Oxford Rd.
                           Bicester.
Mr. R. Jones : 20l, Sheep St.,
                           Bicester

Welfare representative

   R. Newton-Cox
     20l, Oxford Road,
        Bicester. (Fish Scheme)

Action recommended
Need for :-
1. Doctor
2. Nurse
3. Health visitor
4. Chiropodist
5. Physiotherapist
6. O.T.
7. Social worker
8. Voluntary worker
9. Other

Family Tree

○———————⌀ died Nov. 1980

Mrs. R. Higgins   T. Patient
  (b. 1930)   emigrated to
  Kidlington   Australia
  (8 miles   1954
   away)

Other potential hazards

Risk Index
              Medical   Socio-economic
              problems   problems
1.   Nil   Nil
2.   Minor and/or   Minor
3.a Major and   Nil or minor
  b Nil or minor and   Major
④   Major   and   Major
5.   Dependent   -
6.   Wholly dependent

APPENDIX 3.7

COLOUR TAGGING OF N.H.S. MEDICAL RECORDS

In a recent report* the following proposals were made in regard to the colour tagging of N.H.S. medical records:

1. That not more than eight disorders or disease groups be chosen and that these be allotted clear and easily memorised colours.

2. That there be two alternate approved sites for marking records: at the top end of the right edge of the face of the E.C.6, or along the top edge of a projecting insert card or E.C.7 8. For the Scottish form of E.C.6, the left hand top corner is most appropriate, as this place would become the right hand top corner when inserted into the English filing system.

3. That strip-adhesive plastic tape (Sellotape) be the method of choice, ¼" wide tape be applied in ½" lengths on both front and back of insert card or envelope or record envelope. If more than one colour code is applicable the next coloured tape to be inserted alongside as close as possible.

4. These principles are broad enough to cover essentials without the need for an 'interpreter's handbook' whilst leaving the enthusiast free to use striped, matched, spotted or non-primary colours (placed in non-standard sites) for research or administrative purposes of his own without causing confusion to the basic system.

Please turn over for the list of conditions and appropriate colour codes.

*Report on colour tagging by Research Committee of Council J. Coll. gen. Pract., 1964, 8, 84.
**Colour coding Brit. med. J., 1968, 2, 244.

COLOUR TAGGING FOR EIGHT IMPORTANT DISEASE GROUPS

8

RED	1 Sensitivities		(Drug sensitivities, severe toxic drug idiosyncrasies and major allergies)
BROWN	2 Diabetes		
YELLOW	3 Epilepsy		
GREEN	4 Tuberculosis		(Active, arrested or cured)
BLUE	5 Hypertension		(Any variety which has warranted hypotensive therapy)
WHITE	6 Long-term maintenance therapy		(e.g. steroids, thyroid, Vit.B12, antibiotics, etc.)
▓	7 Attempted Suicide		
▓	8 Measles		(To avoid unnecessary immunisation procedures**)

N.B. Users must understand from the onset that the recommended use is positive not negative. The presence of a colour tag means that the disorder so coded is, or has been present; the absence of a tag can never be taken to imply the absence of such a disorder.

Further copies available from the Royal College of General Practitioners, 14 Princes Gate, London, S.W.7.

4 Patient education in general practice

Simon Smail

Education is not that one knows more, but that one behaves differently.

John Ruskin

The World Health Organization (1969) has defined health education as follows: 'Health Education concerns all those experiences of an individual, group, or community that influences beliefs, attitudes, and behaviour with respect to health as well as the processes and efforts of producing change when this is necessary for optimal health.' Thus in practice, patient education is concerned not only with those factors which influence patients' beliefs and attitudes but also with the educational and behavioural strategies that may be used for modifying beliefs, attitudes, and indeed behaviour. Although most definitions of Health Education follow Ruskin's aphorism in emphasizing behaviour change, Gatherer *et al.* (1979) points out that 'it is dangerous as well as too limiting to consider that the only valuable health education is that which can be measured in terms of behavioural change'. Simply imparting information to patients about health is a perfectly legitimate aim (people have a right to know about health) although many would expect some resulting behaviour change as well.

The usual overt aim of education is preventive. In exactly the same way that prevention may be classified as primary, secondary, and tertiary, so health may be linked to such a classification (Tones 1977).

1. Primary prevention: attempts to reduce the incidence (i.e. number of new cases) of disease in a population. Primary health education is therefore concerned with promoting behaviour which will create well-being or avoid disease; for example encouragement of good dietary habits, exercise, the avoidance of accidents.

2. Secondary prevention: attempts to reduce the prevalence of disease (i.e. number of cases present) in a population. Secondary health education therefore is concerned with encouraging both the uptake of screening procedures designed to detect asymptomatic disease and with the efficient use of medical services.

3. Tertiary prevention: aims to reduce disability caused by established disease. Tertiary health education attempts to encourage patients to comply with therapeutic regimens and make use of rehabilitation services.

However, there is another aspect of health education that many feel is of equal importance to the established aims of prevention, and this is the concept of encouraging efficient use of medical services. This is a somewhat difficult and controversial idea from a theoretical point of view, but few practitioners doubt its importance. An editorial in the *Journal of the Royal College of General Practitioners* (1973) stated the idea thus: 'One of the many aims of health education in the future is to synchronize the expectations of the public and the profession'. Patients present in practice who have demands for medical care but many of these patients could be said to have little or no medical need. On the other hand, there are many patients within any practice population who have medical need, which may or nmay not be overt, but who do not present for medical care. Since resources are inevitably finite, it may be necessary to discourage some patients from over-use of services in order to release resources for others and maintain the efficiency of the service.

ETHICAL PROBLEMS IN HEALTH EDUCATION

Underlying most discussion of health education is the assumption that those professionals involved know what is best for the person or population in terms of health behaviour. Yet this assumption cannot be made too readily. Medical history is full of instances of the mistaken beliefs of doctors being thrust upon an unsuspecting public (Comfort 1967). In recent times for example, nutrition education campaigns in the 1940s and 1950s have encouraged people to eat eggs, red meat, and shellfish, whereas at present many would wish to discourage such food habits. Recently many people have become confused and bewildered by the public debate about the value of pertussis immunization. The result has been a dramatic fall not just in pertussis immunization but also in other forms of immunization.

Before any major attempts are made to alter people's behaviour the professionals involved must be able to give clear justification of the reasons behind their proposals. As Cochrane (1972) has pointed out, it may be unethical to proceed with therapeutic strategies that have not been rigorously proven. This principle similarly applies to the preventive strategies of primary health education.

One can enlarge this argument further and apply it to the process of health education. Not only must the proposed behaviour be shown to be more beneficial to the health of the individual or population, but also the method for advocating the behaviour change should do more good than harm. Thus if an educational programme creates an unwarranted degree of anxiety amongst the population screened then it may be judged on ethical criteria alone to be of dubious value.

Another area of difficulty relates to the effect that patient education may have on the doctor's relationship with his patients. Some general practitioners feel nihilistic about health education perhaps on the one hand because they do not see much evidence of effectiveness or on the other because they are wary of creating unwarranted anxiety amongst their patients. There is, however, an increasing demand from patients for information about health and indeed practitioners must be prepared to inform patients about their problems but also must promote individual responsibility for health decisions. Many practitioners find this difficult – particularly if they are used to an authoritarian style and draw some professional satisfaction from patient dependency. The familiar opening phrase 'What can *I* do for you?' may be a token of the real wish of doctors to continue such a relationship with patients. Recent progress in the use of recall registers in practices, including the introduction of computerized systems, may similarly encourage patients to believe that their doctors will take all responsibility for routine paediatric checks, cervical smears, or blood pressure checks. Although such systems can be of great benefit to practice and patient alike, it is always important to ensure that they are used solely as reminder systems, and that the responsibility for attending the surgery for routine checks remains where it belongs – with the patient.

Thus any practitioner who is keen to adopt the principles of health education within his practice may need to take a fresh look at his own objectives and indeed at the relationship that he forms with patients. An authoritarian style will often be unhelpful whereas counselling and advising patients about the significance of health choices facing them will usually be appropriate.

EVALUATION OF HEALTH EDUCATION

Theoretically patient education should follow educational principles. Briefly those applicable to health education can be summarized as follows (Neufeld 1976), and are similar to the principles applicable to any programme of adult education.

1. Individualization: learning is an individual process, accomplished at different rates by different learners; it is not accomplished by magical transmission from the teacher.

2. Feedback: learning is facilitated by rapid individual feedback on the extent to which learning is being accomplished.

3. Relevance: learning is more efficient if the learner perceives the relevance of the subject to himself/herself.

4. Understanding of objectives.

5. Motivation: learning is enhanced if the learner is motivated – particularly by internal motivation.

Evaluation of a programme of health education may concentrate on process – such as whether material is intelligible or remembered – or upon outcome – for example uptake of immunization. Yet in a recent review, Tones (1977) stated 'unfortunately rigorous evaluation of health education programmes is the exception rather than the rule'. However, it is also true that measurement of behaviour change is one of the more difficult and challenging tasks in any educational project. It is relatively easy to measure information imparted but much more difficult to measure beliefs or behaviour. The most fundamental problems are clearly to be found in the measurement of beliefs.

A commonly used measure of patient behaviour in practice is that of compliance. Patients' consulting behaviour has also been used as an overall measure but it is more difficult to relate this to the goals of health education. Thus if a health education activity increases compliance it is held to be a valuable activity, but if it increases – or decreases – consultation rate, how can these effects be said to represent success or failure? In some circumstances consultation rate may be used as a valid end-point, for example in a health education programme to discourage the presentation of minor illness (Morrell *et al.* 1980), but this is the exception rather than the rule.

COMPLIANCE

As outlined above, there is a fundamental assumption in any study of compliance which presupposes that the proposed behaviour change or therapy will act to the good of the patient but which in practice may not always be justified. Nevertheless, one finds in the literature of compliance research a great deal of valuable information which challenges many of the assertions of those practitioners who feel they intuitively know how to persuade patients to follow their advice.

The literature of compliance has been admirably reviewed by Sackett and Haynes (1976) and Haynes *et al.* (1979). These authors have reviewed some 800 referenced original articles on compliance behaviour and derived from them a number of correlations between compliance with advice or treatment given and a number of other features.

The following factors were found to be quite *unrelated* to compliance:
– Severity of symptoms;
– Type of symptoms;
– Duration of symptoms;
– Age and sex of patient.

It was also sobering to find that a doctor's prediction of compliance is unrelated to the behaviour of the patient.

However, a number of features of the proposed therapeutic regime and of the services provided can lead to increased compliance:
– Continuity of doctor;
– Short waiting time for appointment;
– Convenient and efficient surgery facilities;
– Patient satisfaction with doctor;
– Continuing supervision of therapy by doctor;
– Encouragement of self-monitoring by patient;
– Simple therapeutic regime.

Haynes and Sackett reviewed literature relating to compliance both with preventive advice and advice given in illness, although the majority of studies quoted in their review deal with illness. The results, however, do not suggest that a theoretical model of 'illness behaviour' such as that suggested by Suchman (1965) is applicable to compliance behaviour. The inference of such a model is that if a patient experiences a symptom then he assumes a sick role, presents to a doctor, and follows the advice given by the doctor ('dependant' role) before finally relinquishing the patient role to be rehabilitated. Logically such a model suggests that the more severe the symptoms, the more likely is the patient to follow advice, but the studies quoted do not appear to support this.

It has been suggested that a model analogous to the illness behaviour model could be constructed to explain health behaviour (Richards 1975). This would involve (i) symptom perception; (ii) assumption of at-risk role; (iii) preventive visit or test; (iv) co-operative patient; and (v) symptom-free. Again, however, there is little evidence to support such a model of decision-making in relation to health behaviour, despite its superficial attraction to doctors who are used to the analogous illness behaviour model.

The health belief model

Perhaps one of the more useful models of health behaviour for the doctor is the model that has become known as the 'Health Belief Model'. This model was developed by a group of social psychologists in the 1950s working in the United States (Rosenstock 1966) and has since been developed and tested further both in the US (Becker *et al.* 1974, 1979) and in the United Kingdom (Yarnell 1976). The model was developed partly because traditional medical models or 'illness behaviour' models could not satisfactorily explain compliance bahaviour.

The theory behind the model is based on the idea that behaviour may be predicted in terms of the value of an outcome to an individual, and from the individual's expectation that a given action will actually result in that outcome. There are three main ideas embodied in the model. The first of these is that a person's evaluation of a proposed preventive action is dependent upon his or her perceived susceptibility both to the specific disease in question and to disease in general, and also to his or her perception of the probable severity of the subsequent disease. Secondly the person's behaviour will depend upon his or her view of the advocated health activity in terms of its feasibility, and its efficiency – or likelihood of the activity reducing susceptibility to disease. Against this, however, must be set any costs of the proposed activity, in physical, psychological, or financial terms. Thirdly, the model proposes that the person needs some cue to action which may be internal – perhaps the progression of some symptom – or external, such as advice from a friend, nurse, doctor, or a mass-media campaign.

A useful mnemonic for the Health Belief model describes it as the 'three S' model. Compliance with preventive advice will depend upon:

    Perceived Susceptibility

    Perceived Seriousness of disease threat

    Viable Solution proposed.

There have been many retrospective studies in the United States and a few in this country which have attempted to test this model. For example Yarnell (1976) conducted a study of the usefulness of the Health Belief Model in assessing a campaign to improve the uptake of measles immunization in the Bristol area. A group of mothers whose children had been vaccinated after a sustained local publicity campaign were compared with a group whose children had not been vaccinated. Both groups were interviewed after the campaign. Mothers of the vaccinated children were more likely to believe measles vaccination to be safe than those whose children were not vaccinated although mothers in both groups regarded measles as a serious condition. The cues to action for the mothers who attended vaccination clinics were most often from local television publicity and a postcard inviting the child to a specific clinic. Mothers received very little communication from doctors about the campaign.

Similar retrospective studies have found that compliance with advice has usually correlated positively with the following factors:

Patient's perception of:
— the disease as serious,
— susceptibility to the specific disease,
— general susceptibility to disease,
— efficacy of therapy;
Influence of family and friends;
Family stability.

More recently some studies have shown that the Health Belief Model can indeed predict which patients are likely to follow advice. For example Becker *et al.* (1977) found that significant predictions about compliance with advice concerning juvenile obesity could be made just by knowing about the mother's general health concerns. Even more accurate predictions were possible from knowledge of the mother's specific concern about overweight and diet. However, in another study, Taylor (1979) found that compliance of patients with hypotensive therapy could not be predicted at the outset of treatment, but when health beliefs were measured a short time after the onset of therapy, there was a significant correlation between these measures and compliance.

Practical use of the health belief model

Tests of the model have largely been carried out in illness, and there appears to be some evidence that the hypothesis is valid in terms of compliance with therapeutic regimes. Thus its main attraction at present is in terms of secondary and tertiary health education. In future, it may be possible for practitioners to apply specific strategies to improve compliance with therapy for those patients whom one knows will be least likely to follow advice.

The utility of the model in terms of primary prevention is more open to doubt, although Yarnell's study (1976) did make an attempt to assess its value in terms of the acceptance of immunization procedures. There have, however, been few studies which have assessed its usefulness for predicting likely behaviour change in the more fundamental areas of primary prevention such as diet or exercise.

HEALTH EDUCATION STRATEGIES IN PRIMARY CARE

Primary care has often been seen in the past as 'a professional rallying point' for all health professionals involved in health education (Dalzell-Ward 1975). The concept has perhaps been of the surgery or health centre as a focal point for maternal and child health education in a traditional didactic schoolroom style. The provision of a 'health education room' in many health centres bears witness to this approach. Strategies for health education have often been based on those imported from other community education programmes, involving talking to groups of patients, or the use of posters, hand-outs, and leaflets. Such approaches may sometimes be valuable, particularly in terms of imparting information. However, many attempts to provide information by formal means such as lectures or posters have often had little success (Whitfield 1974). Attention has more recently turned to the consultation as a potential vehicle for health education, and it is already clear that previously this potential has been undervalued. In future this is likely to be one of the most successful approaches and indeed the majority of doctors show a preference for health education at the time of the consultation. Few support formal health education within their practices (Pike 1969).

The potential of the consultation

One of the major problems in discussing the consultation has been the lack of a suitable model which can be used to define the components of any consultation. A number of studies attempting to measure consultation behaviour in primary care have been carried out but usually these studies have used special rating scales appropriate to the research objectives of the study which are of limited general application.

Recently, however, a model has been described (Stott and Davis 1979) which, unlike most rating scales, can be used as a *practical* base for discussing the components of the consultation and which may also be used as an *aide mémoire* for the practitioner (see Fig. 2.3, p. 31).

The advantage of this four-part framework is that it can be applied to any consultation to assess not only what took place, but also may be used by the practitioner to elicit the maximum potential from the consultation in terms of content. The first part of the model concerns those activities associated with the management of the presenting problem. The framework also emphasizes the importance of noting any continuing problems the patient may have when they come into the consulting room (Area C). Of particular importance in terms of patient education are the remaining two parts of the model which embody concepts often overlooked in general practice. Area B deals with those aspects of the consultation which may be concerned with modifying the behaviour of the patient in seeking help in the future. For example, doctors may be encouraging continued inappropriate use of resources by prescribing symptomatic remedies for minor self-limiting illness. Marsh (1977) has demonstrated that demand for consultations dropped when his practice adopted a policy of not prescribing symptomatic remedies such as cough medicines, diarrhoea mixtures, or simple analgesics. After appropriate examination the doctors reassured the patients, explaining that no prescription medication was required but they advised the patient how to use common-sense home remedies like lemon and honey or steam for colds.

Lastly, Area D of the framework emphasizes that there is potential for appropriate health promotion at every consultation. Information may be given concerning lifestyle, or screening procedures can be carried out. It has been shown that patients are most receptive to health promotion at the time of the illness interview. Since some 75 per cent of all patients consult at least once per year, the consultation inevitably forms a potential base for both imparting information and also – in terms of the Health Belief Model – acting as a cue to action.

Communication skills and patient education

Efficient communication between doctor and patient in the consultation is associated with not only patient satisfaction but also increased compliance with the advice given by the doctor. For example, Hulka (1979) found that amongst patients with congestive heart failure, efficient communication with the doctor was associated with fewer errors in drug taking, as well as greater patient satisfaction. American studies have found that primary care physicians do spend about 25 per cent of consultation time in counselling and exposition (Bartlett 1980) but deficiencies in simple communication techniques are commonplace (Svarstad 1976; Pendleton 1981).

So how is the doctor to learn these essential communication skills which are clearly of such importance in patient education? Ley *et al.* (1976) taught doctors how to use a number of basic principles in giving instructions and advice to patients which are fully described in the admirable monograph *Communication with the patient* (Ley and Spelmen 1967). They found that when doctors followed these rules, patients' recall of information significantly improved. Briefly, the rules were as follows:

– Give instructions and advice early in the interview.
– Stress the importance of the instructions and advice you give.
– Use short words and short sentences.
– Arrange the information given into clear categories.
– Repeat advice.
– Give specific, detailed, concrete advice rather than general recommendations.

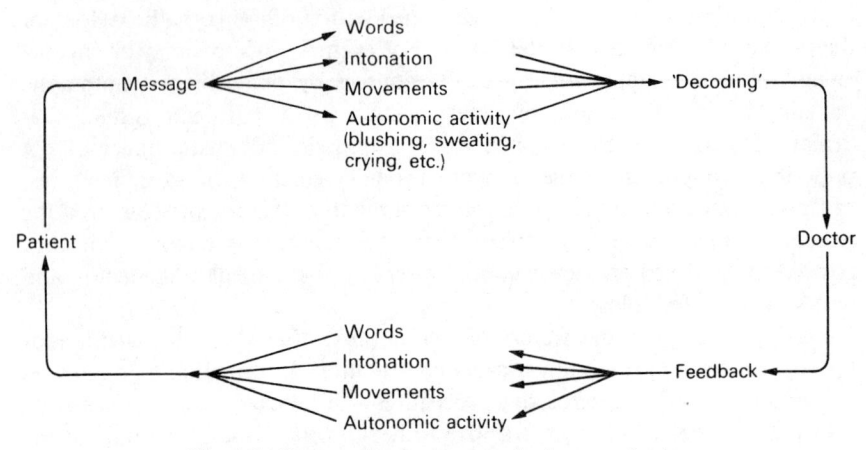

Fig. 4.1. Communication process in the consultation.

However, if the full potential of the consultation is to be achieved it is important to understand the process of consultation behaviour as a two-way process, whereas Ley's approach was more specifically directed to the techniques of giving instructions. Communication consists of a number of modalities apart from simply the words used. Intonation and non-verbal clues are an important part of the whole message that the patient is putting over to the doctor, and similarly a part of the feedback provided by the doctor to the patient. These concepts are illustrated in Fig. 4.1. The importance of doctor and patient feedback cannot be over-emphasized. Both Svarstad and Pendleton found that doctors tend to give advice without eliciting any ideas from the patient about his or her health beliefs. Yet advice will be more effective if it is congruent with the patient's beliefs. Also doctors rarely check that a patient fully understands advice or instructions, but such simple checking can improve both understanding and compliance.

Doctor's can improve their own consultation techniques, for example by using audio-tape recordings. It has also been found that video recordings of consultations have considerable value as a learning and teaching tool (Davis *et al.* 1980). In particular, experienced practitioners' consultation skills have been found to improve when a peer-group reviewed video tape recordings of their interviews (Verby *et al.* 1979).

Many doctors will feel that it is difficult if not impossible to improve consultations as suggested because of the constraints of time. However, this problem can largely be overcome by efficient organization of the practice. Many doctors complain of lack of available time for seeing patients with difficult problems because of the pressure of unnecessary consultations for minor illness yet they are reluctant to use practice nursing staff for routine consultations such as blood-pressure checks, cervical cytology or for consultations for minor problems such as small injuries.

Time can be created by efficient use of other members of the team for routine or minor problems, but patients' expectations can also slowly be changed by a practice policy of refusing placebo remedies for self-limiting illness which will eventually reduce consultations for such problems. The practice income may also be increased by the efficient provision of prophylactic procedures, and by efficiency in claiming for remuneration due for these items, which in turn can be used to employ more staff and so create more available time for the doctors.

Pamphlets, leaflets, and posters

Although much effort has been spent both by government-sponsored bodies and the pharmaceutical industry in producing posters for surgery waiting-rooms, such displays are of little proven value. Some impact can be made by using many copies of the same poster on the same wall, or by carefully co-ordinating the theme of posters. Some doctors have experimented with tape-slide presentations in waiting-rooms, and there is potential for computer-based information systems or viewdata but experiments with such systems in waiting-rooms have been disappointing (Clare *et al.* 1976), almost certainly because the information is not seen by the patient as personally relevant. Greater success, however, has been found with tapes or tape-slide presentations 'prescribed' by the doctor for individual patients.

Ley originally pointed out (1967) that any easy-to-understand leaflet aided comprehension and could indeed aid compliance with advice. There is now considerable evidence that a pamphlet provided by the doctor at the time of the consultation aids compliance with advice. In a study of advice given by doctors to patients to stop smoking Russell *et al.* (1979) found that when a leaflet was given to the patient in addition to verbal advice compliance improved.

Another study has demonstrated the usefulness of providing patients with advice about self-care. There has been wide lay interest both in this country and abroad in books designed to help patients take care of their own health (Sehnert and Eisenberg 1975; Vickery *et al.* 1979; Smail 1980), but Morrell *et al.* (1980) has shown that consultation rates and patient demands for visits can be reduced by providing patients with a very simple guide to home remedies, available in the United Kingdom from the Health Education Council or the Scottish Health Education Group. An important point to which Morrell *et al.* paid a great deal of attention in their study is that leaflets must be easy to read in order to reach the population at large. Generally any writing for patients must use short words and short sentences in the style of the popular tabloid newspapers. Many items of health education literature produced in the past have been unintelligible to the majority of people simply because they have used complicated language.

Fear arousal in communication

A message that arouses some fear in the people who receive it is more effective in changing people's behaviour than a message that arouses no fear or anxiety, or too much. This is an example of the so-called Yerkes–Dodson effect.

In a campaign designed to encourage college students to be vaccinated against mumps, three groups received leaflets designed to generate either low fear, some fear, or high fear. The uptake of vaccination was as follows (Krisher et al. 1973) (Table 4.1).

The implication of the Yerkes–Dodson effect in patient education therefore is that it will be helpful to arouse some fear in the messages one gives, but if too

Table 4.1. *Number of students receiving mumps vaccine*

	Low fear	Medium fear	High fear
Before reminder	2	12	4
After reminder	2	2	2
Not at all	16	6	14

much fear is generated then better results will be achieved by reducing anxiety. If an extreme fear of operations can be reduced by explanation, fewer requests for post-operative analgeisa are received. Judging where an individual patient lies on the 'fear scale', however, must obviously remain an art.

PATIENT EDUCATION AND THE PRIMARY CARE TEAM

Although there is almost uniform agreement amongst primary care workers that patient education is part of the function of the team, there are great differences in the way in which individual teams work. Many doctors see themselves as providing a minimum of education in the consultation but leaving preventive and educational activities to the health visitor. Other doctors may regularly be involved in formal health education programmes such as mothercraft classes. In other centres, the team may involve interested lay groups from outside the practice.

The studies of compliance quoted earlier in this chapter showed that efficient running of a clinic and short waiting time for appointments increased compliance by the patient with advice given. The implication of this for practice managers and receptionists is quite clear.

In the United Kingdom the health visitor is perhaps the team member who is most closely allied to the aims of prevention and patient education in practice, and she will be close to the resources that are available for the team to call upon. On the one hand are the professional resources including the health education officer and his staff, and, providing back-up to the HEC, the Health Educational Council. On the other hand the health visitor may be able to influence relatives, neighbours, and even community leaders to act as local instigators of preventive action. If models such as the Health Belief Model are to be of maximal help to practitioners in the future, a local knowledge of prevalent health beliefs will be vital. The health visitor is most likely to be able to supply such information.

Practical implications for the team

Patient education is a concept which runs through virtually all the interactions the team have with patients. If a primary care team wishes to improve the preventive services it is supplying to patients, the team must therefore agree on the priorities for patient education. It is likely that formal approaches to patient education are less valuable than bearing in mind the following principles at all contacts with patients:

—Ensure that any suggested preventive or therapeutic regime has been *proven* to do more good than harm.

—Encourage patients to take responsibility for their own health and that of their families. Be aware of the risks and problems of undue dependency by patients on medical services.

—Efficient surgery organization and an efficient appointment system improves acceptance of advice by patients.

—Efficient two-way communication in the consultation improves patient satisfaction, and compliance with preventive advice. Elicit patients' health beliefs *before* giving advice. Check that the patient understands what you have said.

—Simple, specific preventive or therapeutic regimes, tailored to individual needs, are more effective than complicated or generalized instructions.

—Written advice in an easy-to-understand format is more effective if it is provided at the time of the consultation rather than left generally accessible to patients.

—Advice is more likely to be accepted if some anxiety is aroused in the patient but too much anxiety is counterproductive.

—Identify patients who do not accept advice. Use reminder cards or other cues to action; explore possible barriers to acceptance of advice, and simplify regime.

—Use other team members to reinforce preventive advice.

REFERENCES

Bartlett, E. E. (1980). Contributions of consumer health education to primary care practice: a review. *Medical Care* 8, 862–71.

Becker, M. H., Maiman, L. A., Kirscht, J. P., Haefner, D. P., and Drachman, R. H. (1977). A test of the Health Belief Model in Obesity. *J. Hlth social Behav.* 18, 348–66.

——, Drachman, R. H., and Kirscht, J. P. (1974). A new approach to explaining sick-role behaviour in low-income populations. *Am. J. publ. Hlth* 64, 205–15.

——, Maiman, L. A., Kirscht, J. P., Haefner, D. P., Drachman, R. H., and Taylor, D. W. (1979). Patient perception and compliance: Recent studies of the Health Belief Model. In *Compliance in health care* (ed. R. B. Haynes, D. W. Taylor, and D. L. Sackett). Johns Hopkins University Press.

Clare, W. D., Engel, C. E., Jolly, B. C., and Meyrick, R. H. (1976). Health education in the doctor's waiting room. *Hlth Educat. J.* 35, 135–41.

Cochrane, A. L. (1972). *Effectiveness and efficiency*. Nuffield Provincial Hospitals Trust, London.

Comfort, A. (1967). *The anxiety makers*. Nelson, London.

Dalzell-Ward, A. J. (1975). The health centre as a focal point for health education. *Hlth Educat. J.* **34**, 48–50.

Davis, R. H., Jenkins, M., and Smail, S. A. (1980). Teaching with audio-visual recordings of consultations. *J. R. Coll. Gen. Pract.* **30**, 333–6.

Journal of the Royal College of General Practitioners (1973). Editorial *J. R. Coll. Gen. practrs* **23**, 235.

Gatherer, A., Parfit, J., Porter, E., and Vessey, M. (1979). *Is health education effective?* Health Education Council Monograph No. 2. London.

Haynes, R. B., Taylor, D. W., and Sackett, D. L. (1979). *Compliance in health care*. Johns Hopkins University Press.

Hulka, B. S. (1979). Patient–clinician interactions and compliance. In *Compliance in health care* (ed. R. B. Haynes, D. W. Taylor, and D. L. Sackett). Johns Hopkins University Press.

Krisher, H. P., Dorley, S. A., and Darley, J. M. (1973). Fear provoking recommendations, intentions to take preventive actions and actual preventive actions. *J. pers. Soc. Psyiat.* **26**, 301–8.

Ley, P. and Spelman, M. S. (1967). *Communicating with the patient*. Staples Press, London.

——, Whitworth, M. A., Skilbeck, C. E., Woodward, R., Pinsent, R. J. F. M., Pilce, L. A., Clarkson, M. G., and Clark, P. B. (1976). Improving doctor–patient communication in general practice. *J. R. Coll. Gen. Practrs* **26**, 720–4.

Marsh, G. N. (1977). 'Curing' minor illness in general practice. *Br. med. J.* **ii**, 1267–9.

Morrell, D. C., Avery, A. J., and Watkins, C. J. (1980). Management of minor illness. *Br. med. J.* **i**, 769–71.

Neufeld, V. R. (1976). Patient education. A critique. In *Compliance with therapeutic regimes* (ed. D. L. Sackett and R. B. Haynes). Johns Hopkins University Press.

Pendleton, D. (1981). Learning communication skills. *Update* May, 1708–14.

Pike, L. A. (1969). Health education in general practice. *J. R. Coll. Gen. Practrs* **17**, 133–4.

Richards, N. D. (1975). Methods and effectiveness of health education. *Social sci. Med.* **9**, 141–56.

Rosenstock, I. M. (1966). Why people use health services. *Millbank Memorial Fund Q.* **44**, 94–124.

Russell, M. A. H., Wilson, C., Taylor, C. and Baker, C. D. (1979). Effects of general practitioners' advice against smoking. *Br. med. J.* **ii**, 231–5.

Sackett, D. L. and Haynes, R. B. (eds.) (1976). *Compliance with therapeutic regimes*. Johns Hopkins University Press.

Sehnert, K. W. and Eisenberg, H. (1975). *How to be your own doctor (sometimes)*. Grosset and Dunlap, New York.

Smail, S. A. (1980). Could clinical algorithms help patients take care of themselves? *Update* April, 903–10.

Stott, N. C. H. and Davis, R. H. (1979). The exceptional potential in each primary care consultation. *J. R. Coll. Gen. Practrs* **29**, 201–5.

Suchman, E. A. (1965). Stages of illness and medical care. *J. Hlth hum. Behav.* **6**, 114.

Svarstad, B. L. (1976). Physician–patient communication and patient conformity with medical advice. In *Growth of bureaucratic medicine*. Wiley, New York.

Taylor, D. W. (1979). A test of the Health Belief Model in hypertension. In *Compliance in health care* (ed. R. E. Haynes, D. W. Taylor, and D. L. Sackett). Johns Hopkins University Press.

Tones, B. K. (1977). *Effectiveness and efficiency in health education.* Scottish Health Education Unit, Edinburgh.

Verby, J., Holden, P., and Davis, R. H. (1979). Peer review of consultations in primary care – the use of audio visual recordings. *Br. med. J.* i, 1686–8.

Vickery, D. M., Fries, J. F., Gray, J. A. M., and Smail, S. A. (1979). *Take care of yourself.* George Allen and Unwin, London.

Whitfield, M. J. (1974). Evaluation of health education in general practice. *Update* April, 965–71.

World Health Organization (1969). *Research in health education. Report of a WHO Scientific Group.* World Health Organization technical report section, 432, Geneva.

Yarnell, J. (1976). Evaluation of health education: the use of a model of preventive health behaviour. *Social Sci. Med.* 10, 393–8.

5 Obstacles to prevention

Muir Gray

In the preceding chapter the general principles of patient education were discussed and these are equally applicable whether the general practitioner is prescribing treatment or advising on prevention. In both contexts the nature and style of the consultation and the manner in which the general practitioner communicates with the person who is consulting him are as important as the message itself in determining the degree of compliance. The emphasis of the preceding chapter was on the principles of communication. The emphasis of this chapter is on the principles which should be borne in mind when composing the message, that is the preventive advice which one wishes to communicate. Some general practitioners are uncertain about the best means of giving advice on prevention but the message is based on the same principles which are used in imparting advice about treatment. In both types of message the risks, benefits, and costs of following the doctor's advice has to be covered.

RISKS, BENEFITS, AND COSTS

In both types of message the person has to be given information about the benefits of treatment, or of changing his behaviour, and about the risks which are entailed. He then compares risks with benefits in what has been termed risk–benefit analysis. For example, a patient with a high blood pressure has to consider both the risk, or probability, that he will have a stroke and the consequences of a stroke, for it is the reduced risk of these which is the benefit of treatment. Analysis of risk may be complicated if the patient exposes himself to a risk to reduce the risk of disease, for example the risk involved in an operation. The patient then has to compare one risk with the other and weigh the resultant risk against the benefit (Fig. 5.1).

One other factor must be brought into the equation – the cost of following advice. The cost of taking medication daily is usually low. However, drug side-effects may be considered as costs, for example the side-effects of antihypertensive drugs. The cost of most surgical operations is greater as operations and the period of recovery may take a considerable time and entail pain and discomfort. These are high costs but are usually acceptable to the person who is advised to have an operation and these costs can be reduced if the person can plan the timing of his operation to fit into his business schedule which is one of the attractions of private medicine. In preventive medicine and health education the influence of costs is even more important because the cost of preventive

Benefit analysis 71

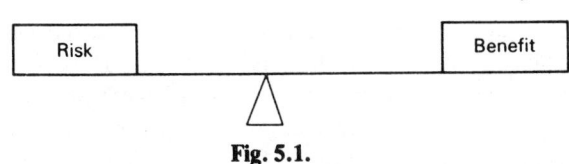

[Diagram: balance scale with "Risk" and "Benefit"]

Fig. 5.1.

advice is often very high. Much of the advice which is given affects enjoyable activities, such as smoking and drinking and eating French food, and it is in this respect that health education, which has as its objective behaviour modification, presents more difficult problems than education which is intended to improve compliance with therapeutic advice. It is often the cost which is the biggest obstacle to the individual trying to change this behaviour or to the doctor trying to influence behaviour.

Benefits, risks, and costs, and the means by which they can be communicated most effectively, will be discussed separately but they are closely inter-related by the individual who has to conduct an extremely sophisticated comparison of the three factors in his cost–risk–benefit analysis (Fig. 5.2).

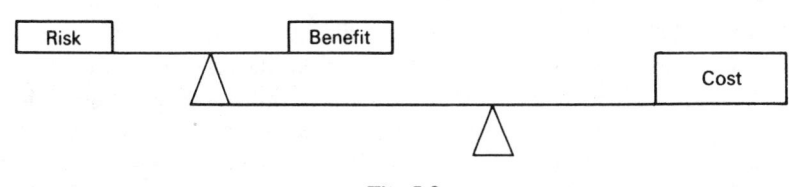

[Diagram: compound balance scale with "Risk", "Benefit" and "Cost"]

Fig. 5.2.

BENEFIT ANALYSIS

Positive and negative benefits

Better health and *less disease*

One point which people involved in the marketing and advertising of commercial products frequently make when criticizing health education is that too much emphasis is given to the absence of disease as the product on offer. This is true because it is the absence of cancer, or the absence of atherosclerosis, or the absence of obesity which is often offered as the benefit rather than a positive reward such as 'better health' or 'feeling well'. One reason why health education has concentrated on disease avoidance rather than health promotion is that we have become disaffected with the all-embracing and vague World Health Organization definition of health as being 'complete physical, social, and mental wellbeing'. Because 'health' cannot be measured accurately, either in individuals or in nations, it is impossible to evaluate the effectiveness of health services and the emphasis has, rightly, shifted to disease as the yardstick by which effectiveness and efficiency can be measured. Various indices of disease such as mortality statistics or, where an individual is being assessed, body weight or blood pressure can be assessed and the medical profession has concentrated its attention on the prevention and treatment of disease rather than on health promotion. It could be argued, however, that we have gone too far in this direction. Patients who are suffering symptoms as a result of disease are influenced by the promise of 'less disease' but the asymptomatic person is much less impressed by the promise of 'less disease' in the future. The Health Education Council and the Scottish Health Education Group have recognized this and have changed the approach of health education with campaigns which, although primarily intended to prevent obesity, coronary heart disease, and bronchial carcinoma, emphasize that people can feel better and look better to members of the opposite sex by modifying their behaviour.

The general practitioner should also be prepared to adopt this approach and throughout the book the importance of emphasizing that the advice given will not only reduce the risk of disease but will also make people look and feel better is stressed.

A long life or a good life

A reduced risk of disease is, of course, attractive but its attraction can be greatly increased if the general practitioner emphasizes that the objectives of preventive medicine are not to increase life span but to help people stay fitter longer. Many people think of geriatric and psychogeriatric wards when told how they can avoid preventive medicine – 'I don't want to live on to be a cabbage'. There is now some epidemiological evidence that the prevention of those diseases which are preventable would not result in a large population of severely disabled 90 year-olds (Fries and Crapo, 1981; Benjamin and Overton 1981). It would, however, result in a much higher proportion of fit and active 50-, 60-, 70-, and 80-year-olds. The effects of preventive medicine is to improve the quality of life not simply to prolong it, and it is this which should be emphasized as the objective of preventive medicine and health education.

It is therefore important to emphasize that preventive medicine offers:
1. A reduced risk of disease.
2. Better health – looking and feeling better.
3. Improved quality of life with less morbidity in middle and old age, not simply a postponement of morbidity and mortality.

Benefits of behaviour change

Finally, people have to be convinced that the change of behaviour or treatment suggested will be effective in reducing risks. The statement that 'smoking causes disease' does not justify the assumption that 'smoking cessation prevents disease' and the individual who is being advised has to be told not only that some aspect of his life increases the risk of disease but that there is evidence that changing his behaviour will reduce the risk of disease. The point is emphasized in the 'health belief model' (see p. 60) (Becker *et al.* 1974, 1979). Therefore the smoker needs to be told that 'stopping smoking will reduce the risk of heart disease and the risk is reduced as soon as you stop smoking', in addition to being told that smoking causes disease.

Telling patients about the benefits of prevention

Semantic problems

It is obviously essential to choose words which are familiar to the individual or group being addressed. It is not sufficient, however, merely to ensure that the words which are chosen are known; it is also necessary to ensure that the meaning of the word is the same for both doctor and the person he is trying to influence. However, the meaning of a word not only includes its literal meaning, as given in a dictionary, but also its implied meaning. For example, it is insufficient merely to ensure that a woman knows that cervical carcinoma is a neoplastic growth which can be detected by cervical cytology. It is equally important to consider how much the person fears cancer, whether or not she associates the term 'cancer' with the term 'incurable' or with 'pain', or whether she believes that cancer is the result of promiscuous intercourse. These and all the other beliefs which a person may have about a disease constitute the implicit meaning of the word used to describe it. The associations which a term has for the person have to be determined by the doctor. The best means of doing this is to ask the person what he or she knows and believes about a disease, for example by saying, 'I don't know how much you know about cancer of the cervix or what you may have heard about it. Perhaps you could tell me so that I don't repeat what you already know'.

The connotation of a term may be different to a doctor and patient not only because their knowledge and beliefs differ; their attitudes towards disease may differ because each views it from a different perspective. To a doctor the connotations of the term 'disease' are unpleasant, doctors are trained to think of the pathology and the symptoms and associate disease with pain, impairment, and disability. To an untrained person who has had little personal experience of serious disease the term may have quite different connotations. To such a person the social consequences of disease – the illness (see p. 22) – may be much more significant than the physical consequences, particularly the more pleasant social consequences – the sympathy and attention which the sick receive from other people and the right to be excused normal obligations such as work or school or military service. General practitioners, of course, are frequently involved in negotiations with people who wish to become patients, for example by being given a sick note. This is usually in the context of a minor disease such as a respiratory tract infection, but a person's attutude to serious disease may be influenced by his experience of minor disease if he has had no close personal contact with the suffering which results from serious disease (Helman 1978).

Consider the problems of trying to educate children about road safety. The person who wishes to promote road safety associates the term 'road traffic accident' with pain, disfigurement, and disability. However, the terms may have different implications to the children he is addressing. Their only experience of the consequences of an accident is usually as spectators who see the injured child as the focus of the school's attention, receiving cards and presents while he is in hospital and being given special privileges and attention when he returns to school using crutches or wearing plaster of Paris. To them a road traffic accident is therefore much less frightening than it is to the educator. Indeed it may appear an exciting proposition.

Grammatical difficulties

The message of the marketing manager of a chocolate bar is simple because he can assure the consumer that he will enjoy the taste. The health educator's message is much more complicated, it often uses the subjunctive mood and frequently has to include conditional clauses to cover certain contingencies; for example, 'if you lose weight then it may be that you won't develop high blood pressure provided that certain other factors are not present'. To people who have not had higher education such complicated messages may be difficult to comprehend or may be completely incomprehensible. It is salutary for a general practitioner who wishes to be a health educator to make regular detailed study of the prose of a number of articles in one of the best-selling daily newspapers to learn how briefly and simply messages have to be worded.

There is, however, another important linguistic difficulty which results from the cultural difference between the people who try to modify behaviour and those at highest risk who are most resistant to the message of health education, namely people in Social Classes IV and V (Hoggart 1957).

One of the most important reasons for such social class differences is that many of the benefits promised to those who change their behaviour in the way which health educators advise are not immediate, as the benefit promised by the man marketing chocolate is immediate, but may be 20 or 30 years in the future. The person who is in a secure, superannuated job and who lives in the security of a mortgaged house which he is sure will come to him at a definite date in the twenty-first century, at which time a number of carefully calculated insurance policies will also come to fruition, thinks about the future in a different manner from the man who is in an insecure job or who is unemployed and who lives in a dwelling which is rented weekly from a landlord who can evict him without notice. To the former the long-term future has a reality which it does not have to the latter to whom the limits of conceivable time may be next Friday. As health educators are found in the former group and the population who are at greatest risk, but who are most resistant to health education, are in the latter this difference in the concepts of time is a major obstacle to preventive medicine. This is not only a grammatical problem of course. The liguistic problem is a reflection of the cultural difference between the two groups each of which lives in its own social reality using its own language (Chu 1966; Gray 1977).

Practical implications

1. The general practitioner should emphasize the positive benefits of his advice as well as the reduction in risk. For example, smokers can be told that they will feel better, smell less, and that they will be more attractive to the majority of the population who are non-smokers. Similarly people can be encouraged to lose weight by telling them that they will look better and be more attractive to members of the opposite sex.

2. It should be emphasized that the result of the advice given is not to keep the person alive for so long that he will become totally dependent and have to enter an institution. It should be emphasized that the objectives of preventive medicine are 'fitness at 50', or 'fitness in retirement'. It may help if the person is assured that there is no guarantee that the advice will help them live any longer but is solely intended to help them stay fitter longer; to add life to years, as the motto of the UN Assembly on Ageing states, not years to life.

3. The words chosen should be familiar to the person or group being addressed.

4. The belief of the person or group about the particular problem being discussed should be determined, and consideration should be given to the connotations of terms such as 'healthy', 'sick', 'ill', and 'disabled'.

5. Every attempt should be made to describe benefits which will be evident within the near future. For example, obese people can be told that their health will improve as soon as they start losing weight and smokers can be told that their lung function will improve within a month of stopping.

RISK ANALYSIS

Attribution of cause
As we have emphasized, the type of preventive measure discussed in this book is primarily that in which a change in the individual's behaviour is the means of reducing his risk of disease. Before a person can be persuaded to change his behaviour he has to accept that his behaviour does affect the risk of disease and that diseases are not solely the result of unknown causes such as fate, or chance, or God's Will, or genes; genetic causation often being expressed as 'it runs in my family', or 'it is due to my glands',

In general people tend to attribute the causes of diseases more to external uncontrollable forces and less to factors over which they have control, such as their smoking or eating habits. The first step is therefore to ask the person about his opinion on the relationship between smoking and disease or between nutrition and disease.

Denial of risk and susceptibility

Many people are still unaware of the risks which they run and one task of health education is simply to inform people about risk. However, some people refuse to accept that the risks described by doctors exist and a common and understandable reason for this is that they perceive that the experts themselves are uncertain. Only a small proportion of people refuse to accept that cigarette smoking increases the risk of disease because the experts are unanimous in their opinion, but their is considerable doubt about the benefits of exercise or of reducing the intake of saturated fats. Advising people on nutrition is particularly difficult not only because experts disagree but also because the public knows that the opinions of the experts have changed over the years and believe that current theories will probably be superseded.

More common, and more difficult to deal with, is the denial of personal susceptibility by the individual who accpts that a risk exists; that is the belief of some people that although there is a risk associated with certain types of behaviour – 'it won't happen to me'. This presents a serious obstacle to the health educator as does another closely related type of belief – the fatalistic belief. Some people are prepared to accept that they might be at risk but refuse to consider changing their behaviour because they believe fatalistically that the risk cannot be reduced. In these instances it is not simply ignorance or doubt which is the obstacle but the person has a well-reasoned argument to justify his opinion that he need not try to modify his behaviour.

Fatalism may be religious in origin, particularly among Moslems who have a very fatalistic view of the future which they believe to be largely under the control of the Will of Allah, and among older people. However, many young people also use fatalistic arguments, for example arguing that 'there is a bullet with your number on it', or 'when your number's up your number's up', or 'it's all in the stars'. These beliefs are not religious in origin but appear to attribute control of events to forces which cannot be influenced and which may be grouped under the general heading of 'fate'.

Some of the young people who are fatalistic hold such a view because they feel impotent and at the mercy of immutable forces and influences in all aspects of their life. This view often results from the economic hopelessness of prolonged unemployment, which is an increasing obstacle to health education. In other young people, however, the fatalistic argument that 'it's all in the stars', or the denial of susceptibility 'it won't happen to me' do not reflect a coherent view of the world in which events are determined by supernatural forces. They are simply arguments which are used to control the individual's anxiety. The fact that people who are very anxious are less likely to change their behaviour than those who are moderately anxious was discussed in the preceding chapter (see p. 65) and this apparent paradox is closely related to the factors which predispose a person to deny that he is at risk or to maintain that everything is controlled by fate.

The probability that an individual will change his behaviour increases as his anxiety increases and a change in behaviour, for example by stopping smoking or losing weight, will reduce the person's anxiety (Dabbs and Leventhal 1966; Janis and Terwilliger 1962; Krisher *et al.* 1973) (Fig. 5.3).

If, however, a person who has been made very anxious is unable to change his behaviour because the cost of doing so would be too high he may have to find other ways of reducing his anxiety (Fig. 5.3). The ways in which this can be done are by denying susceptibility, sometimes citing as evidence a friend or relative who 'has smoked 40 a day for 40 years and is still alive and

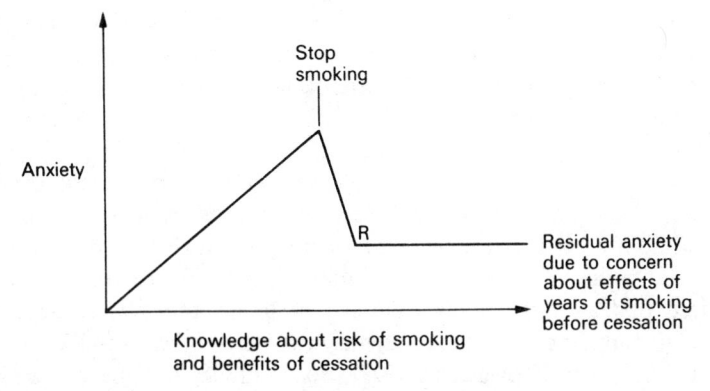

Fig. 5.3. Changes in anxiety levels of a smoker who receives warnings about smoking and then stops.

well', or by maintaining a very fatalistic approach to life or by adopting other types of behaviour, such as a daily dose of Ginseng or laxative and a weekly sauna, which are believed to be protective and health promoting. Anthropologists call such stratagems magic. They are not effective means of solving or preventing problems but they are effective techniques for reducing the anxieties which these problems generate (Gray 1979) (Fig. 5.4). This type of decision

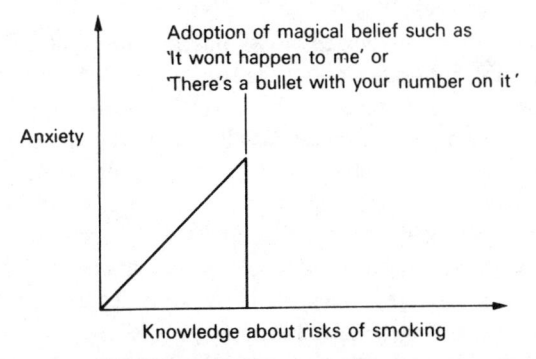

Fig. 5.4. Changes in anxiety level of someone who is unable to change his behaviour but who adopts magical techniques to control his anxiety.

making is not irrational. Although it does not reduce the risk of disease it reduces anxiety and this objective, which is an immediate benefit, may be even more important to the individual than the long-term benefits which may result if he reduces the risk of disease.

Assessing the degree of risk

Having accepted that he is susceptible, the individual must next be given the opportunity to assess the degree to which he is susceptible. This is of great importance for two reasons. Firstly, because there is evidence that people who are contemplating some action which may have unpleasant consequences are influenced to a greater degree by the probability that the unpleasant consequence will occur than they are by the severity of the event. For example, before legislation most car drivers did not wear seat belts because the odds against being killed through not wearing a seat belt are about 1000 to one against. However, most drivers would wear selt belts if there were an evens chance of sustaining minor facial lacerations. Health educators have concentrated on emphasizing the seriousness of the consequences of behaviour such as smoking or obesity or driving without wearing a seat belt but have not given sufficient information on the probability that these consequences may occur. Furthermore, it should be recognized that although many risks appear to be impressively high when viewed nationally or epidemiologically thay may appear very small to the individual who is at risk (Slovic *et al.* 1978). For example, 1000 people are killed and about 12 000 are seriously injured in Britain annually because they were not wearing seat belts, but the type of accident in which a seat belt gives protection occurs only once in every several million trips.

The second reason why it is important to give information about risk is that it is a subject about which many people are ignorant. In addition, there is a tendency to overestimate the risk of uncommon causes of death, such as deaths from lightning, rabies, legionnaires' disease, or tornadoes and to underestimate the risk of common causes of death such as cancer, bronchitis, and coronary heart disease. This bias is largely due to the way in which the media report morbidity and mortality.

Having accepted that the degree of risk has an important influence and that there is considerable ignorance about the risks associated with certain diseases, the general practitioner is faced with the difficulty of choosing a means of expressing the probability comprehensibly. One way is to use words, for example terms such as 'probable' or 'possible', or 'commonly', perhaps qualified by adverbs such as 'very', 'rather', or 'highly'. It has been demonstrated that most people use these terms consistently, for example most people use the term 'probable' to express a higher probability than 'possible', but that there is a considerable range in the probability attributed to each term. Therefore words alone are insufficient and most people also require some numerical expression of risk. The best means of doing this is to try to give the person some idea of relative risk, that is to give him some idea of the risk he is running by behaving in a certain manner compared with the risk he would run if he were not behaving in that way. For example, the Third Report of the Royal College of Physicians – Smoking and Health – emphasized that 'under the age of 65 smokers are about twice as likely to die of coronary heart disease as are non-smokers, and heavy smokers are about three and a half times as likely'. This is useful information. Unfortunately it is not easy for general practitioners to give people a clear idea of the relative risks which are associated with activities such as drinking or obesity because the data collected in epidemiological studies have been unsuitable for the calculation of relative risk; nevertheless it is possible to give some guidelines on expressing risks.

Practical implications

1. The first step in health education should be an attempt to assess the person's beliefs about the risk which is being discussed and about his personal susceptibility. Again a direct question is often the easiest way to open discussion, for example by saying 'I don't know how much you know about the risks associated with smoking or how much you, as an individual, feel at risk'. It is also helpful to obtain some idea of the person's estimates of the risk as opposed to other risks, for example the risk of tetanus or a road traffic accident.

2. Some attempt to assess the person's level of anxiety should also be made because it influences his assessment of his susceptibility. If it reaches too high a level he may adopt a fatalistic approach to life and to risks and thus ignore the advice given him, or he may adopt some ritual which he can believe will offset the risk of smoking.

3. Other causes of anxiety should always be taken into account. For example, it is difficult to help someone stop smoking if he is very anxious about the financial viability of his business, and it may be impossible to persuade an obese woman who is very worried about her adolescent son to weigh up the risks of obesity and plan a diet. In particular it is essential to consider the anxiety which is already present in the consultation before introducing a new anxiety. For example, if a woman is particularly worried about the risks of her oral contraceptive it would be unwise to introduce another anxiety by introducing health education on some unrelated risk factor, such as her alcohol consumption. A useful rule is that no more than one anxiety can be discussed in the one consultation.

4. The person should be given information about the magnitude of the risk in both verbal and, if possible, non-medical terms. Whenever possible the doctor should inform the person he is trying to influence about the relative risk of different diseases even though this is very imprecise. For example, a cigarette smoker can be told that he is hundreds of times more likely to die as a result of his cigarette smoking than he is to die of tetanus.

5. Finally it is important not to discourage practices which reduce anxiety. Many people 'take an apple a day to keep the doctor away', or follow some

other daily ritual which they believe to be important in maintaining their health. It is better to reinforce such behaviour even though there is no evidence that it is effective, provided that it is not causing harm to the person or being used as an excuse for not stopping smoking or taking whatever preventive advice the general practitioner is offering. In fact it is possible to reinforce such behaviour without dishonesty because it does make the person feel better. The fact that the general practitioner believes that the link is psychological and not physical need not be revealed, and a doctor can simply assure the person that the daily dose of Ginseng or vitamin C or whatever is 'good for her health' without compromising his scientific integrity.

COST ANALYSIS

Unfortunately from the health educator's point of view, many of the risk factors in an industrialized society are enjoyable. Few people could have enjoyed drinking water polluted with sewage or inhaling dense and dirty fogs although there was considerable public and political resistance to the measures taken to reduce these risks in nineteenth-century Britain. However, many people enjoy smoking or drinking alcohol or driving their car after having had a few drinks and resist appeals to change their behaviour because they find the cost too high when weighed against the magnitude of the risk and the benefits which may result. The costs of personal prevention may be considered in two groups – social costs and psychological costs – although there is a considerable overlap between the two (Cohen 1972).

Social costs

Drinking, smoking, and eating are social activities although smoking and drinking may also be antisocial. Drinking and eating are usually enjoyed more when they are done with other people, for example when in a pub after work or when eating a Sunday lunch with the family. Of course the taste of both alcohol and food is enjoyable for their own sake and the effects are also appreciated but alcohol, food, and, to a lesser degree, cigarettes are also enjoyed because they contribute to the enjoyment which each member of a group finds in the company of the other members. The buying of a round, the toasting of each other's health, the giving of food to one another and the exchange of cigarettes play a part in binding the members of the group more closely to one another. This may happen when people meet one another for the first time, but if a group meets regularly food, alcohol and cigarettes may become symbolically important and the consumption of the food or the alcohol or cigarettes may become part of the enjoyment of belonging (Janis and Terwilliger 1962; Evans *et al.* 1970; Krisher *et al.* 1973).

Many people who are trying to control their smoking and drinking and overeating often find this most difficult to do when they are with other people who are smoking or drinking or eating. In part this is due to the appetizing effect of the sight and smell of food, drink, or tobacco but the attraction may be social as well as psychological if the group is one in which smoking and drinking or eating are important rituals.

Psychological costs

The psychological costs of behavioural change are often too high for people to be able to modify their behaviour, commonly because the risks have become tranquillizers. Smoking, drinking, and eating help some people to relax. In part this is due to the pharmacological effects of cigarette smoke, alcohol, and, some would argue, food but it is also due to the fact that cigarettes, drinks, and food can become essential elements in relaxation rituals. For example, the act of lighting up a cigarette after she has finished clearing up after the evening meal may act as a signal to a housewife, and to her family, that she has finished work for the moment and should be allowed to sit in peace in front of the television. Not only may the action taken as a whole help the person to relax, the actual act of lighting up, or 'fixing' a drink may help the person relax by giving her purposeful activities to do while she is anxious. Thus behaviour which increases the risk of disease often acts as a tranquillizer but that is not the only psychological benefit which people derive from risky behaviour.

For some people it is the excitement of the behaviour which is attractive. This applies particularly to fast driving which is, of course, not necessarily dangerous, but when combined with alcohol or inexperience, or both, it greatly increases the risk of an accident. The young person who is not interested in sport and who derives no excitement from his job or his studies may find his excitement astride a motorcycle. There are many attractions in fast driving, one of which is the feeling that one is at risk. The combination of excitement and fear is rewarding for some young people and the cost of changing one's behaviour to reduce the risk of disease may be a loss of excitement and this cost may be too high. People in preventive medicine are, in general, cautious prudent people who avoid risk if they can. Many young people on the other hand are not influenced in this way and some actually seek out risk to introduce some excitement to their lives which they believe to be dull and unexciting. The type of education which places too much stress on the danger of certain types of behaviour may increase their attraction.

Often the psychological and the social benefits are intimately related to one another and the clear distinction between social and psychological benefits which has been used in this section is artificial. The less certain that someone is about how he should behave in a group the more difficlut he will find it to refuse a cigarette or drink or the offer of food, not only because he is more anxious and needs the cigarette or drink to reduce his anxiety but also because he feels a greater need to conform and belong than someone who is self-confident. Furthermore, the cigarette or the drink or food offer a useful alternative to either speech or silence to the person who is uncertain what to say next. Pipe smokers have a very good tool for controlling their anxiety because a pipe offers limitless scope for 'fiddling' and for covering the lower part of one's face or for avoiding or delaying speech. Too much has been made of the theory that people seek oral gratification for erotic reasons and not enough of the simpler explanation that cigarettes, drinks, and food are useful to the person who cannot, or does not wish to, speak freely and easily.

Practical implications

1. The person who is being advised to change his behaviour should be asked to try to describe the benefits he receives from that behaviour. Often, however, the person will find it impossible to be accurate until he has tried to make the change. It is only when he attempts to stop smoking or to reduce his food or alcohol intake that the benefits of his behaviour, and therefore the costs of changing it, become evident to him. It is therefore important to arrange an appointment with the person soon after the date on which he has decided that he will try to change his behaviour. If he is succeeding he can be rewarded and praised; if he is having difficulty the particular social situations or times at which he finds his new pattern of behaviour most difficult to sustain can be identified and he can be given on how to cope.

2. If the behaviour which the general practitioner wishes to influence has benefits it may be necessary to offer the person an alternative. It is not difficult just to tell him to stop. The alternative may be teaching a simple technique to help relaxation, or suggesting that he take up a new hobby or interest (see p. 217), or the person may require teaching about foods which are satisfying in bulk but low in energy (see p. 156).

RISK–BENEFIT–COST ANALYSIS

At the end of the consultation it is useful to review the factors involved, to state the risks, emphasize the benefits, and acknowledge the costs which the individual may have to face. The person will make the decision on whether or not he wishes to try to change his behaviour on the basis of the risks and the benefits. Whether or not he will actually succeed in doing so will, however, be influenced more by the third factor in the analysis – the costs involved. The general practitioner will be looked to for advice on all three aspects of the risk–benefit–cost analysis, both when the person is considering a change in behaviour and when he is trying to do so.

PRACTICAL IMPLICATIONS

One way of increasing the effectiveness of communication is to complement the oral advice with written material. The most effective medium would be a summary of the advice given in the consultation written specifically for the individual patient but this is impossible and a leaflet suitable for all people who have a particular condition or problem has to serve instead.

'Leaflets' have, quite rightly, been widely and fiercely criticized but a leaflet prepared in accordance with some simple guidelines can make an effective contribution to both prevention and treatment if it is used to complement the advice given during a consultation. Indeed it can be argued that many consultations are unnecessarily ineffective because the doctor relies exclusively on oral communication. Leaflets have their place in medical practice and that place is not always the wastepaper basket.

THE CONTENT OF THE MESSAGE

The message in any leaflet written to encourage prevention should always emphasize four points.

1. The seriousness of the problem – the aim should be to create concern but not overwhelming anxiety, for example to say that smoking causes lung cancer but not to describe the suffering of a cancer patient in gory detail.

2. The susceptibility of the reader – the statement that there are 185 000 deaths from coronary heart disease in the United Kingdom each year impresses the policy maker or epidemiologist. However, the individual wants to know whether or not he is susceptible, for example by presenting him with a list of risk factors for heart disease which he can use to assess his personal level of risk.

3. The benefits that will result from following the advice – it is insufficient that high blood pressure increases the risk of a stroke. It is also necessary to state that a reduction in blood pressure is associated with a reduction in risk. If there are any other benefits which will follow from following the advice, that is benefits other than reducing the risk of disease, they should be emphasized. For example, by saying that 'if you lose weight you will feel better and fitter and look more attractive' as well as emphasizing the beneficial effects of weight reduction on the metabolic problems of mature-onset diabetes.

4. The difficulties he may face – try to think of the difficulties which the patient may face in following advice and give specific advice on how these may be minimized.

THE STYLE OF THE MESSAGE

Having chosen the facts that are to be included it is essential to set them out clearly. Writing clearly and simply is difficult. It is more difficult than writing long and complicated sentences, with commas and semicolons separating a concatenation of clauses. It takes time and practice to learn how to write simply and clearly but there are a few guidelines which should be observed.

Don't use too many technical terms. When a term is first used it should always be defined. On the other hand, don't use too few technical terms. It is patronizing to use terms like 'tummy' when the technical term is in common use.

Use short sentences.

Use large print; capitals on an ordinary typewriter is a good size of writing for older patients.

Put the most important information at the beginning and then repeat it towards the end of the text, perhaps as a succinct summary of the advice.

Avoid general vague instructions such as, 'take more exercise', or 'eat less fat'. Be specific and precise. If you do not feel that you can be precise while writing a leaflet or handout leave a blank space in the leaflet for specific instructions tailored to the individual's needs. Never be afraid that you will be too detailed in your guidance. Almost always the mistake is to give general exhortations which can aggravate anxiety without changing behaviour. Specific precise instructions reduce anxiety and are more likely to be effective.

The difficulty of writing clearly should not be underestimated. The doctor who wishes to acquire this skill can learn how to draft plain English by reading 'the tabloids' with care and attention to style. Try reading the *Mail* or *Express* or the *Sun, Star,* or *Mirror* carefully at least once a week. Study the leader column for plain prose at its clearest, even if you do not agree with the opinions expressed. An even more effective way of learning, however, is to pilot the leaflet and seek criticism.

PREPARING THE MEDIUM

So much for the message, now for the medium. No amount of care in presentation can improve an incomprehensible message but a clearly written message can be obfuscated by poor presentation.

The rules of leaflet preparation can be summarized simply.

Write in short paragraphs. Use headings to break the text into short sections. If listing a number of facts or points set them in a line and indent them one centimetre to highlight their importance.

Try the question and answer style as one of your drafts. Market research has shown that it is an effective means of keeping the reader's attention.

Leave space for writing in 'personalized' advice. For example, you can give a leaflet on exercise and say that 'there are two points that are particularly important for you to remember so I am going to write them down here'.

Try to find ways in which the reader can use the leaflet to assess his condition or record his progress – self-monitoring improves compliance. For example, leave a space for him to write down what he finds most difficult about following the advice so that he can discuss this with the doctor or health visitor when he consults again.

Pilot your leaflets and try to evaluate its comprehensibility. Remember that many patients are reluctant to criticize anything their general practitioner produces honestly because they are reluctant to hurt his feelings. Try to enlist the help of a medical student or student health visitor or one of the administrative staff in the health centre. Remember that the local research funds of the health authority are able to dispense small sums for this type of action research.

The well-prepared leaflet is a very useful medium for communication which has had a press. If prepared by the general practitioner for his own patients it can make an effective contribution.

REFERENCES

Becker, M. H., Drachman, R. H., and Kirscht, J. P. (1974). A new approach to explaining sick-role behaviour in low-income populations. *Am. J. public Hlth* **64**, 205-15.

——, Becker, M. H., Maiman, L. A., Kirscht, J. P., Haefner, D. P., Drachman, R. H. and Taylor, D. W. (1979). Patient perception and compliance: recent studies of the health belief model. In *Compliance in health care* (ed. R. B. Haynes, D. W. Taylor, and D. L. Sackett). Johns Hopkins University Press.

Benjamin, B. and Overton, E. (1981). Prospects for mortality decline in England and Wales. *Population Trends* 22-8.

Chu, G. (1966). Fear arousal, efficacy and imminency. *J. Pers. Soc. Psychol.* **4**, 517-24.

Cohen, J. (1972). *Psychological probability and the art of doubt*. Allen and Unwin, London.

Dabbs, J. M. and Leventhal, H. (1966). Effects of varying the recommendations in a fear arousing communication. *J. Pers. Soc. Psychol.* **4**, 525-31.

Evans, R. I., Rozelle, R. M., Lancaster, T. M., Dembroski, T. M., and Allen, B. P. (1970). Fear arousal, persuasion and actual versus implied behavioural change. *J. Pers. Soc. Psychol.* **16**, 220-7.

Fries, J. F. and Crapo, L. M. (1981). *Vitality and aging*. Freeman, San Francisco.

Gray, J. A. M. (1977). The failure of preventive medicine. *Lancet* ii, 1338-9.

—— (1979). *Man against disease—preventive medicine*, pp. 145-51. Oxford University Press.

Helman, C. G. (1978). Feed a cold and starve a fever – folk models of infection in an English suburban community and their relation to medical treatment. *Culture Med. Psychiat.* **2**, 107-37.

Hoggart, R. (1957). *The uses of literacy*. Allen Lane, London.

Janis, I. L. and Terwilliger, R. F. (1962). An experimental study of psychological resistance to fear arousing communications. *J. Abnorm. Soc. Psychol.* **65**, 403-10.

Krisher, H. P., Dorley, S. A., and Darley, J. M. (1973). Fear provoking recommendations, intentions to take preventive actions and actual preventive actions. *J. Pers. Soc. Psychol.* **26**, 301-8.

Slovic, P., Fischhoff, B., and Lichenstein, S. (1978). Accident probabilities and seat belt usage: a psychological perspective. *Accident Anal. Prevention* **10**, 281-5.

6 The politics of prevention – the scope for individual action

Michael Daube and Muir Gray

> The only contact I have with doctors in my constituency was when I once phoned up the health centre and invited myself to meet them.
>
> A backbencher with a special interest in smoking.

'The unnerving discovery every Minister of Health makes at, or near the outset of his term of office is that the only subject he is ever destined to discuss with the medical profession is money' (Powell 1966). This may have been true in the early 1960s when Enoch Powell was himself Minister of Health, but in recent years the medical lobby has been active on a variety of issues in preventive medicine. However, when the phrase 'medical profession' or 'medical lobby' is used it normally refers to central representatives of the profession, such as the British Medical Association or the Royal Colleges. Although the efforts of these representatives of the profession in the centre are sometimes effective, politicians who are interested in prevention would welcome much more support in the periphery – the backbencher or Minister who supports activity on a preventive medicine issue is greatly helped by pressure applied at the highest level, but also needs the support of other (on controversial issues a majority) Members of Parliament: for such support to materialize politicians must be lobbied by doctors and other health professionals in their own constituencies. This peripheral lobbying is at present largely missing: the medical profession supports prevention, but its individual members do not take advantage of their many opportunities to promote political action.

'There's no point: he's only a backbencher'; 'It's a waste of time: I know he's against fluoridation'; 'Even Ministers have no real influence: did you see *Yes Minister*?'. Such statements are often made by doctors – and others who feel pessimism about any influence they as individuals might be able to exert over central government.

It is true that a single letter to a Member of Parliament is unlikely either to result in a change in the law (although this has occasionally happened), or to change the mind of a politician who is dogmatically opposed to a specific measure. None the less, a little lobbying goes a long way: Members of Parliament cannot be experts or hold strong views on every topic, and are often surprisingly susceptible to constituency pressures. They can be persuaded to propose, support or oppose, to change their minds, or simply to keep quiet.

CONTACTING MPs

Members of Parliament generally like to reflect and express the prevailing opinion within their constituencies: one of the few means open to them of gauging constituency opinion is through their mailbags. MPs do not conduct local surveys (except when canvassing at elections), and depend on their agents, local committees, surgeries, and mailbags to assess the strength of feeling on any issue.

The letter

Virtually all MPs read all their own constituency letters. Official letters to Ministers will often receive replies from civil servants, but constituency letters are normally dealt with by MPs themselves. Even the Prime Minister is reputed to read all her constituency correspondence, and MPs in office employ secretaries specifically to deal with constituency matters. It may not be far from the truth to suggest – as one activist community physician has done – that for most MPs, 'One letter on a subject is interesting; two are worth noting; three letters on the same theme represent the full force of public opinion'.

The letter is often the most effective means of influencing an MP. It can present facts, arguments, and some impression of feeling in the constituency. MPs are aware that doctors see far more of their constituents than they are likely to do: letters from doctors are all the more likely to be taken seriously.

Timing the letter

If an MP is interested in a topic he/she will welcome letters at any time. Otherwise, the timing of the letter should be carefully considered. There is little point in writing about the Budget in June, or chiding an MP after the event for having failed to participate in an important debate. It is, unfortunately, difficult to find out in advance the precise timing of much Parliamentary business. *The Times* lists each Saturday the principal debates and Select Committee meetings of the following week, but many of the important issues to be discussed in minor debates will not be included in these lists. If a letter is intended to influence a specific action, such as a vote in a debate, it should arrive a few days beforehand. Information as to timing can be obtained from pressure groups such as ASH or the Committee for the Prevention of Child Accidents. Such organizations should also be asked for notification as to when a constituent's letter might be helpful in the future, and they will particularly welcome receiving copies of both letter and response: it is not unknown for an MP to make a commitment in an attempt to placate a constituent that is at variance with his or her public stance.

It is also often appropriate to write to one's MP about some event of national or international significance such as publication of the Royal College of Psychiatrists' report on Alcohol or the Brandt Commission's report (Brandt 1980); similarly, comment may be made on any Governmental or Departmental decision or action. Carefully timed letters can influence not only a decision to participate in a debate, but even the content of a speech: MPs like to represent themselves as being in touch with their constituents, and often do so by reading long extracts from recently received letters.

Style and content

Letters to MPs should be short and to the point, albeit tempered with a little flattery. References are useless to a busy politician, but photocopies of one or two key documents (with relevant parts marked) will be appreciated, together with the offer of further details. Briefings should be factual and include not only one's own case, but an outline and rebuttal of the main opposing arguments. MPs are most likely to act on those letters that specify the action required, whether it be asking a Parliamentary Question or signing an Early Day Motion. Irritation can be caused by letters that display a lack of knowledge of Parliamentary procedure, by, for example, asking an MP to table a bill involving expenditure by Government or requesting a Minister to ask a Parliamentary Question.

Letters should not be too frequent: the crank letter is as obvious to MPs as is the 'rentaquote' MP to the media. It is normally best to concentrate on a few subjects rather than writing on a broad range of issues. Some MPs like to keep a note of their constituents' interests and expertise so that they can ask for occasional advice and briefings; thus it may be appropriate at some stage to describe one's range of interests. A constituent will know that he is considered unimportant or is pestering the MP with too many letters when a response starts, 'Joe Smith MP has asked me to answer your letter . . .' and is signed by the MPs secretary.

Clarity is vital: MPs are busy, and will only scan a letter briefly. Indiscretion, even in a letter marked 'confidential', is inadvisable. One of the authors wrote in confidence to a friendly MP suggesting that he ask a Parliamentary Question – and explaining that the PQ had been privately suggested by a civil servant not unaverse to embarrassing his Minister. The MP read only the first paragraph, and was so sympathetic on the issue that he immediately forwarded a copy of the letter to the relevant Minister demanding action.

MEETING ONE'S MP

On issues about which a doctor feels very strongly, a meeting with the MP can be effective. It is not always possible to arrange a meeting before an important debate takes place, but it is worthwhile trying to arrange to meet one's MP at least once, if only because MPs, like other people, usually take more notice of letters from those they have met. Virtually all MPs hold constituency surgeries; it can also be useful to invite an MP to a health centre or hospital where it is possible for the MP to see the NHS in action and hear the views of those who work in it, and for the doctor to get to know the MP as something more than a political symbol. MPs can of course also be lobbied at Westminster: this is best reserved for emergencies, although on the other hand few MPs will refuse to show their constituents around the House or obtain tickets for a debate.

TELEPHONING THE MP

MPs can be 'phoned at the House of Commons: even if not immediately available, most MPs will return a constituent's call as soon as possible. The House of Commons switchboard (01 219 3000) will take short messages and is efficient. The telephone, however, should not be used for a first contact unless the matter is too urgent for a letter. MPs' secretaries (whether at Westminster or in the constituency) usually have considerable loyalty to both their party and the Member: a few friendly words over the 'phone with the secretary will often ensure that a matter is placed at the top of an MP's agenda.

WHAT CAN AN MP DO?

Some MPs have established a reputation as successful backbench activists, while others are rarely seen in the House. Members of Government cannot ask Parliamentary Questions, but will instead write letters to their Ministerial colleagues. Similarly, the Speaker cannot ask PQs or table Bills – yet those lucky enough to be a Speaker's constituent soon become aware that he can be the most influential MP of all, for courteous letters from the Speaker almost invariably elicit prompt reactions from Ministers only too well aware of the Speaker's procedural powers.

Parliamentary Questions

The humble PQ is often underrated. It draws attention to a subject at least twice (when it is tabled, and when it is answered). It should be tabled in the form of a request for information, but can be used as a platform for lauching a campaign. 'Priority' Questions will be speedily answered, while for maximum publicity an orally answered Question is best. There is a rota according to which each Governement Department answers oral questions in Parliament on a specified day of the week (the Prime Minister takes Questions on Tuesdays and Thursdays at 3.15 p.m.). Some Questions are answered orally, but as time is short only a few at the top of the list can be dealt with each day: the rest are answered in writing. After Questions have been answered orally, MPs can ask supplementary questions – for which the Ministers will have been carefully briefed. It is possible to find out the days on which DHSS Ministers will be answering questions and attempt to ensure that a Question is high up on the Order Paper, but this requires both Parliamentary skill and patience – and even then one's Question may not be reached. The Written Question, however, is an invaluable weapon for a campaigner – or simply for the constituent in search of information. MPs are generally pleased to ask intelligent Questions: it requires no more effort than filling in a form, shows them to be active, and sometimes generates the kind of publicity to which no politicians are averse. MPs can ask up to 40 questions a day: few go to this extreme, but it is not uncommon for an MP to table a series of questions designed to draw out every possible piece of information on a specific theme. Questions will sometimes be amended by the Table Office, but will normally be accepted so long as they are not frivolous or repetitive, and relate to the work of a specific Government Department. Most MPs have only limited opportunities to participate in debates: the Parliamentary Question is a sure-fire method of attracting attention.

Bills

Backbenchers in Britain (as opposed to the United States) have little opportunity to introduce proposals for legislation. There are three main avenues open to MPs who want to present Bills: two will obtain publicity only; the third is literally a matter of chance.

MPs occasionally announce that they are 'introducing a Bill' to ban chocolates or enforce literacy tests for dolphins. The resultant publicity gives the impression that all sweetshops will shortly close down, or that zoos will go bankrupt. In fact, the Bills stand no chance whatever of becoming law.

1. MPs may 'present' bills without obtaining leave from the House. These bills receive a 'first reading' (which essentially means no more than that they have been printed) and then – barring unanimous agreement or a procedural miracle – fall into oblivion. Such bills are useful for publicity purposes, but no more.

2. A 'Ten Minute Rule' bill can be introduced after Question Time on Tuesdays and Thursdays with a speech lasting no more than ten minutes. Again, barring unanimity the bill will go no further, but it brings with it the considerable advantages of a good audience (the House is normally well-attended during Question Time), the opportunity to impress other MPs, and mass media coverage. The opportunity to introduce a Ten Minute Rule bill is obtained on a first-come first-served basis: MPs will sometimes queue from early in the morning to ensure themselves a place.

3. The annual Private Members' ballot provides the best opportunity for an MP to introduce legislation. At the start of each session backbenchers are able to enter a ballot from which 20 names are drawn: the top six are assured of Parliamentary time on specific Fridays for discussion of their bills; the rest stand a chance of being debated, but in reality are unlikely to succeed other than in publicity terms. Even for the top six, the path to legislation is complicated by factors such as the need for Government support (or lack of opposition), filibustering by opponents, and the difficulty of persuading MPs to stay in London for debates on Fridays. None the less, the Private Members' ballot provides a real opportunity for the fortunate half-dozen MPs to introduce legislation. Hardly surprisingly, the winners in the ballot are lobbied extensively by pressure groups.

Other activities

As well as the activities that attract publicity, such as tabling Questions or presenting bills, MPs can also assist their constituents by writing to Ministers: Such letters can cut through red tape, or may be the preferred procedure if an MP is of the Government party and does not wish to embarrass his colleagues with a public disagreement.

Doctors may wish to pressure their Members to vote, to make speeches (for which good briefings are required), to take a particular line in Committee, to speak in the adjournment debate, or to sign an Early Day Motion (a device for drawing attention to and gauging the strength of Parliamentary feeling on an issue). Even unsympathetic MPs can be influenced by letters from doctors. A staunch defender of the tobacco industry or an ardent anti-fluoridationist is unlikely to change his views overnight, but letters from doctors in his constituency may well cool his ardour a little.

It is also worth remembering the House of Lords as a resource. Peers have far less legislative power than MPs, but all Government Departments are represented in the Upper Chamber, where there's much more time for discussion, and 'starred questions' (those followed by a mini-debate) can relatively easily be tabled. Members of the House of Lords are often glad to be asked to take up an issue, may have more time than MPs to follow it through, and can also attract publicity through speeches and comments inside and outside the House.

WRITING TO A MINISTER

Under certain circumstances (such as when the MP is unhelpful or uninfluential) a direct approach to a Minister is indicated, perhaps with a copy of the letter to the constituency MP if it is thought that the subject will be of interest to him. Approaches to a Minister can be made by writing to the civil servant who is responsible for the topic, but if an issue is one on which a doctor holds strong political views, that is views about the action on which Parliament should take, then a direct approach to the Minister may be indicated. The decision to write to a Minister directly can be difficult if the civil servant who is responsible has been helpful and is willing to listen to ideas from outside, because a letter directly to a Minister goes above his head.

Of course the Minister does not consider every letter in detail but even if he only reads it quickly it may influence his private office and senior civil servants. The private secretary to a Minister, who is usually a young high-flier in his late 20s doing the job for a year or 18 months to give him a glimpse of life at the top, is a very useful point of contact. Remember that Ministers receive many brickbats and the occasional bouquet in terms of a letter of support is welcome.

WRITING TO DOWNING STREET

Numbers 10 and 11 may seem remote and unassailable but there are issues on which a letter to the Prime Minister or the Chancellor is appropriate. When an issue involves more than one Department it is the Prime Minister and Chancellor who are key figures. For example, the relative priority given to defence, health, and housing policies is one on which the opinions of the Prime Minister and the Treasury Ministers are critical. Two other decisions which are of great importance to preventive medicine – the level of taxation placed on cigarettes and alcohol – are also decided by the Treasury, whose primary function is to raise money not to prevent disease, and a letter to the Chancellor in the month before the Budget emphasizing the health problems and costs of cigarette smoking and alcohol abuse may influence Treasury opinion.

KNOW YOUR MP

It is both tactically sound and a natural courtesy to find out something about one's MP's views before writing. Back issues of Hansard and local newspapers can be helpful, and local constituency associations will sometimes make available copies of past speeches on, for example, health issues. The House of Commons Register of Members' Interests gives valuable information on MPs' financial backgrounds, while standard reference books such as the *Times Guide to the House of Commons,* or *Vacher's Parliamentary Companion* provide brief biographies. Thus it should be possible to avoid asking a Parliamentary Consultant to the Scotch Whisky Association to lobby for tax increases on alcohol.

CONCLUSION

To write to such remote and busy people as MPs may seem like tilting at windmills, but we believe that such letters have an effect. Political change is often conceived as being the exercise of power, as though there are levers of change which politicians can reach out and pull like a signalman in an old fashioned signal box. Political change, however, is rarely so dramatic or simple. Even the final vote, the pulling of the lever of chance, is only one link in a process of gradual change brought about by the influence exerted from many sides: we may be sure that the commercial and emotional anti-health interest groups understand this process and make every effort to exert their influence. Politics are as much about influence as about power; we believe that doctors underestimate their potential influence.

REFERENCES

Brandt, W. (1980). *North–South: a programme for survival.* The Report of the Independent Commission on International Development Issues under the Chairmanship of Willy Brandt. Pan.

House of Commons Register of Members' Interests. HMSO, London.

Keeswill, A. S. (1981). *Vachers Parliamentary Companion.* HMSO, London.

Powell, J. E. (1966). *A new look at medicine and politics.* Pitman, London.

Times Guide to the House of Commons (1979). Times, London.

7 Screening

Godfrey Fowler

GENERAL PRINCIPLES OF SCREENING

Introduction

Contrary to common belief, the concept of screening for disease is far from new, there being reports of examination of apparently healthy people to detect disease at least as early as the fourteenth century, when prostitutes in the Papal State of Avignon were required to undergo weekly examination to detect 'distempers'. More recently, medical examination of recruits during the two World Wars demonstrated the existence of a substantial amount of previously undetected disease, while between the Wars surveys carried out at the pioneer Peckham Health Centre detected much previously undiagnosed ill-health in the community. Antenatal care, child-health clinics, school medicals, pre-employment medicals, and insurance examinations are all long-established screening procedures.

In the early 1960s with acknowledgement of the 'iceberg of disease' (Last 1963) illustrated in Fig. 2.2 (p. 24), enthusiasm for screening waxed strongly. Prevention became almost synonymous with screening.

This has been followed by a period of more sober assessment of the potential benefits and limitations of the screening approach. Much debate on this issue was provoked by the publication of important reviews of screening (Nuffield Provincial Hospitals Trust 1968) in which criteria for screening were established and in which critical assessment of procedures was conducted in the light of these. The debate continues and views remain divided. On the one hand are those who are enthusiastic – even evangelistic – about the pursuit of undetected disease. On the other, those who remain to be convinced about the benefits of such activity and whose approach to screening is a more cautious one.

Screening and case-finding

As described in Chapter 1, *screening* may be broadly defined as the questioning, examination, or investigation or an asymptomatic individual to determine the presence or absence of disease. *Case-finding* is a form of screening in which the initiative is limited to the opportunistic approach, where the patient seeking advice from the doctor about his symptoms is, at the same time, questioned, examined, or investigated regarding an unrelated condition. This contrasts with the more aggressive pursuit of the uncomplaining individual to which a narrow definition of screening may sometimes be confined and which is a feature of population surveys. The term *anticipatory care* also incorporates case-finding.

The ethics of screening

Screening and case-finding impose obligations on the doctor over and above those to which he is normally subject. In the conventional consultation concerned with illness, the patient seeks the doctor's help and, although the doctor accepts the obligation to try to fulfil this request, there is no commitment to success. In screening or case-finding on the other hand, it is the doctor who takes the initiative and, in so doing, implies that his intervention will be of benefit to the patient. There is a presumption not only that the abnormality which is sought will, if present, be detected, but that such detection will lead to effective treatment. The same consideration applies even if it is the patient who asks for the screening procedure; there being a further presumption on the part of the patient that the availability of a screening procedure implies that its value is established.

Apart from the inconvenience, anxiety, and possible discomfort associated with a screening procedure, there is also the risk that the procedure itself may be harmful. To expose an individual to such a risk is unjustified unless it is clearly established that there is real potential benefit to balance it, even if that risk is simply one of making the patient aware of a suspected disease for which there is no treatment.

The situation is further complicated by the problem of false-positive and false-negative results. A *false-positive* result indicates an abnormality being present when it is not. A *false-negative* result is, conversely, the failure to identify the abnormality when it is present. While a false-positive result will cause unnecessary distress to the individual and expose him to the hazards of treatment which is equally unnecessary, a false-negative result will be followed by erroneous reassurance and failure to treat the abnormality which in fact exists. Even the identification of a true positive has its problems. 'Labelling' of an apparently healthy individual as 'sick' or 'at risk' has profound psychological and social consequences and may itself lead to disability. In one study labelling of patients as hypertensive was found to increase absenteeism regardless of whether the patients were being treated or not (Haynes *et al.* 1978).

The 'costs' to the patient of screening may therefore be:
– inconvenience;
– anxiety;
– discomfort;
– risk that the screening procedure may be harmful;
– risk of labelling as 'sick' or 'at risk'.
The potential benefit must outweigh these.

Scientific basis

Effective screening requires the early detection of disease for which effective treatment is available, but which if left untreated progresses to disability and death. The natural history of the disease, particularly with regard to the latent phase between its onset and the development of symptoms, must therefore be fairly well understood, and so must its subsequent course if left untreated. Ideally the screening procedure should be simple, sensitive in discriminating between those who have and those who have not got the characteristic being sought, and there should be few 'borderline' individuals. It should also be reliable in giving the same result on different occasions in a given individual. Above all, it should be safe.

The criteria for screening have been listed as follows (Wilson 1976):
– The condition screened for should be an important one.
– There should be an acceptable treatment for patients with the disease.
– The facilities for diagnosis and treatment should be available.
– There should be a recognized latent or early symptomatic stage.
– There should be a suitable test or examination.
– The test or examination should be acceptable to the population.
– The natural history of the condition, including the development from a latent to a declared disease, should be adequately understood.
– There should be an agreed policy on whom to treat as patients.
– The cost of case-finding (including diagnosis and subsequent treatment of patients) should be economically balanced in relation to civil expenditure on medical care as a whole.
– Case-finding should be a continual process and not a once for all project.

Economic considerations

Because resources are always limited, the cost–benefit balance of any screening procedure is an important consideration. The inevitable delay, which may be prolonged, between screening and the realization of any potential benefit makes assessment of the value especially difficult. Moreover, because of the large numbers likely to be involved in any screening procedure, financial considerations loom large.

Even if a screening procedure can be shown to be effective as a preventive measure, its feasibility may be excluded by its cost. Because the demand for medical care always exceeds the resources available, the question of priorities is ever present. Economic evaluation of screening is further hindered by the difficulties in measuring both cost and benefit. Apart from the cost of the screening procedure itself, there are indirect ones such as the cost of attending the screening venue and of time lost from work. The benefits in economic terms are even more difficult to evaluate but this problem is not, of course, peculiar to screening. The measurement of economic gain from any medical intervention is rarely simple and the remoteness of the possible benefit from the screening event aggravates this problem.

Screening in the context of general practice

There can be little doubt that if screening in the case-finding sense is worthwhile, the most favourable environment for its performance is general practice. National Health Service general practice ensures that virtually every individual has an identifiable doctor and, more significantly from the case-finding point of view, every general practitioner has a 'list' of patients. Not only does general practice therefore provide ready access to the population at large, especially those less motivated to seek help, but more importantly it is the channel through which management of the problems detected by the screening procedure will be conducted. Screening procedures conducted independently of doctors providing treatment, are likely to be less successful and also suffer from a disadvantage that they are 'once and for all'. This will be particularly so when, as is usually the case, the individual concerned is without symptoms and is required to pursue a course of treatment which not only requires strict compliance but which may also produce symptoms itself.

It is, perhaps, not surprising therefore that the only large scale controlled trial of 'multi-phasic' screening, that of the Californian Kaiser-Permanente Group (Cutler *et al.* 1973) failed to show any significant difference in death rates between screened and controlled groups seven years after the start of the study. Not that such screening has been shown to be effective in general practice either. The only similar study there (South East London Screening Study Group 1977) showed similar results. However, in this latter study some reassurance and perhaps explanation may be sought in the finding that half the abnormalities detected by screening were already known to the general practitioners and 90 per cent of those previously unknown were of a minor nature and neither disabling nor life threatening.

Nevertheless these findings add fuel to the fire of the screening opponents who argue, furthermore, that the time constraint of general practice is a major obstacle to a screening approach in general practice anyway. They emphasize that the mere detection of disease is no guarantee of therapeutic intervention and, what is more, such intervention may not in any case influence the outcome.

If general practitioners are therefore to become more involved in screening and anticipatory care, they will need to be convinced by factual evidence of the benefits of such a shift from their normal demand-orientated approach. Without this the change in philosophical perspective which is necessary will not be achieved. This change in attitude will also need to take place in patients. The usual consumerist approach to medical care implied by the acquisition of a 'remedy for ills' will need to be modified. Indeed the provision of more anticipatory care may require a greater readiness to be more self-reliant in managing minor illness and a greater willingness to receive and implement advice about lifestyle. It would also depend on a more ready acceptance of the roles of the health visitor, nurse, and other members of the primary health care team. But.

in giving such advice, it is important that health professionals do not adopt a moralizing stance.

The reasons why screening (case-finding) should take place in general practice rather than elsewhere are therefore because it:
— provides access to the whole population;
— is in regular contact with the less motivated;
— provides opportunity for screening to be part of the continuing process of medical care rather than 'one off';
— is concerned with the management of any problem detected;
— combines prevention, cure, and care.

Screening in pregnancy, infancy, and childhood

Although this book does not consider in detail prevention in pregnancy and childhood, which are regarded as special subjects, brief reference will be made to antenatal care and neonatal and childhood screening, as illustrating general principles of anticipatory care.

One of the earliest and most widely applied screening procedures to be adopted was antenatal care. Although many of the individual procedures conducted on the pregnant woman remain unevaluated, the benefits of the overall process are generally accepted. Identification of those who are at greater risk of abnormality during pregnancy or confinement is an important function of the initial antenatal examination and physical, psychological, and social factors enter into this assessment. Regular examinations during antenatal care have two broad objectives. One is the early detection of any developing abnormality, for example pre-eclampsia or anaemia; the other is the screening of selected groups at special risk. For example, although rhesus incompatibility is now in theory preventable, examination of the serum of rhesus-negative women for rhesus antibodies will remain a necessary form of secondary prevention because of the possibility that previous sensitization by, for example, an abortion, can be rarely excluded. Moreover, fetal abnormalities can now be detected *in utero*, making early pregnancy termination feasible thanks to the development of methods of screening. An example of this is the measurement of plasma and amniotic fluid levels of alpha-fetoprotein between 15 and 20 weeks of pregnancy, which has facilitated the prediction of open neural-tube defects. Studies have shown the benefits of routine screening but highlighted associated problems. Detection of chromosomal abnormalities, for example, Down's syndrome, poses similar problems.

It may seem self-evident that routine examination of the newborn aimed at detection of congenital abnormalities, for example, dislocation of the hips, is a worthwhile procedure, but evidence justifying such routine procedures is rather flimsy. While such examinations may undoubtedly detect abnormalities present, they may also be falsely reassuring, especially as the experience of examiners varies enormously. Furthermore, although the early detection of some abnormalities, for example, congenital heart lesions, may lead to remedial action, other abnormalities such as unstable hips may revert to normal without intervention and yet others, for example, central nervous system disorders will be irremediable anyway. This is not to deny that early detection, even of irremediable problems, may lead to better mangement, but against this must be set the anxiety which may be created for example, in parents made aware of innocent cardiac murmurs.

Like antenatal detection of fetal abnormalities, neonatal diagnosis of congenital metabolic disorders has been made possible by new scientific developments. For example phenyketonuria, first described in 1934, as a biochemical disorder leading to mental retardation, can be detected by a simple test for phenylalanine in the blood (Guthrie test) and the virtual exclusion of phenylalanine from the diet prevents the development of mental subnormality. Neonatal hypothyroidism is another condition which is easily detected and even more simply treated, but which if left undetected leads to physical and mental retardation.

The value of routine screening examinations in childhood is debatable (Holt 1974) and earlier enthusiasm for regular routine examinations have given way to more selective ones, particularly of hearing, vision, and growth. There are many problems associated with this type of screening. The 'tests' are often imprecise and the knowledge and skills, not to mention enthusiasm of the performer, are crucial. Moreover, proper evaluation of outcome of most of these procedures is entirely lacking.

HYPERTENSION

Significance

High blood pressure has received a good deal of attention in recent years as a condition for which screening may be particularly appropriate. Half the deaths in developed countries are of cardiovascular origin (see Fig. 7.1) and hypertension is a risk factor in cerebrovascular disease (stroke), coronary heart disease, cardiac failure, peripheral arterial disease, and renal disease.

Definitions of hypertension are elusive. Population studies show that levels of blood pressure are distributed continuously and Life Insurance information (see Fig. 7.2) indicates that the risk to life increases as blood pressure rises.

As a screening procedure measurement of blood pressure is attractive because of its apparent precision. There are a number of factors which influence the recording obtained, amongst them the width of the sphygmomanometer cuff in relation to the diameter of the arm, the circumstances under which the measurement is made, the number of occasions on which it is done, the observer error (including 'digit preference'), etc. In measuring diastolic pressures attention should be paid to whether fourth (change in sound) or fifth (disappearance of sound) phases are being recorded.

100 *Screening*

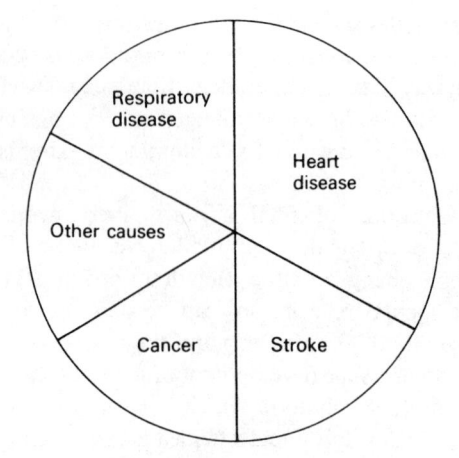

Fig. 7.1. Causes of death in the United Kingdom.

Benefits of treatment

With regard to the important issue of reversibility, that is to say whether treatment and lowering of blood pressure reduces the risk of sequelae, there is now a substantial body of evidence to guide us. Above 180/105 the risk of stroke and left ventricular failure can be substantially reduced by effective hypertensive treatment (Veteran's Administration Study 1972) at least in men below the age of 70 years. The evidence for a reduction in the risk of coronary heart disease is less well established but increasing.

There is also accumulating evidence of the benefits of treating lower levels of blood pressure. Recent studies from America and Australia (Hypertension Detection Follow-up Program 1979; Australian Therapeutic Trial in Mild

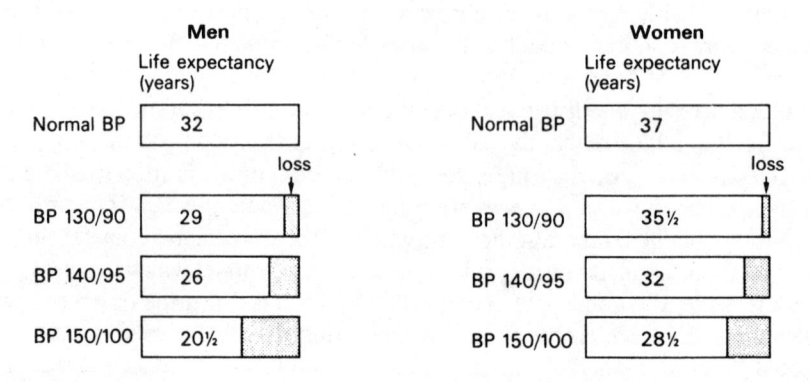

	Men Life expectancy (years)		Women Life expectancy (years)
Normal BP	32	Normal BP	37
	loss ↓		loss ↓
BP 130/90	29	BP 130/90	35½
BP 140/95	26	BP 140/95	32
BP 150/100	20½	BP 150/100	28½

Fig. 7.2. Life expectancy and blood pressure at age 45 years.

Hypertension 1980) have indicated that the benefit of treating hypertension extends to those with diastolic pressures in the range 90 to 105. Other studies of the possible benefits of treating mild hypertension are in progress, notably the Medical Research Council Mild to Moderate Hypertension Trial being conducted in some 100 practices in Britain. The distribution of blood pressure in the population, the associated risk, and the possible benefit from treatment are indicated in Fig. 7.3.

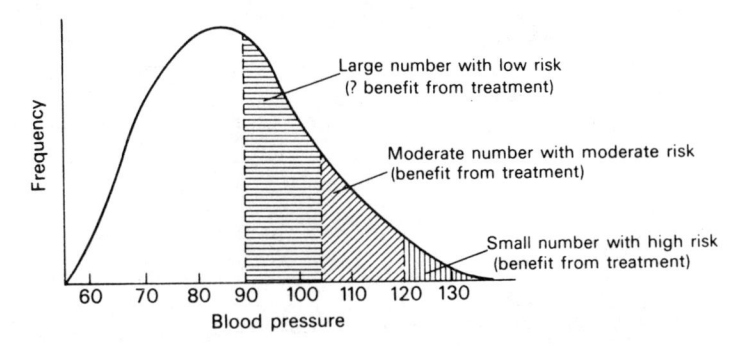

Fig. 7.3. Distribution of blood pressure in population, associated risks, and possible benefit from treatment.

The principal benefit of blood pressure control in these studies has been a reduction in the incidence of stroke, but there is some evidence that it also reduces the risk of coronary heart disease and sudden death. The decline in cardiovascular disease death rate in the United States and Australia over the last decade or so, may – to some extent at least – be attributable to the more vigorous detection and treatment of hypertension which has occurred over this period in these countries (*The Lancet* 1980). This decline is illustrated in Fig. 7.4.

Detection and management

Although about two-thirds of general practitioners think screening for hypertension should be undertaken in general practice (Fulton *et al.* 1979) there appears to be a big gap between this belief and actual performance. A survey of a random sample of patients in Central London showed that only 24 per cent had their blood pressure recorded by a general practitioner during the previous five years, and only 39 per cent of those found to be hypertensive had been followed up. Experience in hospitals doesn't seem to be much better. At two hospitals only 32 per cent of new out-patients had had their blood pressures recorded and only 38 per cent of hypertensives detected were followed up

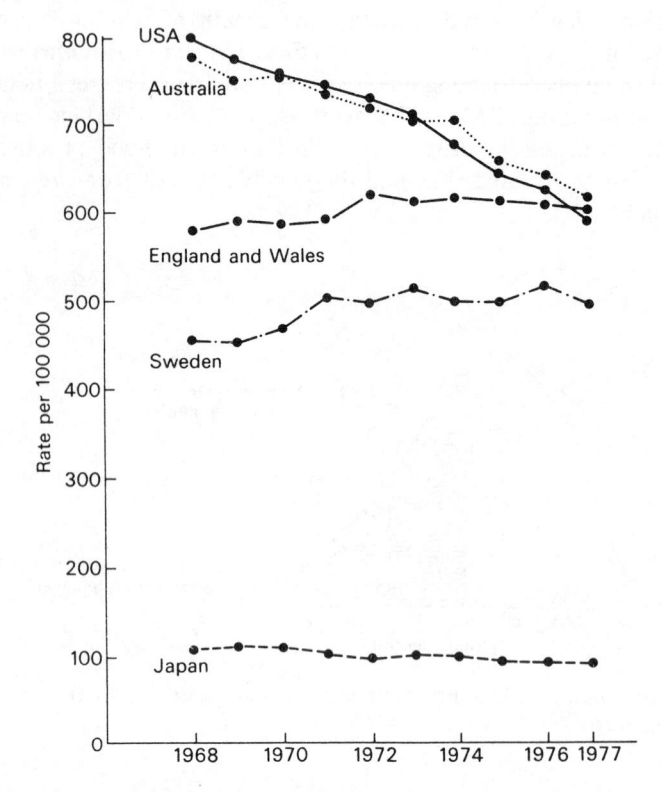

Fig. 7.4. Ischaemic heart disease mortality 1968–77 in the United States, Australia, England and Wales, Sweden. Males 35–74 years. Age-adjusted rates per 100 000.

(Heller and Rose 1977). The rule of halves appears to apply to the management of hypertension in Britain: half of those with the condition are detected; half of those detected are being treated; and half of those being treated are being properly supervized so that their treatment is effective. This is illustrated in Fig. 7.5.

Recommendations

How should the detection and management of hypertension be carried out in general practice? About two-thirds of a practice population consult their general practitioner at least once a year and more than 90 per cent consult within five years. In one population studied, 93 per cent of those with a diastolic pressure greater than 95 had visited their general practitioner within the five-year period (D'Souza *et al.* 1976). Case-finding should therefore be a feasible method, especially given that measuring the blood pressure adds approximately one minute only to the consultation (Buchan and Richardson 1973).

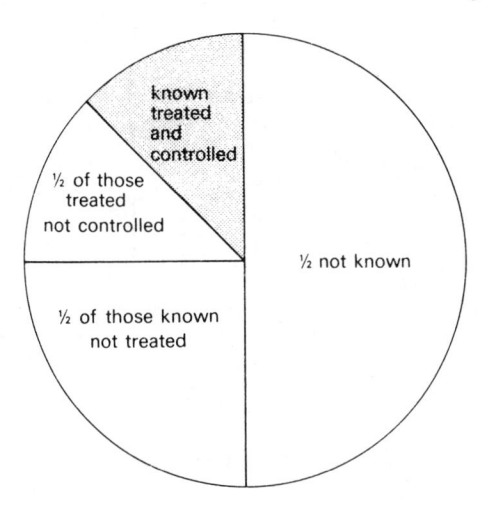

Fig. 7.5. The rule of halves.

It is important that blood pressure measured in this causal case-finding manner is recorded in such a way that the information is easily accessible (see Chapter 3) not only so that comparisons over time may be made, but also so that unnecessary repetition may be avoided. The aim should be to record at least one reading of blood pressure every five years in patients aged 20 to 64 years. Those with a blood pressure at or above 180/105 (this being the mean of three readings and the diastolic recordings being the fifth phase) should be offered treatment and be followed up at intervals not exceeding four months. Under the age of 40 years, this threshold for treatment could reasonably be lowered to 160/100. Taking these levels about 5 per cent of the adult population in this age group will be identified as hypertensive, about 70 patients in an average practice of 2500.

But if the evidence from initial studies of the benefit of treatment of mild hypertension is substantiated, as many as 15 to 20 per cent of the adult population will then be included in this net. These mild hypertensives with blood pressures in the range 150/90 to 180/105 should, for the present, be subject to annual surveillance as well as review of smoking habits and weight. For those with blood pressures less than 150/90, casual five-yearly blood pressure measurements will suffice. One system described by Coope for doing this is the three-box system, illustrated in Fig. 7.6.

Case-finding itself will be only a limited addition to present workload. If a GP with an average list of 2500 patients aims to measure the blood pressure of his adult patients once every five years, he will require to do only one or two blood pressure measurements every day, not as extra consultations, but as opportunistic additions to existing ones. But of course the follow-up of detected hypertensives will impose significant additional burdens. Again, in the average

104 Screening

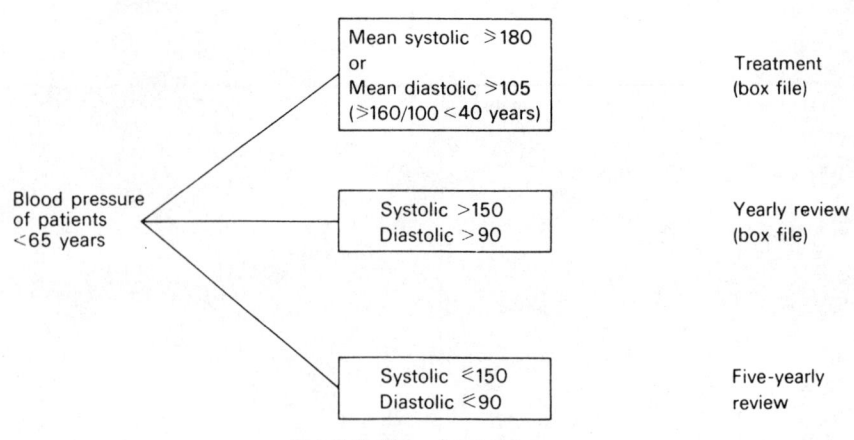

```
                    ┌─────────────────────────┐
                    │ Mean systolic  ⩾180     │
                    │ or                      │    Treatment
                    │ Mean diastolic ⩾105     │    (box file)
                    │ (⩾160/100 <40 years)   │
                    └─────────────────────────┘
Blood pressure      ┌─────────────────────────┐
of patients    ────▶│ Systolic  >150          │    Yearly review
<65 years           │ Diastolic > 90          │    (box file)
                    └─────────────────────────┘
                    ┌─────────────────────────┐
                    │ Systolic  ⩽150          │    Five-yearly
                    │ Diastolic ⩽90           │    review
                    └─────────────────────────┘
```
Fig. 7.6. Three-box system.

practice of 2500 patients, there will, in addition to the 70 or so hypertensives on treatment and requiring surveillance at least three times a year, thus be as many as 150 to 200 mild hypertensives requiring at least annual monitoring.

Some of this work can be delegated to other members of the practice team, notably the practice nurse. It may be appropriate for her to be involved in both case-finding of hypertension and the management of those detected. Newly registered patients should be asked to see the nurse, not only so that she may check their blood pressure, but also to obtain other information for the record 'data base' referred to in Chapter 3. She should also take the opportunity to record the blood pressure of those patients she sees for other reasons whose records show that they have not had this done in the last five years. Furthermore, those mild hypertensives whom it has been agreed to survey annually, can be followed up by the nurse who can, at the same time, check on weight and smoking habits referring the patient to the doctor when necessary on a previously agreed basis. Moreover, even the supervision of those on medication may be shared with the practice nurse. A well-controlled hypertensive needs to be seen by the doctor only once or twice a year, any other follow-up which may help to enhance compliance being conducted by the nurse.

Although it has been customary to consider mainly diastolic pressure as the criterion for diagnosis and treatment, it should be emphasized that the evidence from Framingham and other studies indicates that systolic pressure is a better indicator of prognosis and more reliable when relating treatment to prevention of stroke and heart failure. However, in practice systolic and diastolic pressures are usually closely related.

Finally, the issue of screening for hypertension cannot be left without referring to the problem of compliance with treatment amongst asymptomatic individuals such as hypertensives are. Hypertensives frequently fail to take treatment as prescribed often because it is treatment rather than the hypertension which causes symptoms. Caution should therefore be exercised in translating to the population as a whole the results of studies such as those of the Veteran's Administration which have been conducted on populations specially selected for their compliance. Amongst various methods which may help to improve patient compliance with treatment is the use of patient booklets.

To summarize the recommendations on screening for hypertension:
– An opportunistic approach to taking blood pressure should be adopted.
– The practice nurse should be involved.
– Newly registered adults should have their blood pressure recorded.
– At least one blood pressure every five years should be sought from patients aged 20 to 64.
– Blood pressure must be recorded in such a way that it is easily accessible.

CORONARY HEART DISEASE

More people die from coronary heart disease in developed countries than from any other single cause. Almost half of all male deaths between the ages of 45 and 64 years in Britain are due to this cause, and death is often sudden and unexpected. Furthermore, in spite of the introduction of sophisticated medical facilities such as Coronary Care Units and procedures such as coronary artery bypass surgery, the potential for therapeutic intervention remains severely limited. Is prevention possible, and if so does screening have a role?

Until the last decade or so there has been an inexorable rise in mortality from ischaemic heart disease in developed countries. This 'modern epidemic' appears to be attributable mainly to changes in behaviour. As discussed above, there is evidence, however, of a recent substantial decline in deaths from ischaemic heart disease in the United States and Australia (see Fig. 7.4) and of a more recent, smaller, fall in the UK (*The Lancet* 1980). There has also been a change in the social class distribution of coronary heart disease (Marmot *et al.* 1978, 1981) and these changes are almost certainly due to shifts in behaviour. Until the 1950s coronary heart disease was commoner in upper- and middle-class men than in working men, but this has now changed. Working-class men, particularly those under 50, are now at much greater risk of coronary heart disease than those in the higher social classes. These changes correlate with changes in smoking behaviour and are consistent with the knowledge that cigarette smoking is an important cause of coronary heart disease.

Risk factors

Many epidemiological and other studies have established the concept of risk factors (Dawber *et al.* 1962; Keys 1970). The major risk factors for coronary heart disease are:
– cigarette smoking (see Chapter 6);
– raised blood pressure (see above);
– elevated blood lipids (see Chapter 7).

Others include:
- diabetes;
- physical inactivity;
- type A personality;
- obesity.

Whether obesity is an important independent risk factor is, however, debatable.

Contrary to popular belief, the evidence relating stress to coronary heart disease is poor. The incidence of coronary heart disease amongst so-called type A personalities, characterized by aggressiveness, competitiveness, and preoccupation with time, appears to be greater than that amongst the more phlegmatic type B individuals (Friedman and Rosenman 1959). But even if this is a significant risk factor, the possibility of favourable modification must be limited. Acute stress and adverse life events may be associated with an increased risk of myocardial infarction and their significance is enhanced in those with the risk factors of hypertension and smoking, so that it is such individuals that counselling regarding stress may have value.

Another important risk factor is that of family history of coronary heart disease; although irreversible, its importance lies in identifying those in whom the case-finding approach is particularly valuable. These risk factors are frequently associated one with another, so that more than half the coronary heart disease and sudden heart deaths occur in the 20 per cent or so of individuals with two or more of them.

Benefits of intervention

Although the evidence relating the major risk factors to coronary heart disease morbidity and mortality is conclusive, that demonstrating the beneficial effect of lowering these risks is much less impressive. That for cigarette smokers is best and male doctors between the ages of 34 and 55 years who stopped smoking, reduced their mortality from coronary heart disease by half within five years compared with those doctors who continued to smoke (Doll and Peto 1976). Control of hypertension has not been shown conclusively to reduce the risk of coronary heart disease but this may be because of failure to treat this early enough. There is some evidence, however (Hypertension Detection and Follow-up Program 1977; Puska *et al.* 1979) of falls in coronary heart disease mortality following treatment of mild to moderate hypertension. Again, although abnormalities of lipid metabolism are clearly associated with coronary heart disease, the evidence that dietary change can alter the risk is inconclusive, though there is little dispute about the benefits of achieving an ideal weight and circumstantial evidence in favour of a decrease in saturated fat intake and of some increase of polyunsaturated fats in the diet (see Chapter 7).

But even if these risks are reversible, can they be reversed? Given that they are largely behavioural, motivation, and compliance in the individuals concerned are essential ingredients if changes are to occur and it is encouraging that there is some recent evidence (see Chapter 6) that advice against smoking given during a normal general practice consultation may be effective in helping patients to stop smoking (Russell *et al.* 1979).

But can these risks be reversed in time? Since the underlying atherosclerotic process begins early in life, is middle age too late to try to reverse it?

Not surprisingly there is no consensus on screening for coronary heart disease risks. No control trials have demonstrated the benefits of such screening in general practice, though that showing that screening and correction on a population basis may be beneficial is accumulating (Puska *et al.* 1979). In general practice some enthusiasts have attempted to identify those at risk in their practice populations and to modify their risk factors (Rankin *et al.* 1976). Others remain unconvinced of the value of this.

Recommendations

But few would dispute the value of a case-finding approach. Those with a family history of cardiovascular disease should be subject to special scrutiny, especially if there is a history of coronary heart disease in parents or siblings at an early age. Those who have several risk factors, amongst them family history, hypertension, cigarette smoking, obesity, and indolence, should certainly be offered appropriate advice and help. Known diabetics should be reviewed for these risk factors, especially hypertension and smoking. But enthusiasm should be tempered by the knowledge that the evidence on which to base such activity is limited, though the benefits of stopping smoking and achieving an ideal weight are generally accepted.

To summarize: an opportunistic approach should be adopted to identifying those with risk factors, especially those:
- with a family history of coronary heart disease, especially at an early age;
- with hypertension;
- who are cigarette smokers;
- with diabetes.

CERVICAL CYTOLOGY

Carcinoma of the cervix is the third most common malignancy in women with more than 2000 dying from this disease in Britain each year and accounts for about one quarter of all deaths from cancer in women under the age of 50.

Effectiveness

Cervical cytology introduced by Papnicolau in 1943, was the first screening procedure to be used for the detection of malignant disease. In theory an ideal form of screening, it is only recently that cervical cytology has come to be acknowledged as effective and was therefore introduced as a national programme in Britain in 1964. But some may still dispute this as no controlled trials have been done, nor would they now be ethical.

Screening

There are many reasons for the uncertainty about effectiveness and one of these is the lack of knowledge about the natural history of carcinoma of the cervix. It is now clear that progression from cervical dysplasia through carcinoma *in situ* to carcinoma of the cervix is not an inevitable one. Abnormal cervical smears can revert spontaneously to normal (Kinlen and Spriggs 1978) and there is no absolute evidence that all '*in situ*' lesions will become invasive. This is illustrated in Fig. 7.7. Moreover, the time intervals involved are very variable and may be several decades. In one study the mean ages of diagnosis of carcinoma *in situ* and clinical carcinoma of the cervix were 34 years and 52 years respectively (*Canadian Medical Association Journal* 1976) suggesting a time interval of 10 to 20 years between the development of an '*in situ*' lesion and its progression to frank carcinoma.

Normal ⇌ Dysplasic ⟶ Carcinoma *in situ* ⟶ Carcinoma of cervix

(Unknown what proportion of dysplasic smears return to normal or what proportion of cases of carcinoma *in situ* progress to carcinoma.)

Fig. 7.7. Natural history of cervical cancer.

In spite of the absence of controlled trials, there is circumstantial evidence of the effectiveness of cervical cytology in reducing the incidence of mortality from cervical carcinoma. In Canada and the United States there have been substantial falls in the incidence of carcinoma of the cervix in those areas where intensive screening has been conducted, and there are correlations between screening and declining mortality rates from this condition. In Britain there has also been a fall in recent years in total deaths from carcinoma of the cervix and decline has been greater in two Scottish Regions which have had long-standing screening programmes (MacGregor and Teper 1978), but while there has been a decline in mortality in older women, in younger women it has been increasing.

Practicalities and problems

The increasing incidence of carcinoma of the cervix in younger women has fuelled debate about the age at which screening should be initiated. Each year about two and a half million cervical smears are taken in England and Wales, a quarter of these in women under the age of 25 years and a third of them in the 25 to 34 year age group. The relationship between the age incidence of carcinoma of the cervix and the screening effort are illustrated in Table 7.1.

This distribution of screening effort has been criticized (*British Medical Journal* 1980) as being directed at too young an age group, but the changing incidence of carcinoma of the cervix should strengthen the arguments for early screening. This increase in younger women is associated with changes in sexual bahaviour over the last couple of decades.

There is a reasonable consensus that the first cervical smear in sexually active

Table 7.1. *The relationship between the age incidence of Carcinoma of the cervix and screening effort*

Age (years)	Percentage of all cases of Carcinoma of cervix	Percentage of all smears done
10–19	0	⎫
20–29	3	⎬ 40
30–39	9	20
40–49	23	
50–59	28 ⎫	
60–69	20 ⎬ 88	40
70–79	13 ⎭	
80–89	4	

women should be taken some time between 20 and 25 years, but there is little agreement about the optimal interval between smears. Because of the high false-negative rate which is of the order of 15 per cent, a negative smear should be repeated within a year. Whether the subsequent interval should be three or five years is debatable and will be influenced by the resources available. Ideally women assessed as being at higher risk should be screened at more frequent intervals, and women over the age of 45 years who have been screened regularly have little risk, and for them five-yearly screening should be adequate. There is probably little point in continuing screening beyond the age of 65.

But the main reason for questioning the effectiveness of cervical cytology as a screening procedure is lack of patient compliance, those most at risk being those least likely to be screened. Unwillingness to attend for cervical cytology characterizes many women with the associated risk factors which include:

- low socio-economic status;
- poor hygiene;
- early age of first intercourse and first pregnancy;
- multiplicity of sexual partners;
- multiparity and short intervals between pregnancies.

For these and other reasons, general practice should provide the best opportunities for cervical cytology and it is, after all, the one screening procedure for which general practitioners in British National Health Service practice are paid on an item of service basis. Accepting the desirability of cervical cytology, should it be conducted on a systematic basis, screening the at risk population of a practice or by a case-finding approach amongst those patients attending for another reason? Any systematic screening approach requires the identification of the relevant population in the practice by means of an age/sex register. Using such a register, women in the appropriate age group may be requested to attend a cervical cytology clinic and recalled at agreed intervals. Computerization facilitates such a system, but is of course by no means essential (see Chapter 3). However, responses of patients to such an approach are variable and only a minority of women usually accept such an invitation, generally those at least risk. The help of the practice nurse or health visitor at such clinics is often found to be valuable and, in some practices, the procedure itself has, with success, been delegated to a nurse. But although such cervical smear clinics offer the most systematic method of screening and recall, the case-finding approach should not be neglected. It provides the opportunity to obtain a smear from a patient attending with a gynaecological problem, for obstetric care or for contraception, particularly one who may be at high risk and reluctant to attend a screening clinic. But as with case-finding for hypertension, a review system which ensures that the procedure is repeated regularly is important.

Recommendations

The following recommendations may therefore be made:
 – cervical cytology is a valuable screening procedure;
 – a cervical smear should be taken for the first time between the ages of 20 and 25 in those who are sexually active;
 – all normal first smears should be repeated after one year to minimize the false-negative problem;
 – repeat smears should be taken every five years until the age of 65, or every three years until the age of 45 if resources permit;
 – particular effort should be made to recruit women at high risk into screening programmes, especially when they present for other reasons;
 – all patients with abnormal cervical smears should be referred for gynaecological opinion.

BREAST CANCER

Over 11 000 women die each year from breast cancer in Britain. It is the most frequent malignant disease in women and the commonest cause of death in women between the ages of 25 and 54 years, and the average woman has an approximately 7 per cent chance of developing breast cancer some time in her life. Moreover, in spite of apparent improvements in treatment, the cure rate has not improved and the outlook for women found to have breast cancer is no better now than it was 40 years ago (Baum 1976).

The cause of breast cancer is unknown, but certain women have a higher risk than average and these include those who:
 – are nulliparous;
 – have no children before the age of 30;
 – have a history of other breast disease, usually chronic cystic mastitis;
 – have a family history of breast cancer.

General principles would suggest that early detection should lead to improved prognosis, but there is little evidence to support this contention, though clinical staging has some influence on survival rates. Screening for breast cancer

currently rests therefore on insecure ground. There are four major screening techniques:
- clinical examination by doctor or nurse;
- mammography;
- breast thermography;
- breast self-examination.

Clinical examination by a doctor or nurse is the traditional method of detecting breast lumps. Inspection carried out with the patient in a sitting position, first with the arms at the sides and then with the arms raised, is followed by gentle palpation of the breasts with the flat fingers and examination of the axillae and supraclavivular foci. Such examinations may be conducted during the course of medical examination for other purposes, as a routine periodic examination, at a family planning clinic, in conjunction with cervical cytology or as part of a well woman clinic (Wookey 1971).

Mammography involves taking soft-tissue X-rays of the breasts and studies have shown that, in conjunction with palpation, it may enhance detection of early breast cancer compared with palpation alone.

Breast thermography, a technique of measuring infrared radiation from the breasts, depends on the fact that a neoplasm is usually hotter than normal breast tissue. Although safe, it is subject to high false-positive and false-negative rates and evaluation as a screening procedure is incomplete.

Breast self-examination is simple, but the technique needs to be taught and its regular performance requires a good deal of motivation. It may do more harm than good if it generates a lot of anxiety and canceraphobia. However, many breast lumps are discovered accidently by casual palpation and if a woman wants to carry out regular palpation she should be taught how best to do this and provided with appropriate pamphlets which describe the technique. But there is not, at the present time, a case for urging the universal practice of breast self-examination and it seems very doubtful if other than a small minority of women wish to do it anyway.

Is breast cancer screening beneficial?

The evidence of benefit is inconclusive. The only major study indicating benefit is that of the Health Insurance Plan in New York, the only randomized controlled trial of breast cancer screening so far reported (Shapiro 1977). Between 1963 and 1966, 62 000 women aged 40 to 64, were randomly allocated to a screening group, who were subject to four annual examinations by palpation and mammography and a control group who received normal medical care. Follow-up demonstrated a one-third reduction in mortality over the nine years in the screened group, but the benefits were limited to those aged 50 and over at diagnosis. A controlled trial of clinical examination and mammography in Britain, sponsored by the Department of Health and the Medical Research Council has recently been set up and results of this will be awaited with interest.

One of the major problems with breast cancer screening is that there are a substantial number of false positives, at least half those detected as having possible breast cancer being found to have benign disease and the 'cost' to such patients in anxiety and discomfort is considerable. Moreover, the procedure of mammography is itself a potential hazard, though the radiation dose is very low, the risk of inducing cancer is increased significantly by repetition.

The case for breast cancer screening is therefore unproven. In the light of the delay which occurs before many women who are aware they have a lump seek medical advice (Adam et al. 1980) more information is also needed about the acceptability to women of breast cancer screening.

Recommendations

It is therefore difficult to give any firm recommendations about breast cancer screening, though efforts to reduce the delay in treatment seem justifiable. Self-examination may be encouraged in those motivated to do it and in whom the 'cost' of anxiety is minimal. Inclusion of breast examination routinely in other examinations of female patients, particularly in relation to contraception, pregnancy, and gynaecological problems, on an 'opportunistic' basis also seems reasonable. But there is no case at the present time for 'population screening'.

DIABETES

Diabetes mellitus is a common condition affecting about half a million people in Britain and its prevalence is increasing, especially amongst older adults. It is a major cause of morbidity and mortality.

Enthusiasm for screening for diabetes which was strong in the 1950s has subsequently waned as the belief that early detection and treatment would improve prognosis, although widely held by clinicians, proved hard to substantiate.

The first community survey of diabetes carried out in 1946 showed a total prevalence of 1.4 per cent, half of whom were already known to have diabetes and the other half newly detected (Wilkerson and Krall 1947). Numerous studies elsewhere since have shown a similar pattern with roughly equal numbers of those with symptomatic disease and others who, although asymptomatic, have 'chemical diabetes'. Although some of the latter progress to florid diabetes, in many the glucose tolerance remains unchanged or reverts to normal (Birmingham Diabetes Survey 1970). Such findings, the 'costs' and the uncertainty about whether early treatment modifies the disease have cast doubt on the value of population screening. There is probably more to be gained by screening those at high risk, and these include

- those with a family history of diabetes;
- the obese;
- those with other risk factors for cardiovascular disease, e.g. hypertension;
- those over 50 years;

– women who have had a baby weighing more than 4.5 kg (10 lb).

The criteria for diagnosis of diabetes by screening depend on the definition of the disease, but there is now more general agreement on this and the WHO (1980) criteria are widely accepted. These are
 – in the presence of symptoms a random venous plasma glucose of 11 mmol/l or more or a fasting level of 8 mmol/l or more;
 – in the absence of symptoms a venous plasma glucose level of 11 mmol/l or more two hours after 75 g of oral glucose (those in the range 8–11 mmol/l have 'impaired glucose tolerance' and are at risk of progressing to diabetes).

Examination of the urine for glucose is the traditional screening procedure, but while examination of a post-prandial specimen will reveal most diabetics, the test is unreliable yielding many false positives. Moreover, modern enzyme-strip methods, especially when used in conjunction with a reflectance meter, have made blood-sugar estimation relatively simple and cheap, so that this has tended to replace urine testing and random blood-sugar estimation is a reliable screening method, a venous plasma glucose level of more than 8 mmol/l (or 7 mmol/l fasting) being suggestive of diabetes and warranting of confirmatory diagnostic tests in asymptomatic individuals (WHO Expert Committee on Diabetes 1980).

Apart from the acute metabolic problems associated with diabetes its importance lies in its long-term complications. These include a greatly increased risk of cardiovascular disease and damage to the eyes, kidneys, and nerves. The opportunities for secondary prevention by early diagnosis may therefore be complemented by those for tertiary prevention by regular surveillance of those detected. This will be especially true if recent evidence of the value of careful control of the diabetic state in preventing complications is confirmed.

To summarize the recommendations on screening for diabetes: while there is no case for routine population screening, the diagnosis should be considered (and excluded by random blood-sugar measurement) in:
 – those with symptoms suggestive of diabetes;
 – those with a family history of diabetes;
 – the obese;
 – those with other risk factors for cardiovascular disease;
 – women who have had a baby weighing more than 4.5 kg (10 lb).

GLAUCOMA

Glaucoma is a major cause of blindness accounting for at least 10 per cent of the totally registered blind and a similar proportion of those added to the Register each year – approximately 100 000 and 10 000 respectively in Britain (Sorsby 1972). Chronic simple glaucoma is an insidious disease which, because central vision is not impaired until a late stage, may remain asymptomatic until then and it would therefore seem an appropriate target for screening. Raised intra-ocular pressure causes damage to the optic nerve (with cupping of the disc) and consequent visual-field defects.

Early diagnosis depends on detection of elevation of intra-ocular pressure (above 21 mm Hg) before visual-field defects or disc cupping have developed. In one survey (Bankes *et al.* 1968) about 1 per cent of people over the age of 40 were found to have glaucoma. But population screening based on the measurement of intra-ocular pressure (tonometry) is relatively non-specific. There are large numbers of false positives (in the Bedford Survey 3 per cent had ocular hypertension which on follow-up proved largely benign) and some false negatives (those with 'low-tension glaucoma' with visual-field defects and disc cupping but normal intra-ocular pressure). Moreover, tonometry requires a fair degree of skill.

Attention to high-risk categories rather than a general population screening approach would seem most appropriate.

Those at highest risk are people over the age of 60, especially if there is a family history of the disorder. First-degree relatives are 10 to 15 times more likely to develop glaucoma than the rest of the population and in the Bedford Survey 80 per cent of those detected were over the age of 60 years.

MULTIPHASIC SCREENING

One of the consequences of the increasing enthusiasm for screening in the 1950s was the birth of the concept of multiphasic screening (Breslow 1950). This approach involves submitting individuals to a battery of tests and subjecting those with abnormal findings to further scrutiny. It is a mechanistic form of medicine in which investigation precedes history and examination, the reverse of the usual process, and it has various shortcomings. One of these is the large grey area in which discrimination between normality and abnormality depends on clinical judgement. Another is the tendency to isolate such screening from services concerned with diagnosis, management and surveillance of the problems identified.

Evidence for the effectiveness of multiphasic screening is lacking. A randomized controlled trial by the Kaiser Permanent Medical Care Program in the USA showed no differences in major disabilities between screened and controlled populations on seven-years follow up (Dales *et al.* 1979) and a similar study in Britain produced the same results (South East London Screening Group 1977). The conclusion must therefore be that multiphasic screening is not of proven value.

CONCLUSIONS ON SCREENING IN GENERAL PRACTICE

So, what general conclusions may be drawn about the place of screening in general practice?

Firstly, there is little or no place for 'screening clinics'. If anticipatory care is to be provided, detection must be achieved on an opportunistic, case-finding basis, in patients who have taken the initiative to consult their doctor about some problem, be it unrelated to any preventive activity.

Secondly, the most important conditions to be screened for on this basis are elevated blood pressure and other cardiovascular risk factors, chief of which is smoking. Screening for cervical cancer in women is also worthwhile.

In practice, this means consideration of these conditions should arise in any consultation by a patient in the 30- to 65-year age group.

REFERENCES

Adam, S. A., Horner, J. K., and Vessey, M. P. (1980). *Commun. Med.* **2**, 195.

Bankes, J. L. K., Perkins, E. S., Tsolakis, S., and Wright, J. E. (1968). Bedford Glaucoma Survey. *Br. med. J.* **i**, 791.

Baum, M. (1976). The curability of breast cancer. *Br. med. J.* **i**, 439.

Birmingham Diabetes Survey Working Party (1980). Five year follow-up of Birmingham diabetes survey of 1962. *Br. med. J.* **ii**, 301.

Breslow, L. (1950). Multiphasic screening examinations – an extension of the mass screening technique. *Am. J. publ. Hlth* **40**, 274.

British Medical Journal. (1980). High risk groups and cervical cancer. (Editorial.) *Br. med. J.* **iii**, 629.

Buchan, I. C. and Richardson, I. M. (1973). Time study of consultation in general practice. Scottish Health Service Studies No. 27. Scottish Home and Health Department, Edinburgh.

Canadian Medical Association Journal (1976). Cervical Cancer Screening programs: epidemiology and natural history of carcinoma of the cervix. *Can med. Ass. J.* **114**, 1003.

Cutter, J. L. (1973). *Prevent. Med.* **2**, 197.

Dales, L. G., Friedman, G. D., and Collen, M. F. (1979). Evaluating periodic multiphasic health checkups: a controlled trial. *J. chron. Dis.* **32**, 385.

Dawber, T. R., Kannel, W. B., Revotskie, N., and Kagan, A. (1962). The epidemiology of coronary heart disease – the Framingham enquiry. *Proc. R. Soc. Med.* **55**, 265.

Doll, R. and Peto, R. (1976). Mortality in relation to smoking: twenty years' observation on male British doctors. *Br. med. J.* **ii**, 1515.

D'Souza, M. F., Swann, A. V., and Shannon, D. J. (1976). A longterm controlled trial of screening for hypertension in general practice. *Lancet* **i**, 1228.

Freidman, M. and Rosenman, R. H. (1959). *J. Am. med. Ass.* **169**, 1286.

Fulton, M., Kellet, R. J., and MacLean, D. W. (1979). The management of hypertension – a survey of opinions amongst general practitioners. *J. R. Coll. Gen. Practrs* **29**, 583.

Haynes, R. B., Sackett, D. L., and Taylor, D. W. (1978). Increased absenteeism from work after detection and labelling of hypertension patients. *New Engl. J. Med.* **229**, 741.

Heller, R. F. and Rose, G. A. (1977). Current management of hypertension in general practice and in hospital. *Br. med. J.* **i**, 1441.

Holt, K. S. (1974). Screening for disease – infancy and childhood. *Lancet* **ii**, 1057.

Hypertension Detection and Follow-up Cooperative Group (1979). Reduction in mortality of persons with high blood pressure, including mild hypertension. *J. Am. med. Ass.* **242**, 2562.

Keys, A., Aravanis, C., Blackburn, H., Van Buchem, F. S. P., Buzina, R., Djordjevak, R. Fidanza, F., Karvonen, M. J., Menotti, A., Punnd, V., and Taylor, H. L. (1972). Coronary heart disease: overweight and obesity as risk factors. *Ann. intern. Med.* **77**, 15.

Kinlen, L. J. and Spriggs, A. I. (1978). Women with positive cervical smears but without surgical intervention. *Lancet* **iii**, 463.

The Lancet (1980). Why the American decline in coronary heart disease? (Editorial.) *Lancet* **i**, 183.

Last, J. M. (1963). The clinical iceberg in England and Wales. *Lancet* **ii**, 28.

MacGregor, K. E. and Teper, S. (1978). Mortality from carcinoma of the cervix uteri in Britain. *Lancet* **ii**, 774.

Marmot, M. G., Adelstein, A. M., Robinson, N., and Rose, G. A. (1978). Changing social class distribution of heart disease. *Br. med. J.* **ii**, 1109.

——, Booth, M., and Beral, V. (1981). Changes in heart disease mortality in England and Wales and other countries. *Hlth Trends* **13**, 33.

Nuffield Provincial Hospitals Trust (1968). *Screening in medical care.* Oxford University Press.

Puska Pekka, Jaakko Tuomilehto, Jukka Salonen, Liisa Neittaanmäki, Juhäni Maki, Jarmo Virtamo, Aulikki Nissinen, Kaj Koskela, and Tuula Takalo (1979). Changes in coronary risk factors during comprehensive give year community programme to control cardiovascular diseases (North Karelia Project). *Br. med. J.* **ii**, 1173.

Rankin, H. W. S., Horn, D. B., Mackay, A., and Forgan, C. U. S. (1976). The control of coronary risk factors in general practice: a feasibility study. *Hlth Bull.* **34**, 66.

Russell, M. A. H., Wilson, C., Taylor, C., and Baker, C. D. (1979). Effects of general practitioners[1] advice against amoking. *Br. med. J.* **ii**, 231.

Shapiro, S. (1977). Evidence on screen for breast cancer from a randomized trial. *Cancer* **39**, 2772.

Sorsby, A. (1972). Report on Public Health Subjects No. 128.

South East London Screening Study Group (1977). A controlled trial of multiphasic screening in middle age: results of the South East London Screening Survey. *Int. J. Epidemiol.* **6**, 357.

Veterans Administration Cooperative Study Group on Anti-hypertensive Agents (1972): Effects of treatment on mobidity in hypertension *Circulation* **45**, 991.

Wilkerson, H. L. C. and Krall, L. P. (1947). Diabetes in a New England town. *J. Am. med. Ass.* **135**, 209.

Wilson, J. M. G. (1976). Some principles of early diagnosis and detection. Surveillance and early diagnosis in general practice. Proceedings of Colloquium held at Magdalen College, Oxford, 7 July 1965 (ed. G. Teeling-Smith). Office of Health Economics, London.

Wookey, B. E. P. (1971). *Br. med. J.* **ii**, 31.

8 Resources for prevention

Godfrey Fowler, Muir Gray, Max Blythe, and Elaine Fullard

Prevention has been thought to be a cheap option by some policy makers but there is obviously a need for resources to practise preventive medicine. However, there are a number of problems faced by those who are trying to provide such resources.

Resource problems

A shortage of resources is obviously the central problem but there are a number of associated problems which affect the allocation of resources to preventive medicine.

The problem of marginal costs

The aim in most areas of preventive medicine is to achieve complete coverage of the population at risk but the costs of increasing coverage increase exponential (Fig. 8.1).

Thus the cost of performing a cervical smear on the last 10 per cent of women at risk in a population could well be greater than the cost of covering the previous 90 per cent; the marginal costs rise dramatically as coverage increases. Often, the marginal benefits increase too, for example the women who are last to be screened are often those who are most at risk, and this has an influence on the cost–benefit analysis but the law of diminishing returns has to be taken into account when planning preventive medicine.

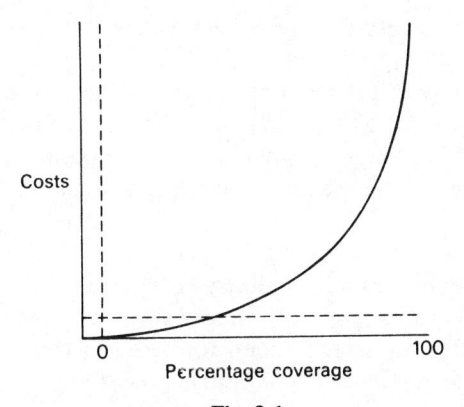

Fig. 8.1.

The problem of delayed benefits

It is rarely possible to invest resources in prevention and achieve rapid returns on the investment. Usually there is a delay of years, or even decades, before the benefits of the investment can be enjoyed. This should not be an insuperable obstacle to investment for it is commonplace to invest resources in hospital building with no prospect of returns for years but this is accepted as inevitable where buidlings are concerned, whereas bids for an investment in prevention are too often considered as impossibly costly in comparison with the immediate returns on investment they offer.

The problem of switching resources

Even if the merit of a preventive programme is accepted there may be difficulty in finding resources for prevention because the service that has to provide the new preventive service is often a different service with a different budget from the service that will benefit from the prevention of the disease. The provision of services to detect spina bifida offers a good example of this type of problem because the services which provide the prevention, obstetric and laboratory, are not those which will benefit, which are surgical, paediatric, urological, housing, social security, and personal social services. For this reason women do not have alpha-fetoprotein screening although cost–benefit analysis of the provision of AFP services has demonstrated that they save resources as well as prevent suffering.

Sources of resources

It is important to distinguish the banker from the true origin of the resources for preventive medicine. While it is true that the Department of Health, the Family Practitioner Committee, and the District Health Authority sanction the use of resources the true sources of those resources are the other services which have been deprived of the resources provided. The bureaucracy merely acts as a bank.

The sources of resources for preventive medicine in general practice and primary care are:

1. New resources provided specifically for preventive health services from other areas of public expenditure such as defence or housing or social security. The main problem being that most would argue that housing and social security are themselves preventive services, and some would argue the same for defence spending.

2. Resources diverted from hospital services.

3. Resources from the insurance industry.

4. Resources from other areas of primary care, for example: (i) resources freed by a reduction in consultations for 'trivial' conditions by patient education; (ii) resources provided by savings in prescribing.

Much can undoubtedly be done within the present constraints but if prevention is to flourish more resources must be devoted to primary care but it is important that these be introduced as part of a plan for prevention in primary care.

PLANNING FOR PRIMARY CARE

Although the United Kingdom has a high quality of general practice and community nursing with complete population coverage there is a danger that we will fail to make the best use of these resources in future because of a lack of planning for primary health care, indeed there is evidence that we are not making the most effective and efficient use of these resources at present. General practitioners are busy providing primary medical care, and community nurses are busy with the provision of important local health services but we are poorly organized to provide a comprehensive pattern of primary health care which, in the words of Dr Halfdan Mahler, 'should fit the life patterns of the community it serves and should meet community needs and demands'. This is not to say that there is no planning of primary health care in the United Kingdom, certain aspects of it are well planned. Nursing officers plan the development of community nursing services; health authority planners work on programmes of health centre and community hospital development; community physicians work at programmes for prevention and an increasing number of general practitioners are trying to set goals and develop operational policies. In addition the Department of Health is aware of the need to plan for primary health care. However, in no more than a few parts of the country is this effort well integrated.

It is easy to identify reasons for the failure to plan for primary care, for example general practitioners are independent contractors, health authority staff work in a large bureaucracy; funds come from different sources; and there are a number of different bodies involved – the Local Medical Committee, the Family Practitioner Committee, the District and Regional Health Authorities, and the Community Health Council to name but the more important. What is needed is to draw together the various organizations with an interest in primary health care, to overcome mistrust and suspicion and to generate an enthusiasm for integrated planning that will overcome problems such as that created by the different status of general practitioners or by the different sources of funds. It must be said that such 'problems' are often more apparent than real and are often used as excuses for not attempting to plan primary health care by professionals and planners who are either reluctant to change or who are unwilling to take on a new area of work when they already feel overloaded.

Principles of planning primary care

The World Health Organization has developed useful principles for planning primary health care and although these were developed with the needs of developing countries in mind as part of the 'Health for All' strategy (WHO 1978, 1981) they are of equal relevance to developed countries: in the planning of primary health care it can be argued that the developed world has more to

120   *Resources for prevention*

learn from the developing world than vice versa. We certainly have good services but their traditions and indeed their quality act as brakes on the process of change. The application of the 'Health for All' principle to European countries was summarized by Dr Leo Kaprio, Regional Director of the WHO's Regional Office in Europe.

1. Health care should be 'needs related', universally accessible, and acceptable.
2. Community participation is essential.
3. Primary health care should be effective and efficient.
4. Primary health care should form part of all national development and of the wider health care system (Kaprio 1979).

So much for the principles; how do we put planning into practice?

Planning in practice

To put these principles into practice requires an initial assessment of needs, both the needs of the community and the needs of the professionals.

The needs of the community can be assessed using data on mortality and morbidity, in consultation with the Community Health Council, patient participation groups if any exist, and with relevant parties, either voluntary associations or professional groups such as the Social Services Department (Fig. 8.2).

The needs of the professionals can be assessed in discussion with the organizations that represent general practice, notably the Local Medical Committee, and the other professionals involved. However, it is important to remember that such organizations cannot represent all shades of opinion and that it is therefore necessary to make contact with all the professionals either by a letter or, much better, by one or more visits. If drug companies find drug reps effective why should we not have health reps?

This type of planning requires time and commitment, but who should do it? The answer will vary from one part of the country to another depending upon local circumstances of which the most important are the interests and attitudes of general practitioners, community physicians, and nursing officers. It cannot be done by either the Family Practitioner Committee or the Local Medical Committee or the Community Services Sector Management Team alone. It needs a group that draws together all these interests and the Community Health Council, a primary health care planning team or a primary care and prevention group. Having drawn up the plan this group should also provide the thrust and drive for implementation (Fig. 8.3).

Motivating

The motivation requires a motivator, a single committed person, and although community physicians have an important part to play general practitioners could do this job very well, provided they were given time and support. Health authorities employ general practitioners in school and child health work but in most authorities they are employed to do no more than deliver a service to a

Planning for primary care 121

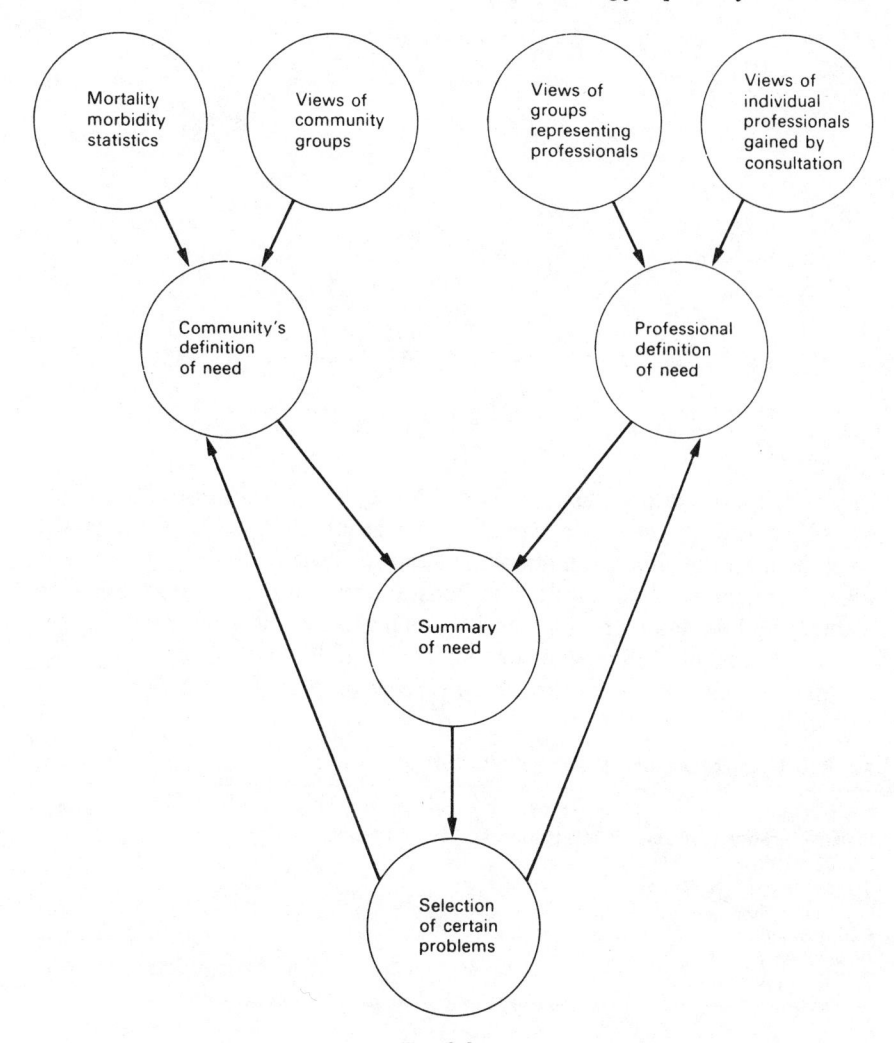

Fig. 8.2.

small number of children. This is obviously important but general practitioners can also make a contribution to health service planning and development. Many do through their membership of health authorities, district management teams, committees and health care planning teams. However, the contribution which they can make to planning is often limited by the time they can afford to spend. Would it not be a more effective use of the time and skills of general practice for a health authority to employ one or two general practitioners to work two sessions a week alongside the community physician and nursing officers closely involved with the planning and promotion of primary health

122 *Resources for prevention*

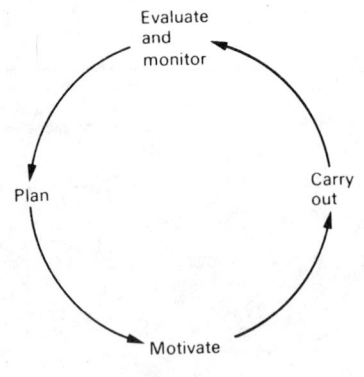

```
        Evaluate
        and
        monitor
           ↑
   Plan         Carry
                out
           ↑
        Motivate
```
Fig. 8.3.

care for children rather than simply employing general practitioners only as school medical officers or to work in child health clinics? The same model could be used for other programmes in primary health care. Why not have a general practitioner working two sessions a week with the responsiblity for planning and promoting primary health care for the people with diabetes or for patients with high blood pressure or for elderly people?

Other examples of primary health care programmes are listed in Table 8.1.

Table 8.1. *Primary health care programmes*

Smoking cessation
Patient education to encourage self-treatment of minor illnesses
Family planning
Prevention of psychiatric disorders
Cervical cytology
Low back pain
Prevention of handicap
Accident prevention

The planning group would have to delegate responsibility for such programmes to smaller groups, and a general practitioner on a sessional contract could play an invaluable part in motivating his colleagues to adopt the aims of the programme. complementing the work of the nursing officer, community physician, and community services administrator.

This may all seem long-term planning because resources are so limited. In the short term a solution would be for the health authority to pay the salary and supporting costs of the Royal College of General Practitioner's Tutors. The tutor is responsible for recurrent education of general practitioners after the period of vocational training is over but most tutors have neither a salary nor adequate secretarial or administrative support. It is obviously important to invest in vocational training but the contrast between the resources available for vocational training and for recurrent education is striking, yet it could be argued that it is the latter who need motivating to a greater degree.

Carrying out the plans

Any plans for primary health care have to be carried out by the primary health care teams but it is important that the individual primary care teams have the appropriate type of support. If, for example, a primary health care plan for the prevention of cancer is developed the health authority could take responsibility for the issue of invitations and recalls to women at risk, leaving the primary care team to concentrate on the delivery of service. If some teams are particularly interested in the prevention and management of musculoskeletal disorders such as low back pain a domiciliary physiotherapist employed by the health authority would complement and supplement the skills of the members of the primary care teams. The responsibility for this aspect of the implementation of the plan should rest with the 'primary care and prevention group' and with the sub-groups responsible for each programme.

Evaluating and monitoring

There is a tendency among those who work in a particular part of the health service to assume that the fact that their work is good and that the good is so self-evident that they have no need of detailed evaluation. This tendency, which is natural, can be detected among those who work in primary health care and preventive medicine as it can in almost all branches of the service but it is very important that we try to collect more detailed information on the way that primary health care services affect the health of the community. New district health authorities are not going to be very impressed by bids for resources supported solely by claims that 'prevention is better than cure' or that 'primary health care is very important'. We have demonstrated what we are doing at present and what we could do given more resources. We can evaluate either by measuring outcome, that is the effect of a programme, for example a reduction in the number of strokes. Alternatively it can be done by measuring the levels of activity, for example the proportion of the population who have had their blood pressure measured and the proportion of people receiving treatment for high blood pressure or the proportion of women at risk who have had a cervical smear.

The collection of data is important because it evaluates the plan as well as providing a basis for future planning and for making bids for new resources. It is also of vital importance because it helps in the implementation of the plan. Being aware of one's actions, and being aware that others are aware, changes behaviour more effectively than any other technique and this is the main benefit of audit. Planning for primary health care and prevention is not a process that runs ahead of, or in parallel with, the provision of services; it is or should be an integral part of primary health care.

RESOURCES WITHIN THE COMMUNITY

Resources for road safety

The specific part which the general practitioner can play in the prevention of road traffic accidents is described later (see Chapter 14) but he may wish to become involved in other aspects of this fascinating problem, in which case he should make contact with the police and the road safety officers of the local authority, who share the responsibility for transport safety education. Road safety is a county council function in the rural counties and a district or borough council function in metropolitan areas.

Road safety officers are very useful sources of information about the pattern of accidents in their area.

Resources for home safety

The health visitor is obviously involved with the prevention of home accidents, but education for home safety is, in fact, the statutory responsibility of the environmental health officer. The environmental health department is an invaluable source of information on all types of hazard in the home and of hazards in the workplace and environment. The Medical Officer for Environmental Health will also be a useful source of information on environmental pollution and infection.

Voluntary groups

In this category fall a very wide range of groups all of which may be useful to the general practitioner and health visitor who are interested in the promotion of preventive medicine. Old people's clubs, the British Red Cross Society, The St John Ambulance Association, the St Andrew's Ambulance Association, Age Concern, and youth clubs are the types of organization which can be drawn into preventive medicine. Obviously this is easier for the general practitioner who is working in the large village or small town for his practice population and the local community are composed of the same people whereas the general practitioner in the city cannot relate to these groups in the same way. He has to depend primarily on 'one-to-one' health education. Nevertheless, community health education, using established community groups, can be practised in cities as well as in small towns.

The University

The local University is an extremely valuable resource and individuals can be found to give advice on the design of research projects, the wording of questionnaires, and the handling of data. The Department of General Practice may be able to advise on whom to approach if there is no one in that department who can give the right type of advice.

The Member of Parliament

If a general practitioner is concerned about some aspect of the environment or some problem which is the responsibility of the local authority it is more diplomatic and usually more effective to approach the relevant local government official in the first place and not the local Councillor. If, however, he is concerned about an issue which is the responsibility of central Government it is more effective to approach the local Member of Parliament. Through him a general practitioner can influence the responsible Minister (see p. 87).

National resources

The Health Education Council and the Scottish Health Education Group are national resources; thay can be used by anyone. They make available a good deal of health education material – posters, leaflets, and audiovisual aids. Some recent literature such as the 'Give Up Smoking' and 'Minor Illness: how to treat it at home' leaflets have been made available specifically for use in general practice. These materials are also available through local Health Education Officers.

The Central Information Service based at the Royal College of General Practitioners is a valuable source of information about many aspects of primary care, especially organization, and the appropriate division in the Department of Health and Social Security and the Scottish Home and Health Department may also provide helpful information on prevention.

On specific subjects advice and information may be obtained from patient organizations, charitable bodies and pressure groups, many of which are listed under Useful Adresses at the end of this chapter.

HEALTH EDUCATION OFFICERS

There are about five hundred health education officers at work in the United KIngdom, serving district Health Authorities and providing local health education services. Their brief is to stimulate the public's interest in health and prevention, and to support and develop the health education being carried out by field workers such as GPs, other doctors, health visitors, nurses, dentists, chiropodists, social workers, and – by no means least – teachers. Health education officers also have a valuable liaison and co-ordination function through their links between local health and social services authorities, also with CHCs and the numerous voluntary bodies concerned with health.

Health education officers are graduates recruited from a variety of professional backgrounds, especially teaching, nursing, and health visiting. Officers receive the necessary additional training in post, some actually starting as trainee health education officers, and most acquire a postgraduate qualification

126 Resources for prevention

by secondment to either a Health Education Diploma Course or one of the M.SC. courses currently on offer. The Health Education Council of England, Wales and Northern Ireland, and the Scottish Health Education Unit are important sponsors of candidates on secondment to these courses. At the present time, the HEC is also financing, with the help of the University of Surrey, a detailed investigation of the continuing education needs of health education officers.

Fully trained health education officers need to be educationalists with a competent view of epidemiology and preventive medicine together with some understanding of people and local cultures they serve. Their skills as communicators and co-ordinators are of immense importance. Each local team, usually closely directed by its District Community Physician to whom it is accountable, is guided in its development and evolution of policy by senior health service, education, social services, and environmental health personnel. The aim in most cases is to seek the widest professional guidance. In addition, there is the broad range of advisory and other support services provided by central agencies such as HEC and Scottish Health Education Unit to help the development of services locally. Thus, the health education officer holds a unique 'middle man' position, providing and regulating a dialogue between expert and layman on health matters. He occupies a difficult but fascinating piece of middle ground on which the future character of health care may well depend.

Since the 1960s, particularly the time of the Cohen Report on Health Education, when health education officers emerged as a separate species within local authority health services, there have been important trends in the evolution of local services. Perhaps most significant has been the move away from propagandist campaigns and towards a much fuller use of the whole spectrum of education to provide continuous and sustained input. Local health education is now more a sustained dialogue about caring: requiring the participation of parents, children at school, school leavers, people at work and people unemployed, people with special needs, not least those who are elderly. It is all the time moving away from the illness models on which health education cut its early teeth. Overall, it is taking on a more ecological flavour, with due concern for all the many factors significant to health rather than remaining perhaps a little too preoccupied with just a few of the tangible dangers.

There are threats to health education services though – and to their success. They require adequate finance. They require professional support because a health education service is only as good as its sponsors, advisors, and professional outlets. Above all though, there is need of the right kind of graduate entrant with the right background skills and capable of specializing in the difficult role of a hybrid, with one foot firmly in health interests and the other persona in education. Given the present cramped career and salary structure this might be too much to hope.

SOME USEFUL ADDRESSES

Action on Smoking and Health,
5-11 Mortimer Street,
London, W1.
Tel. 01-637-9843.

Age Concern,
60 Pitcairn Road,
Mitcham,
Surrey.
Tel. 01-640-5431.

Anorexic Aid,
The Priory Centre,
11 Priory Road,
High Wycombe,
Bucks.

The Arthritis and Rheumatism Council,
41 Eagle Street,
London, WC1 R4Ar.
Tel. 01-405-8572.

Association for Stammerers,
Harold Poster House,
6 Lechmere Road,
London, NW2 5BU.
Tel. 01-459-8521.

BMA/BLAT Film Library,
BMA House,
Tavistock Square,
London, WC1.
Tel. 01-387-4499.

British Dyslexia Association,
4 Hobart Place,
London, SW1 W0HU.
Tel. 01-235-8111.

British Epilepsy Association,
Crowthorne House,
New Wokingham Road,
Wokingham, Berks. RG11 3AY.
Tel. 03-446-3122.

Resources for prevention

The British Heart Foundation,
57 Gloucester Place,
London, W1H 4DH.
Tel. 01-935-0185.

Central Information Service Foundation,
14 Princes Gate,
London, SW7 1PU.
Tel. 01-581-3232.

Centre for Policy on Ageing,
Nuffield Lodge,
Regents Park,
London NW1.
Tel. 01-722-6271.

Coronary Prevention Group,
Central Middlesex Hospital,
London, NW.

Disabled Living Foundation,
346 Kensington High Street,
London.

Family Planning Information Service,
Margaret Pike House,
27–35 Mortimer Street,
London, W1N 7RJ.

Family Welfare Association (publishes *Charities Digest*)
501–503 Kingsland Road,
Dalston,
London, E8 4AV.

Gamblers Anonymous,
17–23 Blantyre Street,
Cheyne Walk,
London, SW10.
Tel. 01-352-3060.

Health Education Council,
78 New Oxford Street
(Resources Centre, 71–75 New Oxford Street),
London, WC1A 1AH.
Tel. 01-637-1881.

Medical and National Councils on Alcoholism,
3 Grosvenor Terrace,
London.

National Council on Alcoholism,
3 Grosvenor Crescent,
London, SW1.
Tel. 01-235-4183.

Royal Institute for the Deaf,
105 Gower Street,
London, WC1 E6AH.
Tel. 01-387-8033.

Royal National Institute for the Blind,
224 Great Portland Street,
London, W1N 6AA.
Tel. 01-388-1266.

Royal Society for the Prevention of Accidents,
4 Priory,
Queensway,
Birmingham, B4 6BS.

Scottish Health Education Group,
Woodburn House,
Canaan Lane,
Edinburgh EH10 4SG.
Tel. 031-447-8044.

Voluntary Council for Handicapped Children,
8 Wakley Street,
Islington, EC1V 7QE.
Tel. 01-278-9441.

OTHER RESOURCES

Health Education and Guide to Voluntary Agencies (Edsall, London. 1980). Available from local Health Education Officers.
King's Fund Directory of Organisations for Patients and Disabled People. Available from local booksellers or The Book Centre, 13 Slaidburn Crescent, Fylde Road, Southport, Merseyside PR9 9YF.

REFERENCES

Kaprio, L. A. (1979). Primary health care in Europe. EURO Reports and Studies No. 14. WHO Regional Office for Europe, Copenhagen.
World Health Organization (1978). Report of the International Conference on Primary Health Care, Alma Ata. Geneva.
—— (1981). *Global strategy for health for all by the year 2000.* Geneva.

Part II

Practising prevention

9 Smoking

Godfrey Fowler

SMOKING AND DISEASE

Introduction

That smoking is a major cause of morbidity and mortality is now beyond dispute. It is without doubt the most important preventable cause of premature death in developed countries. WHO in 1975 declared that 'control of cigarette smoking could do more than any other single action in the field of preventive medicine' and again in 1979 that 'the smoking problem is now a world wide epidemic', and the Report of the Royal College of Physicians 'Smoking or Health' in 1979 estimated that 10 per cent of all deaths were caused by smoking including 25 000 deaths a year in Britain under the age of 65 years.

Mortality of smokers is about twice that of non-smokers and a man under the age of 25 years smoking 20 cigarettes daily shortens his life, on average, by 10 years. At least 55 000 excess deaths a year, more than 1000 each week, are attributable to smoking and mortality from more than 20 diseases is higher in smokers than in non-smokers.

Many studies over the last quarter of a century have demonstrated the relationship between smoking and disease (Hammond 1964; Hirayama 1972; Doll and Peto 1976), the diseases most commonly associated with cigarette smoking being lung cancer, bronchitis and emphysema, ischaemic heart disease, and peripheral arterial disease. In Britain smoking accounts for 90 per cent of lung cancer deaths, 75 per cent of deaths from chronic bronchitis, and 25 per cent of ischaemic heart disease deaths in men under the age of 65 years (Royal College of Physicians 1971). It is also an important cause of morbidity and consequent sick absence (Ashford 1973).

Lung cancer

Lung cancer accounted for nearly 40 000 deaths in the United Kingdom in 1974, more than three-quarters of them in men, and although the death rate from lung cancer in men is now falling, that in women continues to rise. The causal relationship between cigarette smoking and lung cancer is now proven beyond all reasonable doubt. The British Doctors Study (Doll and Peto 1976) demonstrated that those who smoked 25 or more cigarettes daily had more than a 20 times greater chance of dying from lung cancer than non-smokers. There is evidence that this risk is related to the age of starting smoking, the number of cigarettes smoked and to smoking habits, such as frequency of puffs, inhalation, holding the cigarette in the mouth between puffs, etc. The risk is reduced by smoking filter cigarettes and smokers of pipes and cigars suffer much less risk than cigarette smokers, probably because they inhale less. Reduction in tar content of cigarettes has also lessened the risk (Hammond 1977).

As demonstrated by the British Doctors Study, stopping smoking diminishes the risk (as illustrated in Fig. 9.1) so that after about 10 years it reverts almost to that of the life-long non-smoker. The substantial fall in mortality from lung cancer in doctors reflects the drop over the last 30 years in the proportion of doctors who smoke from over 50 per cent to only about 20 per cent at the present time.

Coronary heart disease

Coronary heart disease is the commonest cause of death in developed countries. In Britain about 150 000 people die each year from this cause, a quarter or so of them before the age of 65. As with lung cancer, there is experimental, clinical, and epidemiological evidence that smoking causes ischaemic heart disease. The British Doctors Study quoted above demonstrated that the mortality rate for smokers was about twice that of non-smokers. The association between death

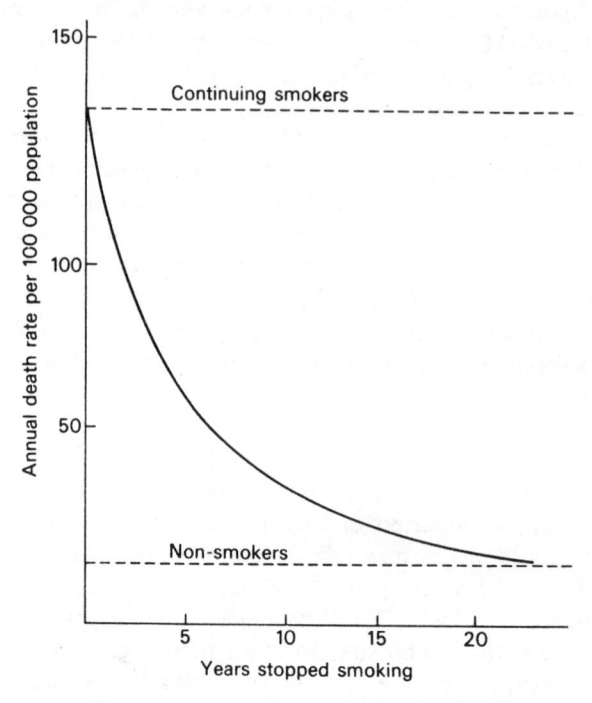

Fig. 9.1. Standardized death rate from lung cancer for cigarette smokers, ex-smokers for various periods, and non-smokers. (From Doll and Hill (1964).)

from heart disease and smoking, though apparently weak, is nevertheless particularly important because coronary heart disease is much more common than lung cancer and therefore the number of coronary heart deaths attributable to smoking is greater than the number of lung cancer deaths attributable to this cause. Moreover, this apparently modest effect of smoking in relation to coronary heart disease conceals a disproportionately greater risk in the younger age group. Those under 45 years smoking 25 or more cigarettes daily have about a 15 times greater risk than non-smokers of dying from coronary heart disease, and, as with lung cancer, the risk depends on the amount smoked.

Stopping smoking results in a rapid reduction in this rsik by about 50 per cent in the first year and then gradually almost to that of the non-smoker by about 10 years. Even *after* a myocardial infarction the risk of a non-fatal recurrence is substantially reduced by stopping smoking (Wilhelmsson et al. 1975). Smoking seems to be particularly important in causing sudden death in men under the age of 50 years.

Coronary heart disease is less common in women than men but mortality from this cause in women is increasing. Smoking greatly increases the risk of coronary heart disease associated with taking the combined oral contraceptive pill and women on the pill who smoke 35 or more cigarettes daily have a 20-fold greater risk of myocardial infarction than those who have never smoked (Mann et al. 1975).

Apart from smoking, the other major risk factors associated with coronary heart disease are raised blood lipids, elevated blood pressure, and diabetes (there are others, but these are the most important ones) and because the risks are multiplicative smoking is particularly hazardous for individuals with these problems and particularly if there is a family history of coronary heart disease (see Chapter 5).

The mechanisms whereby smoking causes ischaematic heart disease and peripheral arterial disease, where the relationship is particularly strong, are uncertain. Increased coronary atheroma has been demonstrated in smokers and there is also evidence of increases in platelet stickiness, of increased concentration of fibrinogen and other coagulation factors and of an increased tendency to arrhythmias in response to catecholamines. Many sudden heart deaths are probably due to arrhythmias, post mortems on such patients demonstrating severe atheroma but no actual arterial occlusion.

Cigarette smoke has been shown to contain some 4000 chemicals of which the most significant appear to be tar products, nicotine, and carbon monoxide. It seems likely that carbon monoxide (which has an affinity for haemoglobin 245 times that of oxygen) may be important here. Reduction of oxygen delivery to the myocardium may result, not only from the formation of carboxyhaemoglobin but also from interference with cell metabolism. Damage to vessel walls may also promote atherosclerosis. Blood carboxyhaemoglobin concentrations have been shown to be a predictor of risk of arterial disease (Wald et al. 1973). Although low-tar cigareetes have been shown to be less damaging to the lungs than high tar ones (so that their introduction has contributed to the decline in lung cancer in men, particularly young adults) neither this change nor the switch from plain to filter cigarettes may have been beneficial in all respects. It is known that filter cigarettes yield more carbon monoxide than plain ones, and if carbon monoxide is a factor in the genesis of cardiovascular disease, this change could be important (Wald *et al.* 1977). There is certainly no evidence that filters reduce the risk of coronary heart disease and even some suggestion that they may be worse in this respect than plain cigarettes (Castelli *et al.* 1981).

Bronchitis and emphysema

Bronchitis and emphysema account for roughly 30 000 deaths a year. They are also very significant causes of morbidity and sick absence, together accounting for 30 million lost working days annually. In the British Doctors Study the certified death rate from chronic obstructive lung disease amongst smokers was 10 times that of non-smokers and mortality from this condition amongst heavy smokers was 46 times that of non-smokers.

Although much of the lung damage caused by smoking is irreversible, benefits nevertheless accrue from stopping. While lung function does not improve, the rate of deterioration of lung function with age reverts to that of the never smoker, rather than following the more rapid decline of the continuing smoker.

Womens' health

Women appear to be just as susceptible to smoking related diseases as men, but as a group have the advantage of having deferred the acquisition of the smoking habit a decade or two, and this delayed increases in the related diseases in women. However, smoking poses peculiar hazards for women.

Smoking during pregnancy causes retarded fetal growth so that babies born to mothers who smoke weigh on average 200 g (half a pound) less than those born to non-smokers. Almost twice as many smokers as non-smokers give birth to 'premature' babies (weighing less than 2500 g) (Butler *et al.* 1972). The mechanism of this growth retardation in babies in unclear but possible explanations are the direct toxic effects of noxious tobacco smoke constituents and the impairment of placental blood flow. Giving up smoking in early pregnancy reduces the risk to those of the non-smoker. The risk of perinatal death is increased by about one-third in the babies of mothers who smoke compared with those of non-smoking mothers, and spontaneous abortion appears to be about twice as common in smokers as non-smokers. There are therefore many reasons for the avoidance of smoking during pregnancy.

The particular hazards of women on the oral contraceptive pill smoking cigarettes have been discussed above. These hazards are particularly significant in women over the age of 30 who should be strongly discouraged from smoking if they wish to continue oral contraception.

Children's health

The harmful effects of maternal smoking referred to above continue, and children of mothers who smoke during pregnancy have been shown to be smaller and less intelligent than those of non-smokers. Moreover, the risk of the infant developing a chest infection in the first year of life is doubled if parents smoke (Colley et al. 1974).

Children of parents who smoke are more likely to smoke themselves and surveys have shown that about a quarter of boys and almost as many girls smoke regularly by the age of 15 and that a third of regular smokers started smoking before the age of nine.

Smoking in children causes persistent and often productive coughing, increased chest infections and reduced ventilatory capacity (Backhouse 1975).

To summarize the ill-effects of smoking on health:

– Smoking causes many diseases, notably lung cancer, chronic bronchitis and emphysema, coronary heart disease, and peripheral arterial disease.

– Additionally, in pregnant women it has harmful effects on the fetus.

– Children are harmed by parental smoking – directly and by encouragement to smoke themselves.

– Passive inhalation of tobacco smoke by non-smokers is harmful to them.

– The risk of harmful effects from smoking is reduced by stopping smoking and the benefit occurs remarkably quickly in the case of coronary heart disease.

– The switch from plain to filter cigarettes has reduced the lung cancer risk but not the coronary heart disease risk (which it may even have increased).

CHANGES IN SMOKING

Prevalence

There have been big changes in the smoking pattern of the community over the last 30 years and particularly during the last decade. In the early 1950s almost two-thirds of men (and two-fifths of women) were regular cigarette smokers. Until recently the proportion of women smokers remained virtually unchanged, while that of men fell substantially, so that the gap between the two has narrowed from about 25 per cent to 5 per cent. This is illustrated in Fig. 9.2.

The latest available figures (General Household Survey 1980) indicate a smoking prevalence in British males of 42 per cent and in females of 37 per cent. In men the fall in prevalence is roughly the same for all age groups and the proportion of ex-smokers and never smokers, especially the former, has risen substantially. In women the recent fall in prevalence is largely confined to the young and middle age groups, with some increase in ex-smokers but no change in never smokers.

But with the decline in the proportion of smokers there has been a substantial increase in the consumption of those who do smoke by roughly 50 per cent in men and more than 100 per cent in women, so that until 1973 there was also a

138 *Smoking*

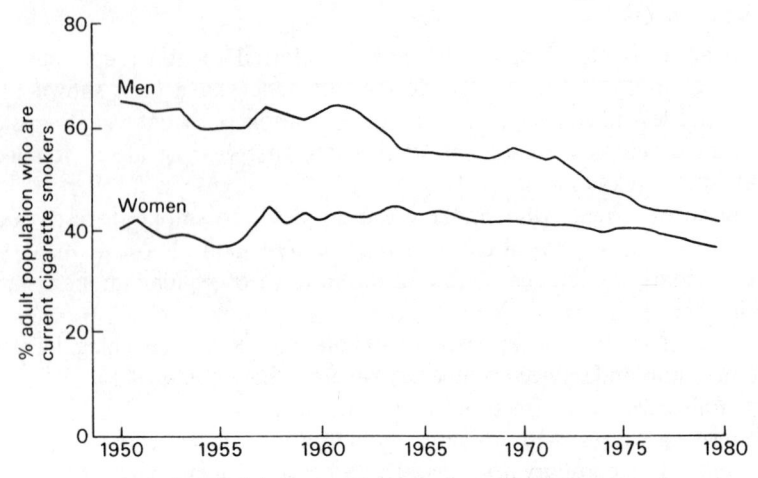

Fig. 9.2. Trends in prevalence in the United Kingdom.

steady increase in the number of cigarettes sold, though because of the big switch from plain to filter cigarettes from the early 1960s there was a fall in tobacco consumption. Since 1973 there has been a fall every year in the number of cigarettes sold, with a particularly dramatic fall in 1981. Over 90 per cent of cigarettes now sold are of the filter variety and there has been a substantial reduction in the tar yield of both plain and filter cigarettes. But while this has important implications for the carcinogenetic aspects of smoking, it is doubtful whether these changes reduce the other noxious effects of smoking, particularly the cardiovascular ones.

Social class

This decline in smoking is largely accounted for by changes in the socio-economic group prevalence of this activity. In 1960 smoking in men (about two-thirds of whom smoked) was more or less equally common in all social classes. By 1972 the proportion of social class V smoking was almost double that of social class I and now it is almost treble. As Fig. 9.3 indicates, a steepening social class gradient has opened up.

As the figure indicates, although there has been some fall in smoking in all groups except women in social class V, this has been particularly impressive in professional males. Translation of this behavioural change to other social groups is the most important challenge for health education and preventive medicine.

Children and smoking

Surveys of children show that the percentage of boys who smoke at least one cigarette a week rises from 4 per cent at the age of 11 to 34 per cent at 15 years.

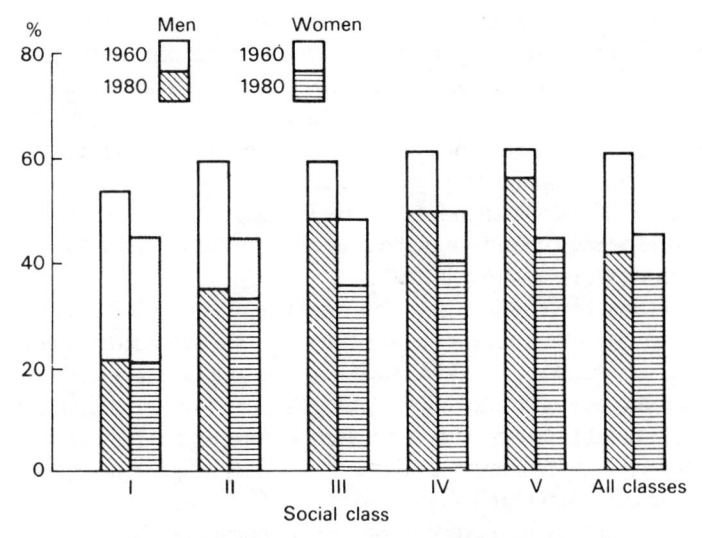

Fig. 9.3. Changes in prevalence with social class.

Figures for girls are about two-thirds those for boys. Of adults who are regular smokers, about one in three started smoking before the age of nine and 80 per cent of children who smoke regularly persist in the habit in adulthood.

Smoking in children occurs as the result of peer-group pressure, but its onset is also influenced by a number of social factors. It is commoner in social classes IV and V, than social classes I and II, and in children of parents who smoke. It is also commoner in schools where teachers smoke.

The reasons why children start smoking include the mimicry of adults, peer-group pressure, the excitement of taking risks, and association of smoking with maturity, sexual attractiveness, and sophistication. Counter-pressures to stop may come from the desire to achieve relationships and improve athletic performance, rather than concern about health. Advice to young people about avoidance of smoking needs to take account of these reasons. Appeals to the young to safeguard their future health will be relatively unrewarding. A more positive approach pointing out current rather than future benefits is likely to be more frutiful.

Passive smoking

Until recently the harmful effects of an individual's smoking was regarded as confined to the individual smoker. But there is now accumulating evidence that passive or involuntary inhalation of tobacco smoke by the non-smoker has harmful effects too. 'Sidestream' smoke (that from the end of a cigarette) is known to contain a much higher concentration of noxious substances including carbon monoxide, nicotine, and nitrosamines (known carcinogens) than does 'mainstream' smoke, i.e. that inhaled by the smoker. It has been shown that non-smokers in a smokey room inhale as much benzpyrene (a tar product) in one hour as they would by smoking four cigarettes. It has also been shown that non-smokers who breath air polluted with tobacco smoke may suffer lung damage. In one recent study non-smokers who had worked alongside smokers for many years had poorer lung function compared with non-smokers without such exposure. Those who had involuntary inhaled tobacco smoke for 20 years had the same degree of damage as those smoking up to 10 cigarettes a day for a similar period (White and Froeb 1980).

It has further been shown that non-smoking women whose husbands are longstanding cigarette smokers die, on average, four years earlier than women married to non-smokers, and that such wives have a higher incidence of lung cancer than those of non-smoking husbands (the risk was about doubled). Over all passive smoking carries with it between a third and a half of the risk of active smoking and involuntary smoking is probably a significant cause of lung cancer in the non-smoker (Hirayama 1981).

These observations have very important implications. No longer can the smoker argue that his smoking harms only himself and that he therefore has the right to pursue his dangerous habit. It is now clear that in doing so he is also harming others than himself. Non-smokers will become increasingly vehement about their right to breath air unpolluted by tobacco smoke.

STOPPING SMOKING

Do smokers want to stop?

Surveys show that the majority of smokers, at least 70 per cent, want to stop smoking. Eighty per cent claim they would stop if advised to do so by their doctors, but only 10 per cent say they have ever been advised to do so. Substantial numbers have succeeded in stopping smoking and already there are at least eight million ex-smokers in Britain (General Household Survey 1976) and it is estimated that there are some 35 million ex-smokers in the USA.

As pointed out above, there have been notable changes in the sex and social class distribution of smoking, the proportion of male smokers having fallen by about one-third while that of women smokers has remained relatively unchanged.

Particularly impressive has been the change in smoking habits of doctors. A survey in 1974 showed that only 21 per cent of general practitioners were current, regular cigarette smokers, and 42 per cent were ex-smokers. This means that two out of three GPs who did smoke have given up. By contrast 48 per cent of nurses were regular smokers and only 12 per cent had given up (Smoking and Professional People 1976).

The fact that large numbers of doctors have succeeded in stopping smoking indicates the potential for people to change their smoking behaviour. What are the factors which have contributed to this behaviour change in such large numbers of doctors? Foremost must surely be awareness of the hazards of cigarette smoking based on knowledge and understanding of the available evidence. The necessary motivation and willpower which are such vital ingredients of behaviour change have followed from this.

There are now increasingly favourable influences. Changing social attitudes towards smoking, restrictions on smoking in public places, and the increasing cost of cigarettes are now also influencing the situation. The media are giving increasing attention to the smoking issue and there are signs of increasing public response. In 1975 half a million people responded to a television programme offering a Quit Smoking Kit, the Health Education Council has been faced with increasing demands for anti-smoking literature, and a recently published small book on smoking achieved 200 000 sales within three months.

How to stop

As has been indicated, large numbers of people have succeeded in stopping smoking. The great majority have done so without any assistance, but do doctors or any other agencies have anything to contribute in helping people to stop smoking? Many approaches have been tried to help people to give up smoking. These include such techniques as individual counselling, group therapy, hypnosis, acupucture, electro-aversive therapy, rapid smoking techniques, and the use of drugs. Amongst these a nicotine substitute in the form of nicotine chewing gum is currently enjoying a new vogue.

The settings for such activities range from routine general practice consultations to special clinics, but whatever the situation or technique the most vital components are the motivation and determination of the individual concerned. But the continuing support of the therapist may also be vital as short-term success rates are often high but the considerable relapse rate means that long-term successes, which are generally regarded as abstinence for a year or more, are more modest.

The potential for the general practitioner to help patients stop smoking is relatively unexplored. There are now more than 26 000 general practitioners, almost 80 per cent of whom are themselves non-smokers, and many of whom are ex-smokers. Collectively they comprise a valuable resource and surveys show that 80 per cent of them feel a responsibility for discouraging people from smoking and 90 per cent believe they could play an important part in anti-smoking education. Bearing in mind that each general practitioner has on his list, on average, some seven or eight hundred patients who smoke – two-thirds of whom consult him at least once a year – the scope for action is considerable. This is particularly so as he has access to those socio-economic groups which include most smokers and who are unlikely to seek help elsewhere. Special smoking withdrawal clinics, on the other hand, are only available in small numbers and necessarily recruit on the basis of motivation. General practice must surely be more relevant for the less educated, lower socio-economic group

142 Smoking

in the population which includes the huge majority of cigarette smokers and face-to-face contact at a time of ill health should provide a major opportunity to influence smoking behaviour.

There have been few studies of attempts by GPs to help patients to stop smoking. In one randomized study, firm advice and an anti-smoking leaflet were given on the occasion of a routine general practice consultation. On six-month follow-up 5 per cent of smokers had given up in both the counselled and the control groups, but the numbers in this study were very small Porter and McCullough 1972). In another general practice study, this time uncontrolled, a 23 per cent success rate was reported on follow-up at one year (Handel 1973). Higher rates have been reported in special screening clinics.

However, a recent study (Russell *et al.* 1979) seems to have demonstrated clearly that simple, firm advice by the general practitioner, given during the course of a normal consultation, and backed up with a leaflet and warning of follow-up, does help patients to stop smoking. In this study 5 per cent of those given such help when compared with a control group who were not, had stopped smoking within a month and were still not smoking when followed up one year later. These may be regarded as long-term successes. The results of this study are illustrated in Fig. 9.4.

This study showed that the effect of such advice was quite specifically on motivation and intention to stop, the proportion of patients who tried to stop being increased, while on the other hand the success rate of those who did try was not increased.

As Russell pointed out, a general practitioner adopting this routine could expect about 25 long-term successes each year and if all GPs did this, about half a million people a year would stop smoking as a result of their general practitioners' help.

So what are the essential features of such advice?

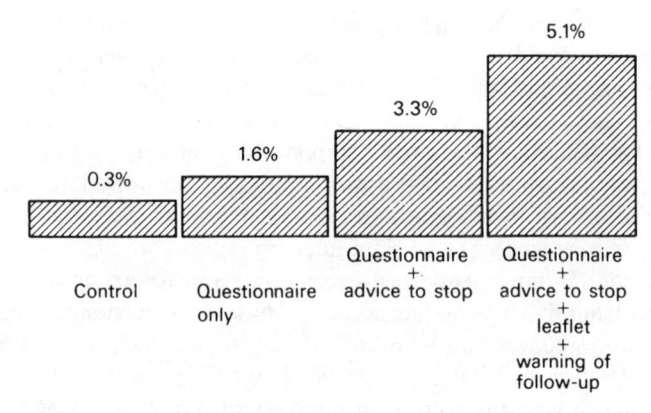

Fig. 9.4. Effect of general practitioners' advice against smoking.

General practitioners' role

Individuals must be made aware of the health hazards of smoking as studies show that smokers seem to be less aware of the health consequences of smoking than non-smokers, or at least to deny such awareness. In one study, two-thirds of non-smokers thought that lung cancer was related to cigarette smoking, but only one-third of smokers thought so, while only about one-third of both smokers and non-smokers thought heart attacks were associated with smoking (Ashton 1979). There is public ignorance of the relationship between smoking and heart disease and the evidence from the Doctors' Study of the 15-fold increase in coronary heart disease mortality amongst heavy smokers under 50 needs wider publicity.

There is also a lack of public awareness of the size of the health risk from smoking and of how this risk compares with other risks. It has, for example, been pointed out (Peto 1980) that about a quarter of all young men who smoke 20 or more cigarettes a day (and who continue to smoke) will die before their time from smoking. This means that of 1000 such young men 250 will be killed by smoking, compared with the six who will be killed at some time on the roads.

But more attention must be paid to the benefits of stopping smoking rather than the harm of continuing to smoke and there may have been undue emphasis on the negative aspects of being a smoker rather than the positive features of being a non-smoker. One obvious benefit is the financial one and the non-smoker now has £5 to £10 more to spend on something else every week than the smoker. Others include better ability to taste and smell, better breathing capacity, and, in many situations, greater social acceptability. The benefits on personal characteristics and athletic performance of being a non-smoker may carry particular weight with young people.

Motivation and willpower are the key to successful smoking cessation and will be influenced by many factors. Health will be one consideration and should be an important one. Concern for health will be determined by the individual's health beliefs which will include his perception of personal vulnerability, how seriously he regards the health consequences of smoking, what benefits of stopping are, and the price to be paid in terms of suffering (see Chapter 4).

People smoke for different reasons, some to relieve tension, some to be sociable, others because it is pleasurable, but many because of dependence on the habit. Three-quarters of those who smoke either want to stop or have tried to but have failed.

Although many people succeed in stopping smoking without any help from doctors and without any special preparation or planning, others do need help and the doctor should be willing to offer this. He should not only be concerned with advising and motivating patients to stop smoking, but helping them to so so. Success depends on all members of the primary care team adopting a committed and informed approach. The health visitor, because of her particular educational role, will be an important ally. Health personnel should not smoke and all should be concerned in advice about smoking. This advice should be offered not only when requested but also whenever opportunity presents in any consultation, especially if it can be related to the presenting medical problem. Printed material such as leaflets is of supplementary value in reinforcing advice, informing the patient and saving the doctor's time, but it does not replace personal advice. Follow-up is necessary to encourage and support abstention from smoking and to advise on coping with the adverse effects of stopping such as irritability and a temporary weight gain.

Advice

There is no single strategy for success, no panacea, and this should be emphasized to the patient. But this must not be taken to mean that no methods are successful and the individual should be helped to plan a personal strategy.

A target date should be set some way ahead, preferably at a relatively stress-free time, such as holiday, or at a time of a change of routine. In the interim motivation may be enhanced by reviewing the reasons for stopping, telling other people about it, and even recruiting a fellow-smoker to join in in giving up. Switching to another brand, recording all cigarettes smoked in one day and when, where and why they were smoked, changing routine, avoiding tea or coffee, and looking for alternatives to smoking, may all be found helpful in preparing to quit.

Generally speaking, sudden, complete withdrawal is more likely to succeed than gradual cutting down in the number of cigarettes smoked, but with some heavy smokers a period of cutting down may be the most effective technique. Conversely some light or moderate smokers may be helped to stop by the so-called 'saturation method' in which cessation is preceded by one or two days smoking two or three times the normal number of cigarettes.

Advice on coping with difficulties after quitting may include having something to nibble, suck, or chew – fruit, nuts, or gum – occupying the hands with a pebble or rubber bands, and learning to relax without a cigarette. Danger times like tea-breaks, after meals, or when having a drink may need careful handling. Avoidance of others who smoke and of smoking environments at these times may be particularly crucial and the co-operation and support of friends and colleagues is vital. Mutual support of spouse is particularly important.

Tension and irritability may cause particular problems and preparation for quitting may well include learning techniques to cope with these. Relaxation exercises, taking deep breaths, and yoga may all be found to be helpful in this respect, but regular physical exercise may be preferable to some.

Advice may be usefully supplemented and reinforced with a leaflet such as the GUS pamphlet (ASH/HEC) and use of such literature has been shown to increase the effectiveness of advice. Follow-up is important to offer continuing help and support as well as advice on managing difficulties. Nicotine chewing gum has recently become available on prescription but not on the NHS, and its usefulness is still being evaluated. There are two ways in which it could help: by providing a substitute oral activity and by relief of withdrawal symptoms due to nicotine dependence. Nicotine is slowly released as the gum is chewed and is absorbed through the buccal mucosa. Use of the gum has been shown to produce blood nicotine levels similar to those occurring during cigarette smoking, but such levels are attained more slowly than by smoking. Careful attention needs to be paid to instructions on the use of the gum.

Although early studies have suggested it may be more effective than other methods in helping people to stop smoking (Raw *et al.* 1980) its usefulness in the general practice setting remains uncertain. Most of the studies to date have been conducted on highly selected smokers attending clinics and have included a substantial group therapy component. No satisfactory trial has yet been conducted in general practice.

In summary, the role of the GP in relation to smoking is to
 – offer advice when requested;
 – seek opportunity to offer advice in any consultation;
 – advise on how to stop;
 – supplement advice with appropriate literature;
 – follow up attempts to stop;
 – offer nicotine chewing gum to those who fail with advice.

The advice offered should include
 – reference to presenting medical problems when possible;
 – information about the health hazards of smoking;
 – emphasis on the benefits of stopping;
 – a reminder that there is no panacea;
 – a plan to include a target date for stopping;
 – ways to prepare for stopping;
 – ways to cope with difficulties after stopping;
 – a warning of the dangers of relapse;
 – explanation of the need for follow-up.

THE POLITICS OF SMOKING

Political, social, and environmental factors profoundly influence attitudes towards smoking and therefore impede or facilitate efforts to stop. This has been particularly true over the last decade with an accelerating shift towards regarding non-smoking rather than smoking as normal behaviour.

Legislation

Recent evidence of the harmfulness of passive smoking has enhanced this change in attitude. The majority of people are, after all, non-smokers and claim the right to breathe air uncontaminated by tobacco smoke – particularly if such smoke may be harmful to them. Public opinion surveys have shown the majority of people support the restriction of smoking in public places and such restrictions are steadily increasing.

Moreover, there are also increasingly strident demands from the medical profession and the public for the abolition of all forms of tobacco advertising. A recent public opinion survey showed that 63 per cent of people were in favour of a total ban. The present voluntary agreement with the tobacco industry in Britain banned advertising on radio and television, limits poster advertising and cinema advertising, requires the printing of health warnings on cigarette packets, and limits cigarette tar yields. However, the irony of allowing promotion by advertisement of a product carrying an obligatory health warning, and which kills at least 1000 people every week, seems likely to be shortlived.

Many countries have banned all forms of tobacco advertisement. Amongst these is Norway, which introduced a Tobacco Act in 1975. This banned all forms of advertising of tobacco, including indirect advertisement, prohibited the sale or giving of cigarettes to those under 16 years, required cigarette packets to carry explicit warnings on the dangers of smoking, and controlled cigarette manufacture. There was much public support for this legislation and a public opinion survey indicated 81 per cent approval of the law. Since the Act the proportion of Norwegian men smoking has dropped from 52 per cent to 43 per cent, while that of young males aged 16 to 24 has fallen from 49 per cent to 33 per cent. There has also been a reduction in the proportion of children who smoke. (Bjartveit 1981).

Taxation of tobacco is an important source of revenue, currently about £4000M in Britain. This, together with the fact that cigarette manufacture is a powerful industry employing almost 50 000 British people, makes smoking an important political issue. Legislation which is likely to reduce revenue and damage the industry is therefore strongly resisted. However, the influence of this levy on the smoking pattern was well illustrated by the rapid increase in the market share of low-tar cigarettes following the imposition in 1974 of an additional tax on those with higher tar yields, and again in 1981 when a 14 per cent increase in duty led to a 10 per cent drop in cigarette sales.

As Sir George Young, Under-Secretary of State at the DHSS, in a speech at the Fourth World Conference on Smoking and Health stated:

> The general proposition that I wish to put to you is that the solution to many of today's medical problems will not be found in the research laboratories of our hospitals, but in our Parliaments. For the prospective patient, the answer may not be cure by incision at the operating table, but prevention by decision at the Cabinet table. If you look at most of the big killer diseases of today they are not caused by nature but by our way of life. I am thinking in particular of cancer, heart attacks, stroke and road accidents. For these illnesses medicine has at best cures which are expensive and partially successful or at worst no cures at all. The answer to these illnesses is not cure but prevention.
>
> My starting point is the assertion that smoking can kill and maim and the ball is in the politician's court. My top priority is to draw up a coherent long-term strategy which has as its own objective the reduction and eventually the elimination of disease caused by

smoking. In developing and implementing this long-term strategy a government must use all weapons at its disposal – price, control over advertising, health education and persuasion.

But the job cannot be left solely for politicians. Doctors and general practitioners especially have an important part to play too, and the success of doctors themselves in giving up smoking is an important asset in this. As the cigarette advertisement warning reminds us: 'think first – most doctors do not smoke'.

REFERENCES

Ashford, J. R. (1973). Illness, sick absence and use of medical services by smokers. *Br. J. prevent. social Med.* **27**, 8.

Ashton, W. D. (1979). Cigarette smoking and associated disease. *J. R. Coll. Gen. Practrs* **29**, 229.

Backhouse, C. I., (1975). Peak expiratory flow in youths with varying cigarette smoking habits. *Br. med. J.* **i**, 360.

Bjartveit, K. (1981). Paper presented at Tenth Anniversary of Action on Smoking and Health, Norwegian Governmental programme on smoking and health (Royal College of Physicians, London, March 1981).

Butler, N. R., Goldstein, H., and Ross, E. M. (1972). Cigarette smoking in pregnancy: its influence on weight and perinatal mortality. *Br. med. J.* **ii**, 127.

Capell, P. J. (1978). Trends in cigarette smoking in the United Kingdom. *Hlth Trends* **10**, 49.

Castelli, W. P., Dawber, T. R., Feinleib, M., Garnson, R. J., McNamara, P. M., and Kannel, W. B. (1981). The filter cigarette and coronary heart disease: the Framingham study. *Lancet* **ii**, 109.

Colley, J. R. T., Holland, W. W., and Corkhill, R. T. (1974). Influence of passive smoking and parental phlegm on pneumonia and bronchitis in early childhood. *Lancet* **ii**, 103.

Doll, R. and Hill, A. B. (1964). Mortality in relation to smoking: ten years' observations of British doctors. *Br. med. J.* **i**, 1399.

—— and Peto, R. (1976). Mortality in relation to smoking: twenty years' observations on male British doctors. *Br. med. J.* **ii**, 1525.

Fletcher, C., Peto, R., Tinker, C., and Speizer, F. E. (1976). *The natural history of chronic bronchitis and emphysema.* Oxford University Press.

General Household Surveys (1978) and (1981), Office of Population Censuses and Surveys. HMSO, London.

Hammond, E. C. (1964). Smoking in relation to mortality and morbidity. *J. Natn Cancer Inst.* **32**, 1161.

——, Garfinkel, L., and Leidman, H. (1977). Some recent findings concerning cigarette Smoking. *Incidence of cancer in humans* (ed. H. H. Hiatt, J. D. Watson, and J. A. Winston). Cold Spring Harbor Laboratory, New York.

Handel, S. (1973). Change in smoking habits in general practice. *Postrad. med. J.* **49**, 679.

Hirayama, T. (1972). Smoking in relation to death rates of a quarter of a million men and women in Japan. Report of Five years follow-up. American Cancer Society's 14th National Science Writers' Seminar.

—— (1981). Non-smoking wives of heavy smokers have a higher risk of lung cancer: a study from Japan. *Br. med. J.* **i**, 183.

Mann, J. I., Vessey, M. P., Thorogood, M., and Doll, R. (1975). Myocardial infarction in young women with special reference to oral contraceptive practice. *Br. med. J.* **ii**, 241.

Peto, R. (1980). *Hlth Education J.* **39**, 45.

Porter, A. M. W. and McCullough, D. M. (1972). Counselling against cigarette smoking: a controlled study from general practice *Practitioner* **209**, 686.

Raw, M., Jarvis, M. J., Feyerabad, C., and Russell, M. A. H. (1980). Comparison of nicotine chewing gum and psychological treatments for dependent smokers. *Br. med. J.* **iii**, 481.

Royal College of Physicians of London (1971). *Smoking and health now a new report and summary on smoking and its effects on health.* Pitman, London.

—— (1977). *Smoking or health: the third report from the Royal College of Physicians, London.* Pitman, London.

Russell, M. A. H., Wilson, C., Taylor, C., and Baker, C. D. (1979). Effect of general practitioners' advice against smoking. *Br. med. J.* **ii**, 231.

Smoking and professional people (1976). DHSS, London.

Social Trends (1979) and (1980). HMSO, London.

Wald, N. J., Howard, S., Smith, P. G., and Kjeldsen, K. (1973). Association between atherosclerotic diseases and carboxyhaemoglobin levels in tobacco smokers. *Br. med. J.* **i**, 761.

——, Idle, M., Smith, P. G., and Bailey, A. (1977). Carboxyhaemoglobin levels in smokers of filter and plain cigarettes. *Lancet* **i**, 110.

World Health Organization (1975). *Technical Report Series* No. 568. WHO, Geneva.

White, J. R. and Froeb, H. F. (1980) Small airways dysfunction in non-smokers chronically exposed to tobacco smoke. *New Engl. J. Med.* **302**, 720.

Wilhelmssen, C., Elmfeldt, D., Vedin, J. A., Tibbling, G., and Wilhelmsen L. (1975). Smoking and myocardial infarction. *Lancet* **i**, 415.

10 Is there a case for dietary change?

Jim Mann and Sue Lousley

INTRODUCTION

A wide range of diseases, which are common in affluent societies and occur rarely in developing countries, has been ascribed in part to aspects of the Western diet. Ischaemic heart disease, diabetes, gall-stones, constipation (and irritable bowel syndrome), diverticular disease of the colon, cancer of the large bowel, dental caries, appendicitis, haemorrhoids, varicose veins, and obesity are probably the most important of these conditions. The features of the Western diet which have been incriminated are an excessive quantity of total and saturated fat (or perhaps a deficiency of certain polyunsaturated fatty acids), excessive amounts of sucrose and other refined carbohydrate, a deficiency of dietary fibre and energy intake in excess of requirements.

I shall summarize the evidence in favour of regarding these conditions as manifestations of malnutrition in affluent societies and consider the arguments for and against recommending dietary change. Of course, specific syndromes associated with nutritional deficiencies do also occur in affluent societies (e.g. rickets in immigrant and underprivileged children, iron deficiency anaemia) but these will not be considered here.

ISCHAEMIC HEART DISEASE

The suggestion that certain dietary practices may be associated with an increased risk of ischaemic heart disease (IHD) is based principally upon epidemiological and animal studies (Mann and Marmot 1983). The epidemiological data are based on the following types of studies:

(i) between-country correlations of IHD rates and food intake;

(ii) prospective observation of subjects for whom individual diet histories are available;

(iii) associations between diet (and changes in diet) and various measures of lipid metabolism known to be associated with IHD.

Between-country correlations of IHD rates and food intake

Most attempts to study dietary determinants of IHD rates have been based on balance sheets of the Food and Agriculture Organization (or, in the United Kingdom, more reliably on household food surveys), and national mortality statistics before 1970 during which time IHD was increasing (at least in men) in most affluent societies. Positive associations with saturated fat, sucrose, animal protein, and coffee and negative correlations with flour (and other complex carbohydrates) and vegetables are some of the best described. However, population food consumption data are notoriously unreliable (they are usually derived from local production figures, imports and exports, with no account of quantities not utilized as food) and the accuracy with which mortality is recorded varies from country to country. Consequently, such data do not provide direct evidence concerning aetiology, only clues for further research. Perhaps more interesting are recent studies from the United States of America, the United Kingdom and Australia which have examined the downward trend of IHD rates in relation to dietary change. There is certainly some association between the falling IHD rates apparent (particularly in males) in these countries and changes in some nutrients, but in view of the strong correlations (positive and negative) among different dietary constituents it is difficult to be sure which dietary factor is principally involved or indeed whether dietary change is simply occurring in parallel with some other more important environmental factor (e.g. increasing physical activity or a reduction in cigarette smoking).

Actual food consumption by people in 16 defined cohorts (in seven countries) and ten-year incidence rates of IHD deaths form the rather more reliable basis for the correlations tested by Keys and co-workers. A strong positive correlation was noted between mean (for each cohort) saturated fat intake and fatal IHD incidence ($r=0.84$). A weaker association was found with dietary sucrose and a later analysis of the data suggested also a positive relationship with intake of polyunsaturated fat. Protein intake appeared to have no effect on IHD incidence and no data were available concerning dietary fibre.

Prospective observation of subjects for whom diet histories are available

In the seven-countries study and several other studies it has not usually been possible to show a relationship between an individual's dietary intake and his subsequent risk of IHD. However, such an association has now been demonstrated in two studies: in one, bank staff, bus drivers, and bus conductors in London completed at least one seven-day weighed dietary record and men with a high intake of dietary fibre from cereals had a lower rate of IHD subsequently than the rest. A high energy intake (apparently reflecting physical activity) and to a lesser extent the presence of a high ratio of polyunsaturated to saturated fatty acids in the diet were also features of men who subsequently remained free of IHD. In another prospective investigation of employees of the Western Electric Company in Chicago, the most striking finding was an inverse association between IHD mortality and consumption of polyunsaturated fat. A positive association was also noted between IHD mortality and dietary cholesterol and with the Keys and Hegsted 'scores' (combined measures of the amount of saturated fat, polyunsaturated fat, and cholesterol in the diet). No association was found between IHD and saturated fat intake considered in isolation. In this study, as in the London study, dietary assessment was very carefully carried out and failure to find similar associations in other prospective studies could be due to insensitivity of their dietary survey techniques.

Diet and lipids

Several measures of lipid metabolism have been associated with an increased risk of IHD. Of these, only total cholesterol has been convincingly shown to be associated with diet. For example, in the study of Keys *et al.* mean concentration of cholesterol in the blood was highly correlated ($r=0.87$) with percentage of total calories from saturated fat. In the Western Electric Study changes from one year to the next in dietary intake of saturated fatty acids and cholesterol were related to changes in serum cholesterol. In the typical Western diet about 40 per cent of energy is provided by fat. A substantial cholesterol reduction is achieved when this is reduced to 30 per cent and the ratio of polyunsaturated to saturated fatty acids increases from 0.2 to 0.8.

The nomadic people of Somalia, Kenya, and Tanzania, whose diets consist mainly of meat, milk, and blood have always aroused particular interest since, despite this diet, they have usually maintained low blood cholesterol levels. It has, however, recently been pointed out that their diet is not in fact habitually high in saturated fat, but that intake is subject to much irregularity in food supply on a seasonal basis. There are other apparently conflicting results, but Epstein has pointed out that these seemingly inconsistent findings do not exclude type and amount of dietary fat as the major determinants of serum cholesterol levels, provided one concedes that these are not the only factors which determine the distribution of serum cholesterol levels within a population. It would seem that a diet which is also excessive in total energy, including that from carbohydrate, is an essential co-requirement. Another factor which may explain the low cholesterol levels in Central Africa is the fact that fat content and composition of animals varies widely. In Uganda, wild buffalo meat contains one-tenth as much lipid as beef from British cattle, and only 2 per cent of the British beef fatty acids are polyunsaturated as compared with 30 per cent of the meat fatty acids from woodland buffalo. Man's tissue lipids approximate the pattern of his dietary fat intake and numerous carefully controlled studies have confirmed the cholesterol-lowering effect of polyunsaturated fatty acids.

In addition to the cholesterol-lowering property of polyunsaturated fatty acids, it is conceivable that the findings from the studies carried out in London and Chicago might be explained by another mechanism: certain long-chain essential polyunsaturated fatty acids, such as linoleic acid, are reported to reduce the thrombotic tendency of the blood. A significantly lower proportion of linoleic acid is present in the adipose tissue of healthy Scots compared with similar men in Stockholm, where the IHD rate is one-third lower than in Scotland. Eskimos who have a high intake of eicosopentanoic acid have prolonged bleeding times and laboratory studies suggest that reduced tendency to platelet aggregation may be explained by the effect of these fatty acids on prostaglandin synthesis.

In summary, epidemiological data do give some credence to the suggestion that diet is related to IHD, possibly via an effect on both atheroma and thrombosis. Certainly, IHD seems to occur very infrequently in communities where the 'Western diet' is not consumed, though of course features other than diet characterize such communities. IHD is now being diagnosed with increasing frequency among the black people of East and Southern Africa amongst whom the disease was previously regarded as exceptionally uncommon and it is the more affluent sections of the community who are principally involved. Further evidence for an aetiological association between diet and IHD is provided by the single factor intervention studies (Mann and Marr 1981). Although, on the whole, these have not shown increased life expectancy, they have demonstrated a reduction in coronary events related to the extent of cholesterol lowering.

Animal studies have yielded some confirmatory data: several research groups have shown that in monkeys it is possible to induce atheromatous lesions by feeding a diet high in saturated fat. The experimental lesions can be reversed by lipid-lowering measures. The process in animals may differ considerably from that in humans, but such findings do nevertheless provide additional evidence concerning the role of diet in atherosclerotic disease.

DIABETES MELLITUS

Diet undoubtedly plays an important aetiological role in non-insulin dependent diabetes (Mann 1980). As early as 1920, Himsworth suggested that excessive energy intake, deficiency of dietary carbohydrate, and possibly an excessive intake of fat might increase the risk of diabetes. His conclusions were based on the following observations: in non-diabetics blood glucose levels following an oral glucose load were lower when eating a high carbohydrate, as compared with a high-fat (low-carbohydrate) diet. When examining mortality rates from diabetes, he found that in countries with high death rates, the diets contained a relatively low proportion of carbohydrate and a high proportion of fat. During the First World War, when death rates from diabetes fell, the main dietary change was a reduction in the proportion of fat and an increase in the proportion of carbohydrate. Finally, when taking diet histories (concerning diet before the onset of symptoms) from newly presenting diabetics, it was found that diabetics in general ate more than non-diabetic controls and fat intake appeared to be especially high.

Controversy has raged subsequently between those who have argued the case for excessive intakes of sugar and others who have suggested a deficiency of dietary fibre as being particularly relevant. The most helpful study has been conducted by West and Kalbfleisch. They used careful survey techniques in 12 countries for studying both diabetes frequency and dietary histories (rather than the much less reliable mortality statistics and population food consumption figures used by other researchers) in an attempt to discover the most important environmental factors in the aetiology of non-insulin-dependent diabetes. Both sugar and fat intake correlated with diabetes frequency, but the most striking association ($r=0.9$) was with energy intake. More detailed analysis of their data suggested that correlations with individual foods were occurring simply as a consequence of the most important factor – energy intake in excess of requirements.

Whilst excessive energy intake seems likely to explain the previously observed correlations between sugar and fat, a protective role of dietary fibre should not be dismissed since there is considerable circumstantial evidence. In Pakistan, diabetes is less common among chapatti (wholewheat unleavened bread) eaters than sections of the population using white flour. In India, the disease occurs less frequently in those areas where unpolished rice is eaten, as compared with the urbanized areas where rice is polished. Diets high in fibre-rich carbohydrate are associated with an improvement in several measures of diabetic control when compared with the standard low carbohydrate diet still in use in most British diabetic clinics. Mice have been shown to develop hyperglycaemia when converted from a diet of 5 to 2 per cent crude fibre. Nevertheless, more research is needed to determine whether any single dietary factor is as important as excessive energy intake in a genetically predisposed individual in determining the risk of developing diabetes. Although diet is important in the management of insulin-dependent diabetes, nutritional factors have not been incriminated as a cause of the disease. Here, genetic and other environmental factors appear to be particularly important.

OBESITY

Of all the conditions associated with overnutrition, obesity is the most obvious and perhaps at the same time one of the least understood. There is little consensus with regard to definition and, consequently, epidemiological data are scanty. There is, however, no doubt about the increased risk of morbidity and mortality associated with marked obesity and it has been suggested that during the past 40 years the average body fat content of the adult population of the United Kingdom has increased by about 10 per cent. Consequently, the prevalence of obesity must also have increased. The precise role of nutritional factors is unclear.

However, in the long term, clearly only a reduction in energy intake or a substantial increase in output will reduce the proportion of overweight people in the population. It is possible that a diet in which carbohydrates are taken in fibre-rich forms will help to reduce obesity by encouraging satiety at a lower level of energy intake.

DIVERTICULAR DISEASE OF THE COLON

The first suggestion that deficiency of dietary fibre may be implicated in the aetiology of diverticular disease of the colon came from the striking geographic variations and the documented increase in the disease rates in several European countries since the 1920s. The variation and trends in rates are certainly compatible with fibre deficiency, but could be explained by several alternative dietary and other environmental factors. The best documented evidence comes from studies of patients with diverticular disease and controls, animal experiments and the effects of treatment with bran. Brodribb and Humphreys obtained diet histories from patients with diverticular disease and controls and found that before the onset of their symptoms the patient reported a lower intake of crude fibre than the controls. However, the patients all had symptoms and this could have modified eating habits and influenced the memory of eating habits before the onset of symptoms. Gear and colleagues carried out barium follow-through investigations on 220 asymptomatic volunteers (including 56 vegetarians) and identified 95 individuals with asymptomatic diverticular disease (Gear et al. 1979). Careful dietary histories were obtained from all participants. The vegetarians, with a substantially higher fibre intake than non-vegetarians, were less prone to diverticular disease (12 versus 33 per cent). In non-vegetarians over the age of 60, dietary fibre intake was 19 g/day in those with diverticular disease and 23 g/day in those without. The difference was more striking in vegetarians with (28 g/day) and without (43 g/day) diverticular disease. Failure to show a significant difference in the under 60s was thought to be due to some of them being in a pre-diverticular state. In this study, differences in total dietary fibre were principally due to differences in intake of cereal fibre and no other dietary constituents differed significantly in subjects with and without diverticular disease. It is of interest that vegetarians with diverticular disease ate more fibre than non-vegetarians without it. Thus, this study which provides strong evidence for a protective role of cereal fibre in diverticular disease, also suggests that factors other than fibre are involved. Animal experiments provide confirmation; for instance an early experiment showed that rats given a low fibre diet develop diverticula and, more recently, rabbits, constipated following a diet of white bread, sugar, and vitamins, developed diverticula after being given prostigmine to induce contractions. An increase in dietary fibre is widely recommended to patients with symptomatic diverticular disease, a treatment justified by at least one double-blind crossover trial and numerous uncontrolled studies.

Plausible theories concerning pathogenesis have been suggested: small hard faeces, undoubtedly features of a fibre deficient diet, are associated with narrowing of the colon and the formation of closed segments in which pressure increases. Additional work is needed by colonic muscles to provide the pressure to move the more solid faeces, producing muscular hypertrophy in addition to the diverticula at sites of weakness where blood vessels penetrate the muscular coat.

Although no formally conducted intervention study in humans has ever shown dietary fibre to be protective against diverticular disease, the evidence in favour of a protective role of dietary fibre seems strong.

CONSTIPATION AND THE IRRITABLE BOWEL SYNDROME

Ninety-nine per cent of a large population sample studied in Britain reported that they defecated at least three times per week. Yet perceived constipation is a frequent complaint. In 1976, 3 per cent of all prescriptions written in the National Health Service (in the United Kingdom) were for purgatives and laxatives, at a cost of around £4 million, and many times this amount was bought over the counter. In another survey, 6 per cent of people aged 18–80 described straining when passing stools. No data are available concerning the frequency of passing small stools. There seems little doubt that constipation is uncommon in populations eating a high-fibre diet. In rural Africa, stool weights are frequently around 500 g daily and bowel transit times around 40 hours. In Britain, stool weights in non-vegetarians are more usually around 100 g (with a very wide range) whereas in vegetarians the average stool weight is over 200 g. Factors other than fibre might be involved, but the fact that British vegetarians and non-vegetarians with average daily intakes of dietary fibre greater than 30 g have transit times of less than 75 hours, whereas those with small fibre intake have transit times ranging from 20 to 124 hours, suggest that fibre must be particularly relevant. There is no doubt that increasing the fibre (in particular cereal fibre) content of the diet relieves the symptoms of constipation, an observation now confirmed by controlled clinical trials. On average, the addition of about 10 g of dietary fibre to the usual daily diet is required (Mann 1979). There is no direct evidence of a causal link between a fibre-depleted diet and the irritable bowel syndrome, but high-fibre diets are widely recommended in the treatment and are believed to be of value in the absence of formal clinical trials.

DENTAL CARIES

Dental caries was exceptionally rare among young people in ancient Britain. In 1975, 80 per cent of five-year-olds required treatment for dental caries and about 10 per cent of all children enter school with more than half their teeth seriously decayed. Some 5 per cent of the adult population in England and Wales and 15 per cent in Scotland are edentulous by the age of 30 years. Careful oral hygiene, fluoridation of the water supply and perhaps, in the future, a vaccine to raise resistance against cariogenic organisms will decrease the frequency of dental caries, but there are impressive data to suggest a nutritional cause. Amongst the indigenous population of many countries where unrefined foods formed the bulk of the diet (e.g. China, Uganda) dental caries had a very low prevalence. Within a few years of the addition of sugar and other refined foods, the frequency showed a rapid increase. A similar change has been shown experimentally in monkeys. In a classical experiment carried out in a Swedish mental hospital, volunteers given toffee apples, chocolate, and caramel, in addition to their control diet, had a 13-fold greater number of tooth surfaces becoming carious each year, compared with those eating the control diet alone.

OTHER DISEASES

Cancer of the large bowel, gall-stones, appendicitis, haemorrhoids, varicose veins, and hiatus hernia all occur frequently in developed countries and rarely in developing countries, but the evidence linking these conditions to a nutritional cause is more tenuous. Gall-stones are undoubtedly associated with obesity and, in the case of both gall-stones and appendicitis, there are some rather indirect data suggesting an association with fibre deficiency or excessive quantities of refined carbohydrate. The addition of bran to the diet can make bile less saturated and experimentally induced gall-stones in animals tend to be reduced if fibre-rich food is given. Data from the United Kingdom and South Africa taken together provide interesting information concerning appendicitis: appendicitis rates were compared in two matched South African Caucasian groups, the privileged group living in University halls of residence and the other living in establishments for the more indigent where the diets contained more fibre. Annual rates were 7.8 and 1.8 per 1000 respectively. Of course, factors other than diet might explain this, but the similarity in rates to those found in an almost identical study in Bristol (7.6/1000 in a public school and 0.8/1000 in an orphanage) are very striking.

THE CASE FOR DIETARY CHANGE

Ischaemic heart disease, non-insulin-dependent diabetes, diverticular disease, constipation, dental caries, and obesity are conditions in which malnutrition plays a definite role in aetiology. It is of some interest to consider the frequency of these diseases. The first three accounted for approximately 10 per cent of all hospital admissions to acute hospitals in the Oxford region in 1978. Ischaemic heart disease and diabetes accounted for 40 per cent of all deaths in men aged 45–54 years in England and Wales in the same year.

The case for recommending dietary change hinges on (i) the importance of these conditions in affluent societies; (ii) the strong evidence for a nutrional aetiology in a substantial number of the disease; (iii) the evidence from clinical trials that cholesterol lowering (of the order of magnitude that can be achieved by dietary means) reduces the risk of non-fatal IHD; (iv) the evidence from animal atheroma, and perhaps other diseases of disordered nutrition, might be reversible. Numerous official and semi-official bodies have suggested dietary change (Select Committee 1977). The great majority have been aimed at reducing the frequency of IHD and have centred around increasing the proportion of fat coming from polyunsaturated sources, with or without a reduction in total fat. More recently, advice has been offered concerning a more generally 'prudent diet' than the typical British diet, which comprises 45 per cent of calories from carbohydrate (substantially refined and low in fibre), 44 per cent from fat, and 11 per cent from protein (Mann 1979). Criticisms of this approach have been (i) lack of conclusive evidence concerning the beneficial effects of such change; (ii) possible harmful effects of dietary change; (iii) infringement of personal liberties; (iv) the fact that dietary modification would not be compatible with traditional dietary practices in many affluent societies (Ahren 1979). The two latter objections are of less relevance to scientific arguments since recommendations themselves do not affect individual rights – certainly no more than present national policies determined by political considerations (e.g. the subsidy of butter and other dairy products). The most difficult issue when recommending dietary change is the lack of conclusive evidence, i.e. from adequately conducted clinical trials. It is necessary to point out that in view of the very considerable costs such trials will probably never be conducted and the evidence will perhaps only come from natural experiments – observations of disease rates in which populations or sections of populations do change their dietary practicies. A little of this kind of evidence is already available from the fall in IHD mortality rates in the United States of America, which appears to be at least to some extent associated with the dietary change which has occurred in that country. The suggestion that dietary change might be harmful is chiefly based on the observation that very low levels of total or LDL cholesterol are associated with an increased risk of non-cardiovascular death (chiefly cancer). Studies in two populations (in London and Paris) indicate that this inverse association is confined to deaths in the very early years of follow up. Thus, a low cholesterol may be a metabolic consequence of cancer, present but unsuspected at the time of examination. The question must remain not fully resolved, but from the point of view of dietary prevention, it is worth pointing out that the shift of cholesterol likely to result from the suggested changes is unlikely to reach the range where an increased risk of cancer has been observed. One of the difficulties has been the sectional interests of many of the bodies making recommendations and those criticizing them. Even the recommendations by the Food and Nutrition Committee of the National Academy of Sciences have been criticized because of the substantial representation on the Committee of the Food Industry.

Despite this, there would appear to be a few general recommendations which are likely to be reasonably free of controversy and may be beneficial to the health of affluent societies. The importance of maintaining ideal body weight is perhaps the only entirely non-controversial suggestion. There does, in addition, seem to be quite a strong case to recommend an increase in complex fibre-rich carbohydrate, especially wholegrain cereals, dried beans, and unprocessed fruit and vegetables at the expense of fats, simple sugars, and refined carbohydrate. This represents, for many affluent societies, a trend towards past eating habits and certainly a trend towards the diet of populations where the diseases of affluence occur very infrequently. It should be stressed that there is no single clinical trial which has confirmed the benefits of such modifications and consequently it is impossible to give a precise proportion of total daily energy which might be derived from carbohydrate, but 55 per cent, rather than 45 per cent at present, is the most frequently quoted suggestion, together of course with a radical change in the type of carbohydrate. Dietary fibre intake in

158   *Is there a case for dietary change?*

the United Kingdom is currently 20 g/day and, at least as far as gastrointestinal function is concerned, it would seem from the data on bowel transit times that intake should be at least 30 g/day (Gear *et al.* 1981). Possible adverse effects of increasing dietary fibre do need to be considered. Calcium, iron, and zinc absorption could be impaired chiefly as a result of the cation-binding effect of phytate in cereal fibre. In vulnerable groups such as the elderly and Asian immigrants supplementation of the diet with calcium-rich foods might be necessary. In vegetarians there is at least a theoretical possibility of iron and zinc deficiency (since meat is a particularly good source of both) but his has not been evident in a recent study of vegetarians, suggesting that such deficiencies, if they do exist, must be uncommon and probably need not act as a deterrent from recommending a general increase in fibre-rich carbohydrate.

An increase in complex carbohydrate will need to be associated with a reduction in total fat in order to avoid obesity. If carbohydrate is increased to 55 per cent total energy, fat will need to be reduced from the current level of 44 per cent total energy to 30–35 per cent. Controversy surrounds any recommendations relating to the nature of the dietary fat. Currently the ratio of polyunsaturated to saturated fatty acids (p/s) is 0.3. The early studies of IHD prevention (and also the earliest recommendations) increased this ratio to two in the context of an overall 40 per cent fat diet. Such change increased the risk of gall-stones and it is now known that a p/s ratio of about 0.8 (in a diet where fat provides 30–35 per cent total energy) can produce long-term cholesterol lowering of about 10 per cent in well-motivated freely living adults. For this reason a p/s ratio of 0.8 to 1.0 is suggested in more recent recommendations for a 'prudent diet'. It is, however, criticized on the one hand by those who claim that this proportion of polyunsaturated fat has not been tested in any clinical trial and on the other hand by enthusiasts for the suggestion that polyunsaturated fatty acids may have an antithrombotic effect who presumably feel that while this ratio may be adequate to lower cholesterol, it may not be sufficient to exert the antithrombotic effect. Clearly, the situation is unresolved. To this writer it would seem that a ratio of 0.8 is a reasonable compromise; it would certainly aid cholesterol lowering, it may be sufficient to produce some antithrombotic effect (though, of course, the addition of eieosopentanoate, present only in very small amounts in the present diet may be necessary for this) and it is more unlikely to be harmful (it is certainly below the amounts taken naturally by people in many parts of the world).

Dietary change along the lines suggested here is possible, but it would represent a fairly substantial change from the 'typical' British diet. It could not be achieved without a substantial reduction of meat and dairy products (which account for the present relatively high fat intake) and an increase in vegetable protein and fibre-rich cereals. Furthermore, major changes would be required in agricultural policy which, in the United Kingdom and many other countries, favours the dairy industry.

Dietary recommendations made by various official bodies have ranged from a 'no change' policy to far more wide-ranging recommendations than offered here (e.g. to include reduction in salt intake in the hope of reducing frequency of hypertension; and concerning fluoridation, breast-feeding, alcohol, food-additives, and measures to reduce the incidence of iron-deficiency anaemia, rickets, and oesteomalacia). All these recommendations have been criticized. There is, therefore, considerable advantage in suggesting the simple changes mentioned above concerning the major nutrients. Such manipulation is likely to have the greatest effect on the health of entire populations. These suggestions imply a trend back towards an eating pattern which was prevalent in the United Kingdom and other European countries earlier in the century. Although fairly similar recommendations have been made by the Health Education Council of the United Kingdom, there is, as yet, no information concerning the best means by which people might be persuaded to change their diets. Work of this kind should be a priority amongst general practitioners and others with a special interest in prevention.

REFERENCES

Ahrens, E. H. (1979). Dietary fats and coronary heart disease: unfinished business. *Lancet* **ii**, 1345-8.

Gear, J., Brodribb, A. J. M., Ware, A., and Mann, J. I. (1981). Fibre and bowel transit times. *Br. J. Nutrit.* **45**, 77-82.

—— Ware, A., Fursdon, P., Mann, J. I., Nolan, D. J., Brodribb, A., and Vessey, M. P. (1979). Asymptomatic diverticular disease and intake of dietary fibre. *Lancet* **i**, 511-14.

Mann, J. I. (1979). A prudent diet for the nation. *J. hum. Nutrit.* **33**, 57-63.

—— (1980). Diet and diabetes. *Diabetologia* **18**, 89-95.

—— and Marmot, M. G. (1983). The epidemiology of ischaemic heart disease. In *The Oxford textbook of medicine* (ed. J. G. G. Ledingham, D. J. Weatherall, and D. J. Warrell). Oxford University Press.

—— and Marr, J. W. (1981). Chapter 12. In *Lipoproteins, atherosclerosis and coronary heart disease* (ed. W. E. Miller and B. Lewis). Elsevier/North Holland, Amsterdam.

Medical Aspects of Dietary Fibre. A summary of a report from the Royal College of Physicians, London. Pitman, London.

Select Committee on Nutrition and Human Needs. US Senate. US Government Printing Office. December, 1977. Stock No. 052-070-03913-2.

11 Exercise in the prevention of disease and disability

Archie Young

There is nothing new about the idea that ill health may be prevented by regular physical exercise. What is new is the increasing body of evidence which confirms the salubrious effects of exercise or at least indicates that exercise has physiological effects which are potentially beneficial (Fentem and Bassey 1978; Fentem et al. 1979).

Increasing awareness of the health benefits of regular exercise has led to a variety of campaigns intended to encourage the general public to adopt a more active lifestyle. Public reaction to these has been mixed. There are cynics who assume that if official bodies are advocating exercise, there must be a flaw. Their arguments are fuelled by newspaper stories of the more bizarre hazards of jogging, such as being struck by lightning or developing penile frostbite. A Member of Parliament has even gone so far as to recommend that tracksuits should carry a Government health warning 'Danger – jogging can kill', seeming to imply that regular physical activity should be equated with cigarette smoking. In contrast, a growing number of people seems interested in the idea that exercise might not only promote good health but that it might also be fun to do. This response has been much more marked in the upper social classes, just as they have responded best to education about the health hazards of smoking.

People are now approaching their general practitioner with a request for advice on the relationship between exercise and health. In order to answer these questions effectively, the general practitioner must not only be up to date on the available scientific evidence but must also be aware of the prevailing popular beliefs or 'myths' about exercise. For example, a widely-held, lay view is that exercise which causes breathlessness is intrinsically harmful!

GENERAL BENEFITS OF REGULAR EXERCISE

Regular exercise can increase endurance, strength, suppleness, and skill. This reduces the disturbance of the resting state which is required to perform everyday activities, thereby also reducing the subjective sense of effort. The nature of the training exercise determines the nature of the adaptations which occur.

Improved endurance

Aerobic (or oxygen-using) exercise is exercise conducted at a submaximal intensity for periods upwards of five minutes. Repeated bouts of such exercise constitute 'endurance training' and produce adaptations throughout the oxygen transport system. These are both central and peripheral adaptations. Physiologists delight in debating their relative importance.

Centrally there is little or no change in lung volumes (at least in the adult) but the heart gets both larger and stronger and ventricular emptying during exercise becomes more complete. Blood volume and total body haemoglobin both increase; the latter change is sometimes partially obscured by a slightly greater change in the former.

Peripherally, there is an increase in the ability of the working muscles to extract oxygen from their blood supply. Contributing factors include an increase in muscle capillarity and an increase in the oxidative enzyme content of the muscle fibres. The latter is reflected morphologically by an increase in the number, size, and complexity of muscle mitochondria. These changes are more pronounced in the muscles, and even in the individual muscle fibres, which were used most during the training exercise.

The same intensity of exercise will therefore require a smaller flow of blood through the working muscles and correspondingly less diversion of blood away from the splanchnic bed. There will be a smaller rise in peripheral resistance and a correspondingly smaller increment in arterial blood pressure.

Unless there has been an improvement in skill or exercise technique, a given intensity of aerobic exercise will require the same level of oxygen uptake post-training as it did pre-training. This level of oxygen uptake, however, will be achieved with a lower ventilation and a lower heart rate after training than before and the sensation of effort is less for a given work rate after training.

Increased strength

Appropriate training can increase the strength of a muscle. Strength-training comprises a relatively small number of maximal or near-maximal muscle contractions. Except for the specialist athlete, it is probably of little importance whether these contractions are isometric or isotonic – that is whether the muscle's length is unchanged or whether the force is unchanged. There are two possible exceptions to this: (i) isometric contractions may sometimes be preferable in order to produce a training effect without irritating a painful joint or a soft-tissue injury; (ii) isometric contractions may sometimes be relatively contraindicated on account of their tendency to produce large elevations of blood pressure; this will be discussed in more detail later.

Increased suppleness and skill

Regular repetition of appropriate types of movement will also improve suppleness and neuromuscular co-ordination (skill). As with strength and endurance these benefits will be specific to the nature of the training exercise.

They can be demonstrated in extreme situations, such as following a stroke but would be hard to confirm statistically in normal subjects. Nevertheless, they are prominent among the subjective benefits described by people taking regular exercise. It also seems likely that they contribute to the prevention of the 'musculoskeletal strain syndrome' – i.e. the spectrum of common, but ill-defined, conditions presenting as 'fibrositis', neck or shoulder pain, etc.

Benefits in old age

Regular exercise is no elixir of youth, but it can go a long way towards reducing the level of impairment which is all too readily accepted as being synonymous with old age. For example, loss of muscle strength (especially in the presence of joint disease) may mean that an elderly person is no longer able to use a bath unaided or is unable to avoid a fall if he stumbles on an uneven surface. Diminished aerobic fitness may mean that climbing the hill to the shops produces an unacceptable degree of tachycardia and tachypnoea. Appropriate physical training, however, can increase the elderly person's strength and/or aerobic exercise capacity at least as readily as in young people.

Hypothermia is an important cause of mortality and morbidity among elderly people. The elevation of the metabolic rate which persists after the cessation of exercise may well reduce the risk of hypothermia.

Regular physical exercise is not merely beneficial for elderly people. It may be critical for some in determining whether or not they retain their independence (Bassey 1978).

Benefits of exercise when chronic disease is present

Physical training reverses the effects of inactivity due to the typical, modern life-style. In patients with chronic disease, however, the effects of immobility can be even more severe; patients may have been immobilized by doctors or by their own perception and (mis)understanding of their symptoms. For example, if a patient's disease is such that symptoms occur during exercise (e.g. dyspnoea in chronic bronchitis) he will tend to avoid physical activity (Fig. 11.1). The loss of physical fitness which results from his inactivity results in the occurrence of symptoms at progressively lower levels of exercise, even though the fundamental physical impairment due to the disease remains unchanged (i.e. he gets breathless more easily, despite an unchanged peak expiratory flow rate). This 'vicious circle' can spiral through so many revolutions that a patient with only moderate disease becomes severely disabled by his low exercise tolerance. Such a 'vicious circle' applies in many different situations, but can be seen very clearly when dealing with patients with chronic airways obstruction, angina or peripheral arterial insufficiency. As doctors, we are insufficiently alert to the extent to which the physiological effects of immobility contribute to our patients' symptoms and disabilities.

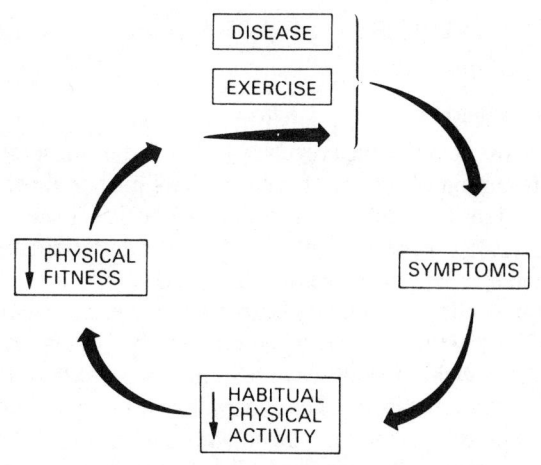

Fig. 11.1. 'Vicious circle' that may ensnare patients with exercise-related symptoms, with the result that their symptoms are provoked by progressively lower levels of exercise. (Reproduced, with the publisher's permission, from Young (1981).)

Psychological benefits of exercise

Physical training has been incorporated into therapeutic programmes for patients with recognized psychiatric disorders. For example, it has been argued that 'any rational, safe, and effective treatment regime for depression should include a prescription for vigorous exercise'. Physical recreation is also rewarding for many mentally handicapped people. Nevertheless, I believe that the major psychiatric role for regular exercise (preferably as recreational sport) is not so much in the treatment of established psychopathology, but rather in the prevention of anxiety, depression, boredom, and self-deprecation in the 'normal' population. In addition, exercise with a team or club ensures important opportunities for informal psychological support.

This is one of the most difficult areas in which to conduct satisfactory scientific studies to validate the claims made for exercise. Nevertheless, there is reasonably good evidence that regular aerobic exercise may result in improved sleep, reduced anxiety, and reduced depression. These changes are seen at their best in patients participating in a therapeutic exercise programme and whose anxiety and depression are related to the physical impairment resulting from their medical condition. For example, following myocardial infarction one of the principal justifications for the inclusion of physical exercise in a rehabilitation programme is the improvement which it produces in confidence and self-esteem (Hackett and Cassem 1973).

At a time when 10–20 per cent of the adult population receive at least one prescription per year for a psychotropic drug, the title of an article by Professor Peter Fentem sets a very relevant question: 'Tracksuits or tranquillizers?'

SPECIFIC PREVENTIVE BENEFITS OF REGULAR EXERCISE
Exercise in primary prevention
Ischaemic heart disease

This is probably the area in which regular exercise has its most important role in the primary prevention of disease. Recent reviews include those by The Royal College of Physicians of London and the British Cardiac Society (1976), Morris (1979), Clarke (1979), Froelicher *et al.* (1980), and Paffenbarger and Hyde (1980). The evidence will never be absolutely complete; a controlled trial of exercise in the prevention of coronary heart disease would mean totally dictating the life-style of several thousand people for at least five to ten years.

There is a great weight of evidence in favour of a protective effect of exercise against coronary heart disease and I consider the case proven 'beyond reasonable doubt'. Those who disagree usually do so with one of three arguments. I shall comment on each of these in turn.

The classical studies of Morris and his colleagues into the exercise habits and ischaemic heart disease experience of transport workers and civil servants and of Paffenbarger and his colleagues with San Francisco dockworkers showed that men whose daily life involved vigorous physical activity were less likely to suffer myocardial infarctions and were even less likely to die from them. This kind of study can easily be criticized on the grounds that men with undiagnosed, premorbid ischaemic heart disease might have tended to select lighter jobs and leisure activities. Morris has now gone a long way towards discrediting this counter-argument with his demonstration that eight years after the survey, those men who had reported participation in vigorous exercise continue to have a more favourable coronary heart disease experience (Morris *et al.* 1980).

Secondly, it is sometimes claimed that inactivity, if statistically isolated from all other influences, seems to be a relatively weak 'risk factor' for coronary heart disease. In fact, the studies of Paffenbarger and of Morris indicate that inadequate exercise has a similar valency to other major risk factors. Moreover, this kind of analysis, by definition, only evaluates a hypothetical, intrinsic effect of exercise itself. It does not take into account the fact that physical training influences several other risk factors, changing all of them in a 'protective' direction. Thus, physical training may lower the circulating concentrations of 'pathogenic', very-low-density-lipoprotein triglyceride and low-density-lipoprotein cholesterol, may increase 'protective' high-density-lipoprotein cholesterol, increases the fibrinolytic response to vascular occlusion, may lower blood pressure slightly, decreases ventricular ectopic activity, reduces the myocardial oxygen consumption required to perform a standard amount of external physical work, helps to regulate weight, improves glucose tolerance and perhaps even discourages the wish to smoke.

Thirdly, it is sometimes argued that there is no point in encouraging a patient to exercise if the 'risk factor' dice are already loaded against him. Why bother persuading him to start swimming if he is not going to stop smoking? Once again, Morris has the answer to this attitude – 'In virtually every situation we have studied, favourable or unfavourable, men engaged in vigorous sports or recreations . . . had about half the coronary attack rates of their fellows.' This is also borne out by Paffenbarger's work.

Exercise in secondary and tertiary prevention

Physical training allows a given level of external work to be performed at a lower heart rate and a lower arterial blood pressure than before training. Physical training therefore reduces the oxygen requirements of the myocardium and thus allows a greater level of external work to be performed before the onset of angina.

The importance of physical training for the post-coronary patient is more controversial (Shephard 1981). Nevertheless, authoritative opinion is in favour of exercise training, on the grounds that angina of effort can be improved or relieved, exercise tolerance increased, the psychological sequelae of a heart attack (principally anxiety and depression) reduced, and a sense of well-being produced. (Royal College of Physicians of London and the British Cardiac Society 1975). Supervised exercise in a group may be particularly useful since it allows the patient convenient and informal access to the 'health professional' running the class. Many patients also derive considerable psychological support from membership of a group of people who have been confronted with similar problems.

Supervised, group rehabilitation involving regular attendance at a hospital gymnasium would usually be prohibitively expensive. It is probably also unnecessary for all but a few patients. An arrangement which is more widely applicable is that the group should train at a local sports-centre, under the guidance of a general practitioner. It is surely better for a man's self-image that he should attend a public sports-centre rather than a hospital. There might also be a better chance that he will continue to be physically active. In one such scheme, the 'graduates' from the class meet during a public session immediately before the class. This maintains their contact with the class and also encourages those who have just joined the class.

Peripheral arterial insufficiency

Patients with longstanding, intermittent claudication can increase their claudication distance by following a programme of regular walking exercise (e.g. Larsen and Lassen 1966). The beneficial effect of regular exercise in a patient with stable peripheral arterial insufficiency is not due to an increase in calf muscle blood-flow during submaximal work. It is due to the trained muscle's greater ability to extract oxygen from its blood supply – the same adaptation that endurance training produces in normal muscle.

166 *Exercise in the prevention of disease and disability*

Hypertension

Mild or moderate hypertension is ameliorated by regular aerobic exercise. The subject is discussed by Denolin and Mallion (1977) and by Scheuer and Tipton (1977). It is not known whether the sequelae of hypertension are more or less frequent when the pressure has been reduced by exercise than when it has been reduced by drugs. At least regular exercise does not cause impotence, diabetes, and cold extremities.

There are two points to remember about drugs, hypertension, and exercise: (i) Normal doses of sympatholytic drugs do not prevent the sudden and large increase in blood pressure which can be produced by isometric exercise (vd. 'Hazards'); (ii) The heart rate cannot be used as a guide to the intensity of exercise in a patient being treated with a beta-blocker.

Airways obstruction

Once again, the emphasis is on tertiary prevention. The beneficial effects of regular physical exercise for patients with chronic airways obstruction are well described in the literature (e.g. Grimby and Skoogh 1980; Editorial 1980) and their value in tertiary prevention was underlined by a recent report from the Royal College of Physicians of London (1981). There is also a useful pamphlet for patients (McGavin *et al.* 1979).

The benefits are probably due to a combination of reversal of the effects of inactivity, reduction of the fatiguability of the respiratory muscles themselves, and an increased psychological tolerance of breathlessness. Grimby calls the last of these mechanisms 'physical habituation' rather than 'physical training'. Its importance must not be underestimated; even if it is 'only a placebo effect' to the physiologist, it still represents a major reduction in the patient's disability.

It is also important that the child with asthma should be able to enjoy the general benefits of improved physical fitness and be relieved of the stigma of seeming less able than his peers. In addition, there is some evidence, alberit rather weak, which suggests that children with asthma may also derive other, more specifically therapeutic, benefits from regular swimming training, e.g. a lower bronchodilator consumption and a lower frequency of exacerbations.

In order that the child with asthma may participate to the full in physical recreation, it may well be necessary for his doctor to give appropriate advice on the choice of sporting activity and the optimal use of drugs in order to prevent exercise-induced asthma. In most patients, exercise-induced bronchoconstriction can be prevented by the inhalation of salbutamol or disodium cromoglycate during the half-hour preceding exercise. Games with an intermittent pattern of running (e.g. football, hockey, etc.) are usually rather less asthmogenic than continuous running and, since exercise-induced bronchoconstriction is precipitated by heat loss through the bronchial mucosa, the warm humid atmosphere in an indoor swimming pool greatly reduces the likelihood of provoking an attack. Many young people with asthma have been able to achieve international success as swimmers. Exercise is also of great benefit to adults with asthma (Young 1981), even to those who are steroid-dependent (Afzelius-Frisk et al. 1971).

Obesity

Regular exercise assists weight regulation in all but the most severely obese (e.g. Editorial 1976; Björntorp 1978; Bray 1978).

Weight reduction programmes which include both dietary restriction and regular physical activity are more acceptable (and therefore more effective) than those which concentrate on dietary restriction alone, since the severity of dietary restriction can be less. It is not only during exercise itself that calorie expenditure is elevated, the metabolic rate may be elevated for several hours after the cessation of exercise. This becomes particularly important if the exercise occurs regularly and frequently. Body fat can be significantly reduced by an exercise programme comprising 40 minutes vigorous walking four times a week.

Diabetes mellitus

Immobility results in impairment of glucose tolerance. Physical training restores this to normal. Further training of normal subjects does not increase glucose tolerance any further, but enhances peripheral insulin sensitivity, i.e. it has an 'insulin-sparing' effect. Practical experience is that the control of maturity-onset diabetes may be improved by regular physical activity. It seems likely that this may be due to a training-induced increase in insulin sensitivity, since insulin-resistance (rather than insulin-deficiency) is the major cause of hyperglycaemia.

Exercise also has beneficial metabolic effects for the patient whose diabetes is well controlled with insulin; it should be an integral part of his management (e.g. Felig and Koivisto 1979). Exercise may, however, aggravate the hyperglycaemia and hyperketonaemia of the insulin-requiring diabetic whose condition is poorly controlled (e.g. Berger et al. 1977).

Patients requiring insulin for the control of their diabetes also meet some practical problems when exercising. In particular, exercise may greatly increase the absorption of insulin from subcutaneous injection sites in the exercising limb. Absorption from other subcutaneous sites is unchanged or even reduced and the use of a non-exercised site is recommended to reduce exercise-induced hypoglycaemia. The adjustment of insulin dose and carbohydrate intake for periods of exercise lasting over an hour should be made with specialist guidance.

Osteoporosis

Disuse results in a loss of strength in bone. When a limb is immobilized in plaster, it takes only a few months for localized osteoporosis to become apparent.

Regular physical training can be used to increase the strength of the skeleton. For example, calcium loss from the os calcis was prevented during the third Skylab mission by requiring the astronauts to perform an exercise which entailed the repeated application of force to the bone by strong, resisted contractions of the triceps surae (Whittle 1979). Similarly, considering a problem more closely related to everyday life, it seems that regular exercise may reduce the loss of calcium from bone in post-menopausal women (Aloia *et al.* 1978). This extremely important conclusion is based on only a single study (with nine experimental subjects and nine controls) but it seems likely to be correct.

Arthritis

Of all the significantly disabled people aged 15–65 years, nearly one-third owe their disability to some form of arthritis. It is unlikely that exercise can make much contribution to primary prevention in this area. There may, however, be some scope for secondary and tertiary prevention. For example, it is widely accepted that the worst degrees of spinal deformity in ankylosing spondylitis can be prevented by adherence to a regular programme of stretching and mobilizing exercises, ideally in combination with regular swimming.

Muscular weakness is a common clinical problem in the presence of joint disease. It may contribute to further joint injury. Isometric exercises, as prescribed by physiotherapists, can increase muscle strength, even in the presence of rheumatoid arthritis. Isometric exercise is used in the expectation that dynamic exercise would aggravate joint pain and inflammation. Nevertheless, a group of patients with ankylosing spondylitis reported diminished pain and joint stiffness after a four-week course of intensive, dynamic, physical training, viz. 3–5 hours daily of swimming, gymnastics, hiking, cross-country skiing, horseback riding, and spinal exercises. It seems likely that we could safely encourage patients with arthritis to participate more fully in recreational sport, provided they choose activities which will not jar painful joints. This would help to prevent a 'disabled' self-image and to restore muscle strength and aerobic fitness without damaging the joint.

Back pain

A large, prospective study of Los Angeles firemen showed that back 'injuries' (undefined) were more common the lower the level of physical 'fitness' (defined as a composite score including measures of aerobic performance, lifting strength and spinal mobility) (Cady *et al.* 1979). It is not clear, however, which component of fitness contributes most to the prevention of back injury. Nor is it known to what extent these findings may be extrapolated to people in sedentary occupations. There have been no good experiments to test the efficacy of exercise in preventing or treating low back pain. There is evidence that treatment with isometric flexion exercises is better than treatment with either flexion/mobilization or extensor-strengthening exercises but it is not known if it is any better than no treatment at all. Nevertheless Nachemson (1976) has pointed out, 'It is known that . . . when lifting and carrying heavy objects . . . contraction of abdominal and costal muscles will help to relieve some of the load of the lumbar spine'. Moreover, the quadriceps take more weight in 'correct' lifting than in 'incorrect' lifting. Therefore, the logical inference is that strengthening abdominal, costal, and quadriceps muscles will relieve the load on the lumbar spine and so contribute to the prevention or amelioration of low back pain. Accordingly, many rheumatologists advise patients with recurring low back pain to take up regular swimming.

HAZARDS OF EXERCISE

Sudden death

How big a risk?

In addition to extolling the benefits to be derived from recreational exercise, it is important that this chapter should also examine the possibility that vigorous exercise may be associated with an increased risk of unwanted side effects, the most important of which is sudden death. Much of the evidence has been reviewed by Vuori *et al.* (1978) and by Tunstall-Pedoe (1979). An analysis of British military experience has been published by Lynch (1980)

Deaths associated with vigorous exercise are most commonly due to ischaemic heart disease, subarachnoid haemorrhage, or congenital abnormalities of the coronary and great vessels. In Lynch's study deaths from subarachnoid haemorrhage were seldom related to formal sport but more to sudden bursts of heavy work which probably produced a sharp rise in blood pressure. There is little that could be done to avoid these deaths.

Of greater importance for the general population is whether vigoraous exercise can cause sudden death from ischaemic heart disease. The evidence is difficult to evaluate. For example, an excessive number of deaths may be reported as associated with non-exercise because premonitory symptoms caused the victim to avoid exercise. Conversely, an excess of 'exercise deaths' may be reported since epidemiological practice dictates that sudden death can be said to be associated with vigorous exercise if it occurs within 24 hours of exercise. Thus Lynch reported that over a ten-year period, 12 per cent of the deaths due to ischaemic heart disease among British soldiers were associated with sport or other strenuous exercise within the preceding 24 hours. Yet his paper also points out that 'most soldiers undertake near-maximum exercise on most days of the week'.

Exercise associated with extremes of temperature probably ought to be avoided. This is illustrated by the relatively high death rate recorded by Vuori in respect of sauna baths and by others in respect of hot showers following exercise.

The estimates of the importance of viral myocarditis as a cause of exercise-associated sudden death vary considerably from report to report. There is good experimental evidence from work with animals to suggest that it would be unwise to exercise while suffering a viral infection since this may activate an otherwise transient, subclinical myocarditis.

The place of exercise electrocardiography in prevention

There is a widespread belief in both medical and lay circles that the safety of exercise can be increased by undergoing an electrocardiographically-monitored exercise test before starting training. This is fallacious and the reasons have been very clearly set out by Epstein (1979): 'In patients who, by history, have a high pre-test likelihood of coronary-artery disease: 1. a positive electrocardiographic exercise-test result is of marginal diagnostic importance because it only slightly increases an already high likelihood of coronary disease; 2. a negative result in these same patients is valueless clinically because of the very high percentage of patients with false-negative results.' Moreover, with subjects who have a low pre-test likelihood of coronary artery disease, a positive response is often false-positive and a negative response does not rule out the presence of significant disease. In the present context, the practical consequences of these conclusions are: first, that the public must be educated to recognize for themselves whether they are 'at risk' from coronary heart disease, and, if the answer is yes, to seek medical advice; secondly that a normal exercise ECG is not a licence to ignore the advice to start gently and build up gradually.

The place of public education in prevention

If the average, untrained individual does indeed run a slight risk when he takes vigorous exercise, it seems likely that the level of risk can be greatly reduced by starting the training programme with a very light level of exercise and making only small and gradual increments. Thus, as fitness improves, the relative strain imposed on the body increases very slowly indeed; any suggestion of untoward symptoms can be noted and acted upon. It is important that the lay public is educated to recognize the signs of an ischaemic myocardium being exercised too close to its limits. This is an area where family practitioners and national bodies responsible for health education must combine forces. It is essential that the jogger knows to seek medical advice if he experiences syncope or chest pain during exercise, palpitations associated with shortness of breath or chest pain during exercise or shortly afterwards.

The Royal College of Physicians of London and the British Cardiac Society (1976) stated that 'Few need to consult their doctors before making a graded increase in their physical activity'. It is important that those who do need to consult their doctor can be identified or, more properly, can identify themselves (e.g. Fig. 11.2). They can then be given any particular advice which is necessary for them to exercise safely, effectively, and enjoyably.

CONSULT YOUR DOCTOR IF:

1. You are under regular or recent medical treatment

OR 2. You've ever had high blood pressure, heart disease, chest pain, or an irregular heartbeat

OR 3. A close blood relative has had a stroke or a heart attack under the age of 50

OR 4. You're more than three stones overweight

OR 5. You smoke

OR 6. You're worried whether exercise may affect any other aspect of your health

Fig. 11.2. Suggested guidelines to permit self-identification of those who should consult their doctors before making a graded increase in their physical activity.

Hazards of isometric exercise

Isometric exercise involves muscle contraction without movement, e.g. holding a heavy weight or trying to push an immovable object. It is often advised that isometric exercise should be avoided by those who might be thought to be susceptible to ischaemic heart disease or cerebrovascular problems. This is because isometric work produces a very large rise in blood pressure.

It must be remembered, however, that the concomitant increase in heart rate is very small and, as a result, the increase in the rate × pressure product is actually smaller during high-intensity isometric work with small muscle groups than with submaximal dynamic work with large muscle groups even though the increase in arterial blood pressure may be greater with isometric exercise. Since myocardial oxygen consumption depends more on the rate × pressure product than on the blood pressure alone, it is probably increased less by the isometric exercise.

It may be that isometric work is less dangerous for the myocardium than is usually stated. Nevertheless, isometric exercise can still produce two potential hazards: (i) when performing isometric exercise it is no longer appropriate to use the heart rate as a guide to myocardial oxygen consumption although this can be done during dynamic work; (ii) myocardial oxygen consumption can be pushed very high indeed by a combination of isometric exercise with a small muscle group (e.g. hand grip) and dynamic work performed with large muscle groups (e.g. brisk walking). Classically, this arises when the middle-aged, obese, hypertensive, aggressive business-executive tries to hurry through an airport terminal carrying his suitcase.

Muscular hazards

Stiffness

Muscle stiffness 24–48 hours after unaccustomed exercise seems to be due to the occurrence of 'microtrauma'. The important practical points are that muscle stiffness can be minimized by making only a slow and gradual increase in the level of exercise and being particularly cautious about the amount of exercise involving eccentric muscle contractions (i.e. contractions in which the muscle is being lengthened despite being active . . . e.g. the quadriceps during the landing phase of squat-jumps). The most effective cure for such muscle stiffness is the performance of gentle rhythmic exercise. Drug treatment is not indicated.

Cramp

Additional salt is probably completely irrelevant for the prophylaxis of the vast majority of muscle cramps experienced in temperate climates. From a practical point of view, the important things to know are (i) cramp can usually be relieved by stretching the muscle and (ii) regular training seems to reduce the incidence of muscle cramps.

Rhabdomyolysis

Severe rhabdomyolysis is an extremely rare, but potentially catastrophic, muscular complication of exercise. The resulting myoglobinuria may cause tubular necrosis and renal failure.

It is seen most commonly in military recruits made to perform many repetitions of an unaccustomed exercise which puts a very high stress on a limited number of muscles. The patient with the so-called 'squat-jump syndrome' complains of painful 'stiff' muscles, is unwell and passes 'Coca-Cola'-coloured urine or may already be anuric. He should be managed by measures to encourage a large output of alkaline urine while arrangements are being made for his immediate transfer to hospital.

Over-use syndromes

Excessively severe training, or an attempt to increase the training load too rapidly, can result in one or more of a variety of 'over-use' syndromes. Since running is the commonest form of exercise for 'keep-fit' athletes, the lower limbs are commonly affected (Fig. 11.3).

In the acute phase, these injuries should be treated by cessation of exercise and the prescription of a non-steroidal anti-inflammatory agent for a few days. Exercise should then be resumed at a much lower intensity and should be increased more slowly than before. Very occasionally, additional treatment may be advised using, for example, ultrasound or the local infiltration of steroids.

Once established, over-use injuries can prove difficult to shake off and it is therefore preferable that they should be prevented. As already indicated, the most important factor in preventing over-use injuries is careful control of the rate of increase of the training load. Recurrent problems are an indication for a close examination of the athlete's technique.

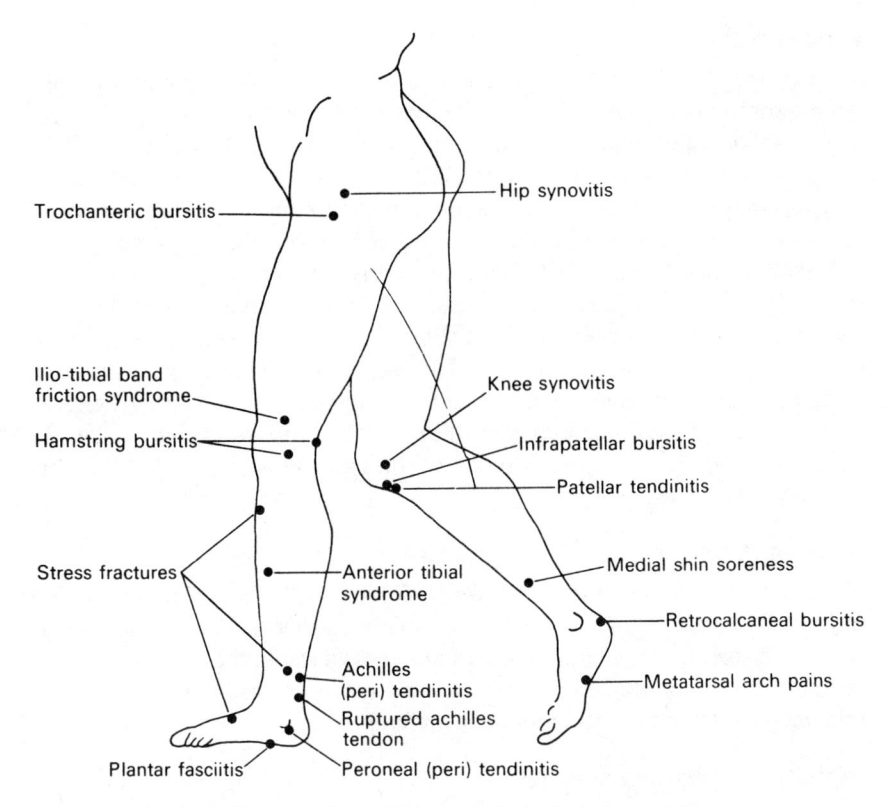

Fig. 11.3. Common sites of overuse injuries in joggers and runners.

Head injuries

The medical profession has an important role in the prevention of sports injuries due directly or indirectly to features of the equipment or the tactics (legal or illegal) used. The association between injuries sustained in rugby football and illegal practices is a good example (Davies and Gibson 1978).

How long will it be until the medical officers of sports such as rugby football and soccer, insist on players waiting four weeks after loss of consciousness before participating again – the rule which applies in amateur boxing? Such a step is overdue since it has been clearly shown that psychological function is impaired for two to three weeks after injuries producing even just a brief period of unconsciousness and that the effects of repeated injuries of this sort are cumulative.

THE EXERCISE PRESCRIPTION

Form of exercise

Most of the health benefits of exercise result from activities which train the oxygen transport system. These are activities which use large muscle groups and whose performance requires a large proportion of the maximal capacity of the oxygen transport system. This means brisk walking (progressing gradually to jogging and perhaps even to running), cycling, swimming, or a programme of 'physical jerks' such as the Canadian Air Force 5BX and XBX systems.

Although they too can bring their problems, the repetitive movements of swimming and cycling cause much less trouble than running since the body weight is supported in both these activities. This is particularly important for people who are overweight or who have a history of back or other joint symptoms. Even for those who are not overweight, weight-bearing exercises should mean the use of shoes with a thick, shock-absorbing cushion under the heel. Similarly, joggers should avoid hard surfaces and, wherever possible, run on grass.

Duration of exercise

The first few minutes of exercise are performed with the aid of the body's oxygen stores and by using the body's ability to exercise for a brief period without the use of oxygen (anaerobic exercise). As a result, the oxygen transport system can only be trained by exercise which lasts for more than just a few minutes – a minimum of ten minutes is preferable.

Intensity and frequency of exercise

A significant, aerobic-training effect can be achieved without exercising at the limit of capacity. Excessive zeal results in injuries which, although trivial in themselves, effectively prevent any further training for a week or two.

An endurance training programme should be started at an extremely low level of exercise – so low that the former athlete may be embarrassed by it. Over the age of 30 years, the first two to three weeks of a jogging programme should consist of nothing more strenuous than walking. Ten to twenty minutes of brisk walking three times a week will produce a significant training effect. Subsequently, brief periods of jogging can be introduced at intervals during the walk. The relative proportions of jogging and walking can then be gradually reversed.

Once a basic level of aerobic fitness has been achieved, the training exercise should be performed at some 60–70 per cent of the maximal oxygen uptake. During submaximal dynamic exercise, the heart rate (expressed as a function of the individual's resting and maximum heart rates) is a reliable indicator of the percentage of his maximal oxygen uptake being utilized. The heart rate can therefore be used to check whether the training exercise is sufficiently, but not excessively, vigorous (American College of Sports Medicine 1975).

This sort of approach is commonly advocated in the literature spawned by the current jogging boom in North America. I feel, however, that it is unduly introspective and, moreover, there is evidence that it is not very reliable in practice. A perfectly adequate guideline for most people is that the exercise should be sufficiently strenuous for them to be aware that they are breathing more heavily. In the words of the Royal College of Physicians of London and the British Cardiac Society (1976) 'Getting breathless some time every day is a good habit'. The level of exercise which will be achieved by someone following this guideline will cross the training threshold sufficiently often for the desired effect to be achieved.

In order to ensure that the training intensity is not excessive, it is necessary also to have a guide to the upper limit of exercise intensity which should be attempted by someone unaccustomed to exercise. The Sports Council's guideline – 'Run at talking pace' – is very satisfactory. Ventilation during exercise should not be so great as to prevent the athlete from carrying on a conversation while continuing to exercise.

The frequency with which endurance training should be performed depends to a large extent on the intensity and duration of each exercise session. For someone pacing himself as described above, the exercise should be continued for at least 10 minutes at a time, three times a week. Some may choose to fit their training exercise into the normal working day. Certainly it should not be too difficult to include a minimum of ten minutes of deliberately brisk walking on three occasions in the working week. This is not to say that important benefits might not be gained from less exercise, although they might be hard to confirm statistically. It is important that we are not too dogmatic in our assertion of the minimum amount of training exercise; some exercise is better than no exercise.

If the chief purpose of the exercise programme is to aid weight-loss, the intensity of activity may remain fairly low if the individual bouts are longer and more frequent. This might mean walking for an hour a day, five days a week.

'Behaviour modification' and the prescription of therapeutic exercise

The prescription of graded physical training is an important part of tertiary prevention for many patients. Motivation, however, can be a problem. It is often difficult to persuade a patient that he really will benefit from physical training. Sometimes, an increased level of 'exercise behaviour' can be encouraged by applying the elementary principles of 'behaviour modification' (Series and Lincoln 1978). Any therapeutic exercise 'class', whether in general practice or in hospital, should be planned in such a way that attention, test and feedback of progress may all be used as 'reinforcers' to increase the frequency of 'exercise behaviour'. The length and severity of the work periods in each patient's exercise prescription should be adjusted so that, for example, a rest period is a 'reward' for the successful completion of a period of exercise, rather than being the consequence of an inability to continue the exercise. This rarely happens in current hospital practice.

In a person who has been inactive for a long time, the physiological effects of even a small amount of training may be dramatic. Fitness-testing can therefore be used to provide the patient with evidence of progress and so reinforce his exercise behaviour.

THE GENERAL PRACTIONER'S CONTRIBUTION

If the medical profession accepts that there are significant health benefits to be gained from regular physical exercise, then it is morally bound to try and influence popular behaviour accordingly. 'Preventive medicine' becomes virtually synonymous with 'health education'. The public must be informed about the various ways in which regular exercise promotes health and the wide range of people (including patients) who can benefit.

The major public-health argument for advocating an increase in physical activity is the contribution that this would make to reversing the epidemic of coronary heart disease. I doubt, however, whether the individual layman would see this as a sufficiently powerful argument for him to change his own, personal level of physical inactivity. A guarantee of immunity would be ideal, but a mere reduction in the likelihood of suffering a catastrophe at some unspecified time in the future is not an effective 'sales pitch'. Instead (in addition to informing the public about the role of exercise in the prevention of coronary heart disease) we should stress the early, positive benefits which can be guaranteed to come from physical training.

Having convinced people that they, personally, stand to gain something from regular exercise, the next responsibility is to ensure that they may exercise safely and that they continue to exercise. Newcomers to exercise must be educated in the recognition of untoward, exercise-related symptoms and the action to take if they occur. They must be taught how to avoid the troublesome aches and pains that may result from misguided enthusiasm or inappropriate equipment. Doctors must be able to give the right advice and guidance.

Acknowledgements

I am very grateful to several friends who were kind enough to criticize an early draft of this chapter, viz. Professor J. N. Morris and, in general practice, Drs K. and E. M. Armstrong and Drs J. and A. L. Noble. I also thank the Department of Health and Social Security for financial support.

REFERENCES

Afzelius-Frisk, I., Grimby, G., and Lindholm, N. (1977). Physical training in patients with asthma. *Le Poumon et le Coeur* **33**, 33–7.

References

Aloia, J. S., Cohn, S. H., Ostinu, J. A., Cane, R., and Ellis, K. (1978). Prevention of involutional bone loss by exercise. *Ann. int. Med.* **89**, 356–8.

American College of Sports Medicine (1975). *Guidelines for graded exercise testing and exercise prescription.* Lea and Febiger, Philadelphia.

Bassey, E. J. (1978). Age, inactivity and some physiological responses to exercise. *Gerontology* **24**, 66–77.

Berger, M., Berchtold, P., Cüppers, H. J., Drost, H., Kley, H. K., Müller, W. A., Wiegelmann, W., Zimmermann-Telschow, H., Gries, F. A., Krüskemper, H. L., and Zimmermann, H. (1977). Metabolic and hormonal effects of muscular exercise in juvenile type diabetics. *Diabetologia* **13**, 355–65.

Björntorp, P. (1978). Physical training in the treatment of obesity. *Int. J. Obesity* **2**, 149–56.

Bray, G. A. (Ed.) (1978). *Recent Advances in Obesity Research—II.* Proceedings of the 2nd International Congress on Obesity. Newman, London.

Cady, L. D., Bischoff, D. P., O'Connell, E. R., Thomas, P. C., and Allan, J. H. (1979). Strength and fitness and subsequent back injuries in firefighters. *J. occup. Med.* **21**, 269–72.

Clarke, H. H. (ed.) (1979). Update: physical activity and coronary heart disease. *Physical Fitness Research Digest*, Series 9, No. 2. President's Council on Physical Fitness and Sports, Washington DC.

Davies, J. E., and Gibson, T. (1978). Injuries in Rugby Union football. *Br. med. J.* **2**, 1759–61.

Denolin, H. and Mallion, J. (1977). Hypertension and exercise. In *The role of exercise in internal medicine* (ed. D. Brunner and E. Jokl). *Medicine and Sport* **10**, 97–117. Karger, Basel.

Editorial (1976). Effect of exercise alone on obesity. *Br. med. J.* **1**, 417–18.

Editorial (1980). Exercise and the breathless brochitic. *Lancet* **ii**, 514–15.

Epstein, S. E. (1979). Limitations of electrocardiographic exercise testing. *New Engl. J. Med.* **301**, 264–5.

Felig, P. and Koivisto, V. (1979). The metabolic response to exercise: implications for diabetes. In *Therapeutics through exercise* (ed. D. T. Lowenthal, K. Bharadwaja, and W. O. Oaks), pp. 3–20. Grune and Stratton, New York.

Fentem, P. H. and Bassey, E. J. (1978). *The case for exercise.* Research working paper No. 8. The Sports Council, London.

—— Bassey, E. J. and Blecher, A. (1979). *Exercise and health—a bibliography*, The Sports Council, London. (A bibliography of 1334 references collected during a literature search for evidence that exercise is of benefit to health.)

Froelicher, V., Battler, A., and McKirnan, M. D. (1980). Physical activity and coronary heart disease. *Cardiology* **65**, 153–90.

Grimby, G. and Skoogh, B.-E. (1980). Rehabilitation of the respiratory patient. In *Recent advances in respiratory medicine,* No. 2 (ed. D. A. Fenley), pp. 225–35. Churchill Livingstone, Edinburgh.

Hackett, T. P. and Cassem, N. H. (1973). Psychological adaptation to convalescence in myocardial infarction patients. In *Airlie conference on exercise testing and training of coronary patients* (ed. J. Naughton and K. K. Hellerstein), pp. 253–62. Academic Press, New York.

Larsen, O. A. and Lassen, N. A. (1966). Effect of daily muscular exercise in patients with intermittent claudication. *Lancet* **ii**, 1093–6.

Lynch, P. (1980). Soldiers, sport and sudden death. *Lancet* **i**, 1235–7.

McGavin, C. R., McHardy, G. J. R., and Lloyd, E. L. (1979). *Exercise can help your breathlessness.* Chest, Heart, and Stroke Association, London.

Morris, J. N. (1979). Evidence for the benefits of exercise from epidemiological studies. *Br. J. Sports Med.* **12**, 220–2.

Morris, J. N., Everitt, M. G., Pollard, R., Chave, S. P. W., and Semmence, A. M. (1980). Vigorous exercise in leisure time: protection against coronary heart disease. *Lancet* ii, 1207–10.

Nachemson, A. (1976). A critical look at conservative treatment for low back pain. In *The lumbar spine and back pain* (ed. M. Jayson), pp. 355–65. Pitman Medical, London.

Paffenbarger, R. S. and Hyde, R. T. (1980). Exercise as protection against heart attack. *New Engl. J. Med.* **302**, 1026–7.

Royal College of Physicians of London and British Cardiac Society (1975). Cardiac rehabilitation 1975. *J. R. Coll. Phys. Lond.* **9**, 281–346.

—— (1976). Prevention of coronary heart disease. *J. R. Coll. Phys. London* **10**, 213–375.

Royal College of Physicians of London (1981). Disabling chest disease: prevention and care. *J. R. Coll. Phys. Lond.* **15**, 69–87.

Scheuer, J. and Tipton, C. M. (1977). Cardiovascular adaptations to physical training. *Ann. Rev. Physiol.* **39**, 221–51.

Series, C. and Lincoln, N. (1978). Behaviour modification in physical rehabilitation. *Br. J. Occup. Therapy* **41**, 222–4.

Shephard, R. J. (1981). *Ischaemic heart disease and exercise.* Croom Helm, London.

Tunstall-Pedoe, D. (1979). Exercise and sudden death. *Br. J. Sports Med.* **12**, 215–19.

Vuori, I., Mäkäräinen, M., and Jääskeläinen, A. (1978). Sudden death and physical activity. *Cardiology* **63**, 287–304.

Whittle, M. W. (1979). Exercise and the astronauts. *Medisport* **1** (6), 12–15.

Young, A. (1981). But of course, exercise wouldn't help me! – physical conditioning for patients and normal subjects. In *Good health—is there a choice?* (ed. P. H. Fentem), pp. 37–50. Macmillan, London.

12 Alcohol

Peter Anderson

ALCOHOL AND DISEASE

Introduction

Over the last 20 years alcohol consumption in Britain has roughly doubled (Fig. 12.1) and the same trend has been seen in most Western countries (Produktschap voor Gedistilleerde Dranken 1981). Associated with the increase in consumption there has been an increase in the many forms of individual and social damage associated with alcohol and the World Health Organization now regards alcohol problems as amongst the world's major public health concerns (WHO 1980). In many countries cirrhosis ranks among the five leading causes of adult death and is one of the most rapidly increasing causes of death for the population over 25 years of age (Schmidt 1977).

Heavy drinkers and alcoholics have a mortality over twice that of the normal population (Brunn *et al.* 1975) and in Britain, although only 3000 death certificates a year mention alcohol the true premature mortality is probably in the order of 5000 to 10 000 a year (Office of Health Economics 1981). The Office of Health Economics also estimate that in England and Wales 150 000 or 0.4 per cent of the total adult population are dependent on alcohol, 700 000 or 2 per cent have problems related to alcohol, and 3 000 000 or 8 per cent are heavy drinkers showing detectable biochemical abnormalities. Men with alcohol problems outnumber women roughly by five to one.

It is difficult to obtain figures for the prevalence of alcohol problems in general practice. In the second national study of morbidity, 0.9 per 1000 patients consulted for alcoholism and drug dependence, a rate of 1.1 for the age group 25–44 and 1.7 for those aged 45–64 with a consultation rate per 1000 population of 4.5 and 6.5 respectively (OPCS 1979). Wilkins (1974) estimated a prevalence rate of 11.1 per 1000 population aged 15–65 for present alcoholics in his practice.

Before considering the damage related to alcohol use we should remember that the majority of the adult population of this country who regularly drink alcoholic beverages do so without appearing to suffer major harm.

Furthermore, a number of studies have reported that light drinkers experience a lower total mortality than abstainers. Setting the mortality for those drinking up to two drinks a day at 1.00, the Kaiser Permanente Study found that mortality ratios were 1.40 for non-drinkers, 1.40 for those drinking 3–5 drinks a day, and 2.02 for those drinking six or more drinks a day (Klatsky *et al.* 1981).

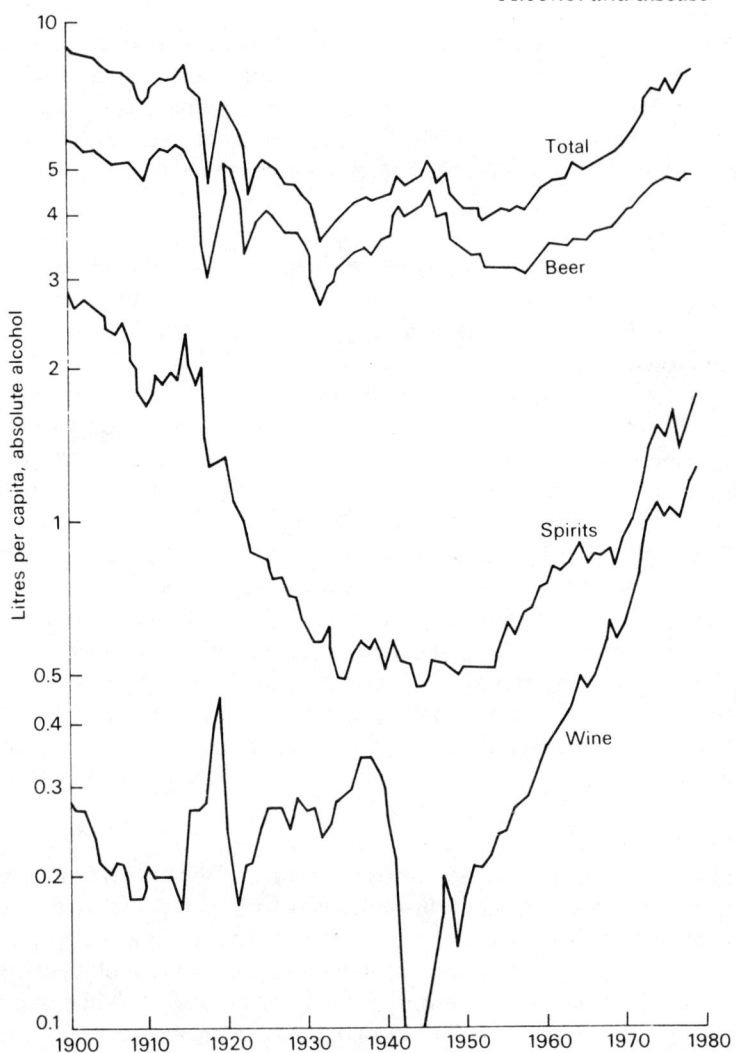

Fig. 12.1. Alcohol consumption by type. United Kingdom 1900–79. (From Office of Health Economics (1981).)

The excess mortality of the abstainers was largely due to an increase in cardiovascular deaths and was independent of smoking.

Accidents

The role of alcohol in road traffic accidents is widely recognized. One in three drivers killed on the roads have blood alcohol levels over the legal limit, a proportion which increases to two in three at night (Department of the Environment 1976). Alcohol is a significant cause of other accidents (Office of Health

Economics 1981). Excluding traffic accidents, nearly two-thirds of male admissions to accident emergency facilities with head injuries have blood alcohol levels equivalent to having drunk six or more pints of beer. About a third of home accidents are alcohol related and heavy drinkers have an accident rate at work three times higher than normal (Observer and Maxwell 1959).

Brain damage

Some 9 per cent of alcoholics admitted to a treatment unit have chronic organic brain syndromes (see Sherlock 1982). The frequency of these syndromes is higher in women (21 per cent) than men (6.6 per cent) and increases with age and duration of drinking in both sexes.

Only a quarter of those with clinical evidence of brain damage have the classical Wernicke–Korsakoff's syndrome. The remainder probably have brain damage due to cortical atrophy. In men without clinical evidence of brain damage, CAT scans demonstrate an increased sulcal width in about 40 per cent. Significant changes occur in alcoholics below the age of 40, but surprisingly the duration of drinking and the quantity of alcohol consumed do not correlate significantly with the severity of the radiological abnormalities.

As many as half of superficially intact alcoholics have specific disabilities of cognition and memory on formal psychological testing (see Sherlock 1982). The disabilities only partially recover with abstinence and age and length of drinking history increase the degree of impairment and slow the rate of recovery. There is very little relation between the severity of CAT scan changes and the degree of cognitive impairment.

Cancer

A heavy alcohol intake increases the risk of cancer of the mouth (excluding lip) and pharynx three-fold, larynx four-fold, and oesophagus two-fold (see Sherlock 1982). This effect is irrespective of the type of beverage and independent of smoking. However, the effects of alcohol and smoking are multiplicative: the relative risk for cancer of the oesophagus may be increased 150-fold in a heavy drinker and heavy smoker. A high alcohol intake increases the risk of primary hepatocellular carcinoma (PHC) two-fold and the reported risk of PHC in alcoholic cirrhosis ranges from 3–15 per cent.

Circulatory system

It has already been mentioned that light alcohol consumption may decrease the risk of coronary heart disease. There is also an association between high alcohol consumption and coronary heart disease although it is not known how much this excess is due to associated cigarette smoking (Bruun *et al.* 1975). There is a strong relationship between alcohol consumption and hypertension and the blood pressures of alcoholics are raised and fall on abstention (Saunders *et al.* 1981a). The Yugoslavia cardiovascular disease study demonstrated that high alcohol consumption was associated with a two-fold increased risk of death from strokes, an effect which was accounted for by increased blood pressure (Kozararevic et al. 1980).

Alcohol directly causes a congestive type cardiomyopathy, which may develop in well-nourished men after consuming half a bottle of whisky a day for several months (see Sherlock 1982).

Gastrointestinal

Alcohol exacerbates heartburn and is a common cause of gastritis. Although cirrhotic patients have a high frequency of peptic ulcer, it does not seem that the ulceration is actually caused by the alcohol intake. Nor do those who continue to consume alcohol have noticeably different healing or relapse rates of their gastric ulcers than those who do not (see Sherlock 1982).

Haemopoiesis

Alcohol has a direct toxic effect on the developing erythroblast leading to macrocytosis which occurs in about 90 per cent of alcoholics (see Sherlock 1982). Alcohol also inhibits the production and function of white blood cells, contributing to an increased susceptibility to infection. A megaloblastic anaemia occurs only in those who have nutritional folate deficiency. Megaloblastic anaemia is more common in those with a poor dietary intake and in wine and spirit drinkers which contain negligible amounts of folic acid, whereas beer contains 100 µg/l.

Liver

Mortality from liver disease is raised 10 times above average in alcoholics. The liver injury is unrelated to the type of beverage consumed; it is related only to its alcoholic content. The steady daily imbiber is more at risk than the spree drinker whose total alcoholic intake may be no less (see Sherlock 1982). In two studies on defined populations in France the relative risk of cirrhosis compared to an alcohol consumption of 0–20 g/day (10 G or one unit is the equivalent of ½ pint beer, a single spirits, or glass of sherry or wine) was six times greater at 40–60 g/day and 14 times greater at 60–80 g/day (Pequinot et al. 1978).

Alcoholism of shorter duration may be compensated by a higher daily dose and vice versa. Women develop alcoholic liver disease after a shorter and lighter exposure than men and at presentation seem to have relatively more severe liver disease (Saunders et al. 1981b).

Only about 10 per cent of alcoholics develop cirrhosis, liver function tests show severe damage in a quarter and less damage in a half. Genetic influences probably determine susceptibility.

Nutrition

Alcohol provides 7.1 kcal/g so that a standard bottle of 70° proof spirit will provide 1500 kcal. Alcohol, however, does not provide equivalent caloric food value when compared with carbohydrate. Thus, although among many moderate drinkers alcohol contributes to obesity, when alcohol is consumed rather than carbohydrate, body weight is reduced. Chronic alcoholics commonly show evidence of malnutrition and reduced levels of circulating vitamins. Although poor dietary intake and poor socio-economic background contribute to malnutrition, this is not the whole story. In a study of middle-aged, middle-class alcoholics, 29 per cent showed evidence of malnutrition (see Sherlock 1982). However, there was no relationship between nutritional status and dietary intake or the severity of liver disease. Impaired intestinal absorption is well documented in alcoholics and this may be due to impaired intestinal function and inhibited biliary and pancreatic secretions. The malnutrition contributes to many of the alcohol-related diseases.

Pancreatitis

There is an association between alcohol consumption and chronic panceatitis but the role of alcohol, if any, in the aetiology of acute pancreatitis is unclear (see Sherlock 1982).

Pregnancy

Few babies are born to severely alcoholic women: the main reason is that cirrhosis leads to amenorrhoea. Moderate alcohol consumption is associated with an increased risk of fetal or neonatal death (see Sherlock 1982). In a recent study which was controlled for the effects of cigarette smoking, the relative risks for spontaneous abortion during the second trimester was 1.03, 1.98, and 3.53 for women taking less than one, 1–2, and more than three drinks daily compared with non-drinkers (Harlap and Shiono 1980).

Heavy alcohol intake in pregnancy is associated with the fetal alcohol syndrome (mental deficiency, microcephaly, reduced body weight, and characteristic facies), which occurs in about a third of the children born to mothers drinking the equivalent of half a bottle of whisky a day.

Even moderate alcohol intake is associated with an increase in minor birth defects, especially of the mouth and genitourinary systems and in minor brain damage. The most vulnerable period for alcohol-related brain damage is around 4–10 weeks after conception and its incidence seems to be increased by binge drinking. Alcohol consumption is also related to intrauterine growth retardation. The increased risk of babies small for dates is 4.6 per cent greater for non-smoking alcoholic mothers, 2.6 per cent greater for smoking non-alcoholics, and 9.2 per cent greater for smoking alcoholics.

Psychological illness

Alcohol use is clearly related to depression and sexual difficulty. Suicide rates in male alcoholics have been reported up to 80 times higher than expected, but an underlying depression may contribute in some cases (Office of Health Economics 1981). Alcohol is commonly used either before or during acts of self-poisoning or self-injury (Hawton *et al.* 1982).

Sexual function

Loss of libido, reduced sexual activity, gynaecomastia, and testicular atrophy occur in about a half of alcoholics irrespective of liver damage (see Sherlock 1982).

Even moderate amounts of alcohol consumption (50 g/day) are related to male infertility. Many chronic alcoholic women complain of sexual difficulty and of menstrual problems such as cycle irregularities, menorrhagia, and amenorrhoea.

Alcohol and drugs

Acute alcohol use prolongs the effect of tranquillizers (particularly diazepam), antipsychotic, and antidepressant drugs. Drugs such as barbiturates, beta-blockers, and antihistamines impair psychomotor performances when taken even with a little alcohol. Sulphanylureas and metronidazole may cause a disulfiram-like reaction. In the chronic alcoholic, as a result of enzyme induction the metabolism of anticonvulsants, diazepam, warfarin, and sulphanylureas is increased. If cirrhosis develops, then the metabolism of many drugs will again become slowed.

Alcohol dependency

Anyone could, in given combinations of circumstances, become alcohol dependent; the main factor is exposure to prolonged heavy doses of alcohol. The symptoms of alcohol dependence in a typical order of occurrence are listed in Table 12.1. Essentially the subject's life becomes more and more focused on

Table 12.1. *Symptoms of alcohol dependence in a typical order of occurrence*

Completely unable to keep to a drink limit
Needing more drink than companions
Difficulty preventing getting drunk
Spending more time drinking
Missing meals drinking
Blackout, memory loss
Giving up interests because drinking interferes
Restless without a drink
Changing to drinking same on a work day as a day off
Organizing day to ensure supply
Change to drinking same amount whatever mood
Passing out while drinking in public
Trembling after drinking day before
Times when can't think of anything but getting a drink
Morning retching or vomiting
Sweating excessively at night
Withdrawal fit
Morning drinking
Decreased tolerance
Waking up panicking or frightened
Hallucinations

Source: Chick and Duffy (1980).

Alcohol

alcohol consumption, and the maintenance of alcohol supply becomes seen as a central necessity with destruction of work, family, and other supportive social relationships.

CONSUMPTION PATTERNS

Alcohol consumption

During the last 20 years alcohol consumption has roughly doubled. Figure 12.2 shows how the quantity of alcoholic drink consumed has changed. Beer consumption has increased by 40 per cent, wine by over 250 per cent and spirits by

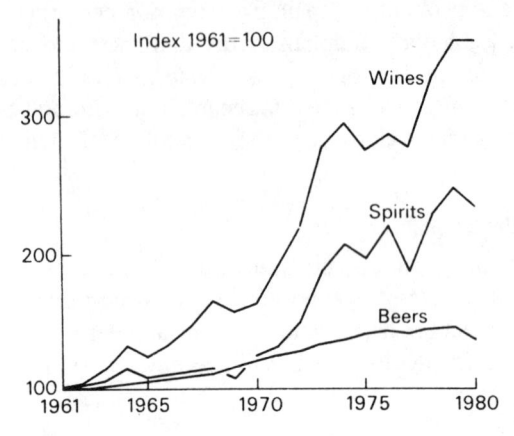

Fig. 12.2. Volume of consumption of beers, wines, and spirits. (From Central Statistical Office (1981).)

135 per cent. In 1980 the British population drank the equivalent of nine pints of beer per week for each individual over the age of 16 and spent £10 200 million to do so; this represents 7.5 per cent of all consumer expenditure which includes expenditure on housing, food, clothing, cars, etc., and is the same as the total expenditure on the Health and Personal Social Services. It should be remembered, however, that the present increase in alcohol consumption started from an historical low point in the period 1930–1960 (Fig. 12.1) and there have been periods of much higher consumption. In the 1680s, for instance (Fig. 12.3) beer consumption reached an estimated peak level of 2.3 pints per person per day, four times the present figure.

Current drinking habits

Our knowledge about current drinking habits derives from surveys which record people's self-reported alcohol consumption in a given period. Such surveys usually show only about half of the alcohol consumption known to

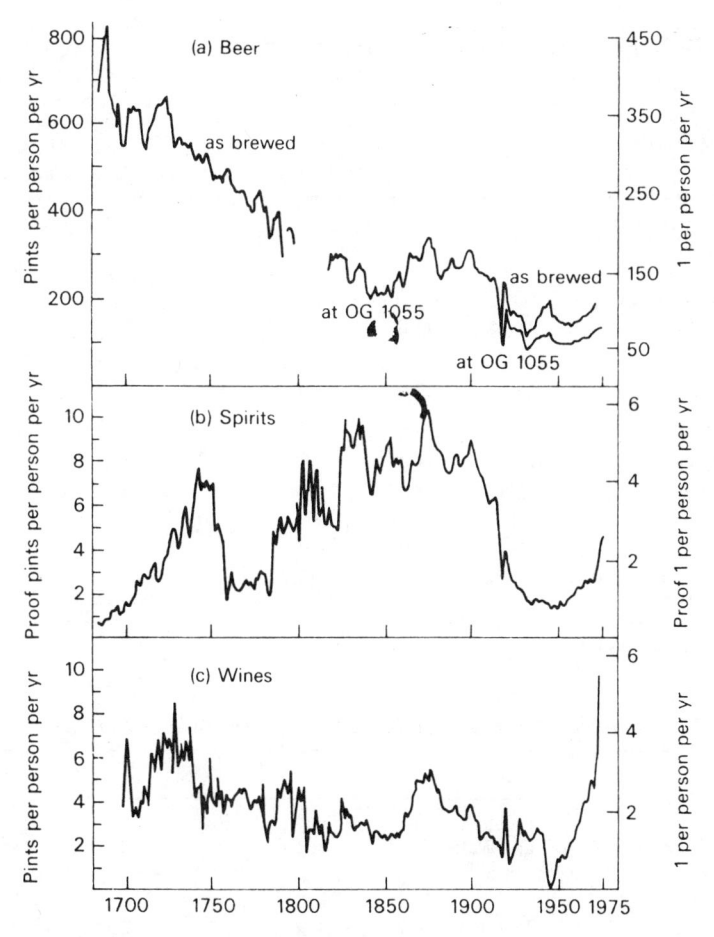

Fig. 12.3. Beer, spirits, and wine available per person in the United Kingdom. (From Spring and Buss (1977).)

take place in the community according to taxation figures (see Sherlock 1982). The reasons include under-recording of drinking due to forgetfulness or embarrassment but also biased sampling in that heavy drinkers are likely to be not available or non-responders. Tables 12.2 and 12.3 present the most recent data on United Kingdom drinking levels measured in standard units (one unit is equivalent to half a pint of beer, a single of spirits, a glass of wine and a glass of sherry and contains about 10 g, 1 ml, of alcohol). The highest consumption is by the young age groups, particularly men. In Scotland high consumption continues amongst young men for longer than in England, Wales, and Northern Ireland.

Alcohol

Table 12.2. *Percentage consuming standard units of alcohol per week*

	Men aged 20 or over			Women aged 20 or over		
	England and Wales	Scotland	N. Ireland	England and Wales	Scotland	N. Ireland
Nothing (and nothing in the last year, i.e. teetotal)	6.0	7.0	31.0	11.0	11.0	53.0
Nothing (but had had a drink in the last year)	18.0	15.0	23.0	32.0	34.0	27.0
1– 5 units	20.0	21.0	14.0	34.0	33.0	14.0
6–10 units	14.0	12.0	11.0	10.0	3.0	3.0
11–20 units	16.0	18.0	12.0	10.0	7.0	1.0
21–35 units	13.0	14.0	5.0	2.0	3.0	1.0
36–50 units	8.0	8.0	1.0			
51 units or more	6.0	6.0	3.0	1.0	0.0	1.0
Average consumption of drinkers last week	19.6	19.5	14.5	7.0	6.2	6.5

Source: Wilson (1980*a*).

Table 12.3. *Consumption of standard units of alcohol last week, by sex*

	Men			Women		
	England and Wales	Scotland	N. Ireland	England and Wales	Scotland	N. Ireland
Age						
20–27	26.6	26.2	18.9	9.7	7.7	7.0
28–37	19.7	24.9	15.2	6.4	6.3	6.9
38–47	19.5	20.9	14.4	7.7	6.2	
48–57	20.1	16.1	12.3	7.2	6.1	
58–67	15.5	13.5	9.9	4.4	3.9	5.4
68+	11.7	6.4		5.0		
all aged 20+	19.6	19.5	14.5	7.0	6.2	6.5

Source: Wilson (1980*a*).

Drinking was concentrated into fewer days in Scotland, so that 40 per cent of all adult male drinkers in Scotland had drunk eight units or more on one day compared with 27 per cent of English adult male drinkers. There appeared to be no major overall variations in alcohol consumption between the main social groupings.

Alcohol and women

In the past decade the longstanding gap between men's and women's consumption is diminishing. A repeat survey in the Lothian region of Scotland found that whereas there was no increase in the proportion of heavy male drinkers, 11 per cent of women in 1978 consumed 11 or more units a week compared to 4 per cent in 1972 (see Sherlock 1982). The increase was accounted for chiefly by younger, single women and may be due to a variety of factors: greater female employment and higher earnings; increased availability of alcohol in supermarkets; advertising aimed specifically at women; growing numbers of women employed in public houses and clubs; blurring of traditional sex differences in both leisure and work activities. As problems related to alcohol consumption have increased amongst men, so they have amongst women (Shaw 1980).

Alcohol and the young

Children come into contact with alcohol very quickly. Forty per cent of Glaswegian six-year-old schoolchildren have tried alcohol (Jahoda and Cramond 1972). Many teenagers drink furtively and most are drinking before they reach the age when legally allowed into pubs (Davies and Stacey 1972). A recent study of 1036 Scottish 15–16-year-olds showed that many were drinking and many were, as a result, suffering health and social problems: 70 per cent of the boys and 61 per cent of the girls had at some time been merry, a little bit drunk, or very drunk. Forty per cent of the boys and 27 per cent of the girls had had an upset stomach from drinking and 3 per cent of the boys and 2 per cent of the girls had lost a day's schooling because of drinking (Plant *et al.* 1982)

Alcohol and occupation

There are links between occupations and alcohol problems as demonstrated by mortality from cirrhosis of the liver (Plant 1981). Publicans have a rate of 15 times higher than the average and fishermen six times higher (Table 12.4).

There are several reasons for this association: availability of alcohol at work, social pressure to drink, separation from normal social or sexual relationships, freedom from supervision and pre-selection of high-risk people.

In the 1978 England and Wales survey, workers from the construction industry had the highest proportion of men drinking over 50 units/week (19 per cent compared to 6 per cent for the whole male population) and men from the drinks industry had the highest average per person consumption (38 units per week compared to 20 for the whole population) (Wilson 1980*b*).

Plant (1979) studied workers in some Edinburgh breweries and distilleries and noted that the drink trade was attracting men who were already heavy drinkers; also as some workers changed their jobs, so they changed their drinking habits. Some heavy drinkers in the drink trade deliberately changed their jobs to drink less and succeeded in doing so.

190   Alcohol

Table 12.4. *Liver cirrhosis mortality (England and Wales 1970–2)*

Occupation	Standardized mortality ratio
Publicans, innkeepers	1576
Deck officers, engineering officers, ships' pilots	781
Barmen, barmaids	633
Deck and engine-room ratings, barge and boatmen	628
Fishermen	595
Proprietors and managers in boarding houses and hotels	506
Finance brokers, insurance brokers, financial agents	392
Restaurateurs	385
Lorry drivers' mates, van guards	377
Armed forces (British and overseas)	367
Cooks	354
Shunters, pointsmen	323
Winders, reelers	319
Electrical engineers	319
Authors, journalists, and related workers	314
Medical practitioners	311
Garage proprietors	294
Signalmen and railway-crossing keepers	290
Maids, valets, and related service workers	281
Tobacco preparers and product makers	269
Metallurgists	266

Source: Plant (1981).

Relationship between consumption and damage

One of the clear results from studies of the drinking patterns of many groups is that the graphs showing how much people drink are always unimodal; there is no discrete population of individuals who drink more than everybody else. This suggests that the more alcohol a society consumes the more heavy drinkers there should be.

Cartwright *et al.* (1978) compared surveys carried out on different sampling frames in South London in 1965 and 1974. The mean consumption of respondents in the second survey was 47 per cent greater than in the first. The proportion of individuals drinking over 50 units/week increased from 1.3 to 4 per cent.

There is good evidence linking the changes in alcohol consumption with changes in alcohol related disorders (Fig. 12.4). The relationship between alcohol and cirrhosis mortality is clearly established. From a death rate of 23/million in 1950 it rose by 3 per cent a year to 44/million in 1979.

Comparing alcohol consumption and deaths from cirrhosis in various countries provides further evidence of the link between consumption and damage (Fig. 12.5).

Causes of harmful drinking

There are a number of factors that influence alcohol consumption and the morbidity that arises from consumption. Some have already been mentioned

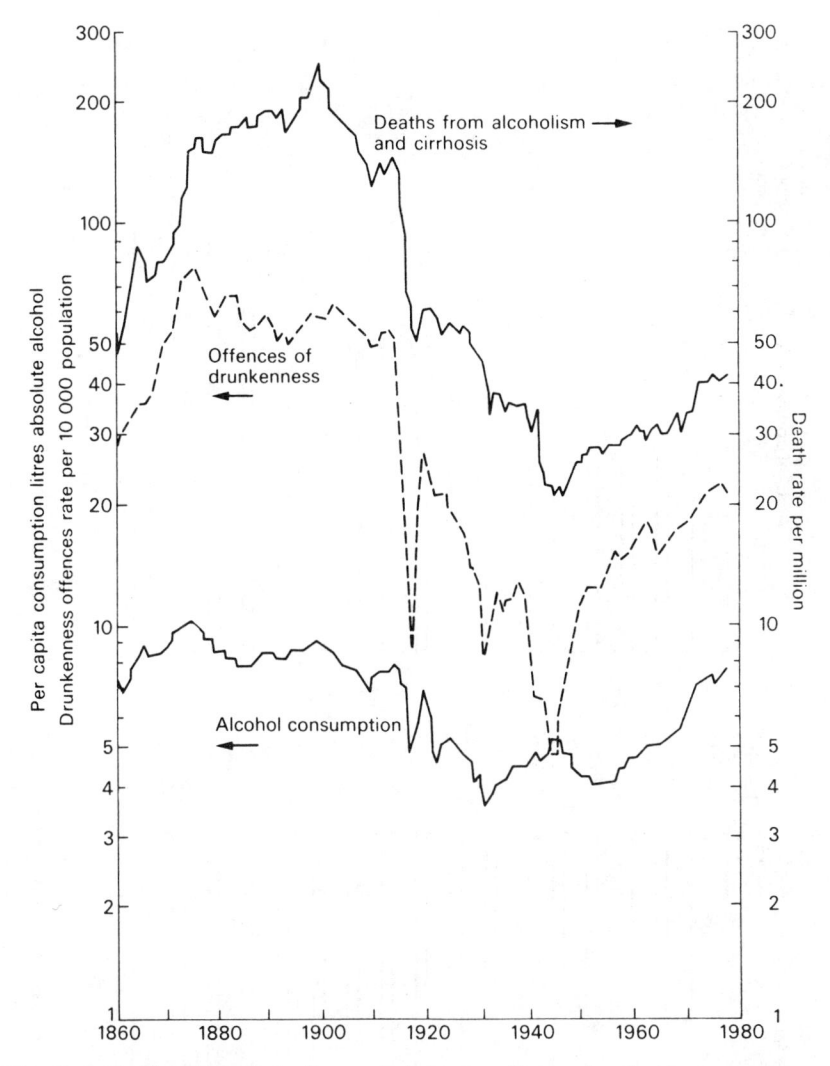

Fig. 12.4. Deaths from alcoholism and cirrhosis, offences for drunkenness and consumption of alcohol, England and Wales 1860–1978. (From Office of Health Economics (1981).)

including age, sex, and occupation. Other influences include price, availability of alcohol, and advertising. On an individual level several factors are involved.

Informal social controls are a major determinant of drinking patterns. The quantity which a person drinks on any occasion will be determined not only by the amount of money he has in his pocket and by licensing laws, but also by whether social mores deem it to be an appropriate time of day for drinking and

192 *Alcohol*

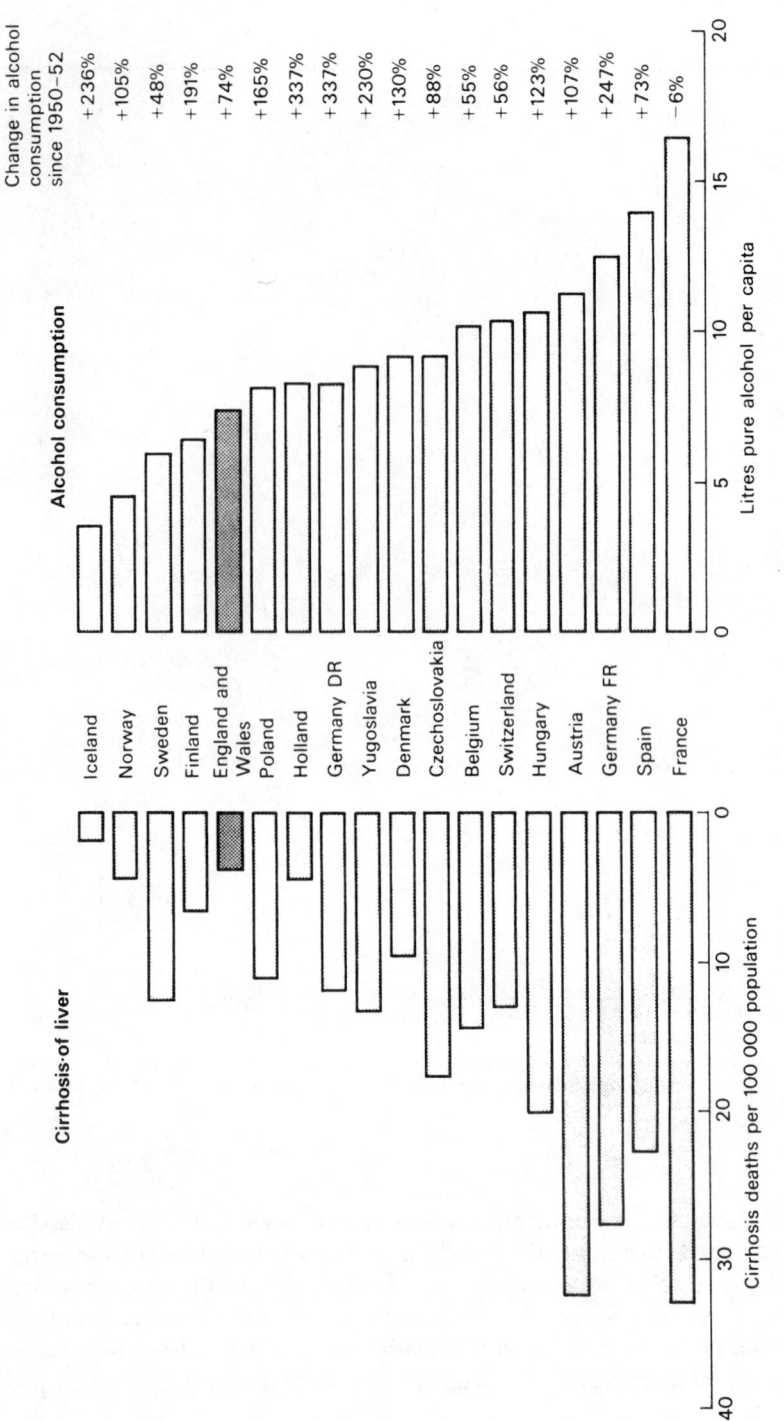

Fig. 12.5. Liver cirrhosis, mortality, and alcohol consumption, selected countries mid 1970s. (From Office of Health Economics (1981).)

whether it is generally appropriate when drinking to take alcohol in moderate quantities or to drink to inebriety and so on.

Some communities seem to be able to protect their members from alcohol harm despite its general availability. In Jewish society drinking is learnt in a controlled manner in the family circle with overt intoxication being frowned on (Snyder 1958). On the other hand there is evidence that the children of people who are teetotal, yet who are raised in societies that permit drinking are at an increased risk of problem drinking and of ultimately becoming dependent (O'Connor 1978).

Certain personality traits are predictive of harm from drinking. When cohorts of young men are followed into adult life those who were impulsive, gregarious, and rebellious as teenagers are more likely to have subsequent problems from drinking. Amongst working men, impulsivity, rebelliousness, and carelessness predict problems even when consumption is held constant, as do early separations from mother or father (see Sherlock 1982).

Parents have a strong influence on the development of drinking behaviour and the rates of dependence are considerably raised amongst those with an alcohol-dependent parent. The first drinking experience usually takes place in the family and children tend to follow their parents' drinking patterns. Parents, however, seem to be pessimistic about their influence (Aitken and Leather 1981).

From the early teens onwards more drinking takes place outside the home. The importance of friends' influence grows parallel with this shift in location and peer group pressure and the need for peer-group standing appear to be strong influences upon adolescent drinking (Davies and Stacey 1972).

REDUCING DRINKING

Natural history of drinking

There is good evidence that heavy and problem drinkers want to cut down on their drinking and that when treatment facilities are offered people come forward for help. Following both the Scottish Health Education Group campaign in 1976 and the Health Educational Council campaigns in the North East of England, there were good responses from people coming forward to seek advice about drinking problems (Plant *et al.* 1979; Cust 1980).

There is also good evidence that patients with alcohol problems treat themselves and people are able to move out of alcohol dependence by drinking less.

Vaillant (1980) has reported the preliminary results of a longitudinal study of 456 Boston 14 year olds followed up for 35 years from 1940. During this 35 years 110 developed symptoms of alcohol abuse. Of that 110, 48 subsequently achieved at least one year of abstinence and 22 were able to return to social drinking. About a third of the 49 who became abstinent and nine of the 22 men who returned to social drinking did so with the aid of professional treatment and about a third who became abstinent had also been helped by Alcoholics Anonymous. Most, however, helped themselves and there were a number of factors that helped the men return to abstinence: firstly, 53 per cent found help by substituting for alcohol food, cannabis, gambling, meditation, three packets of cigarettes a day, or compulsive hobbies. Secondly, 48 per cent developed a medical problem that was instantly made worse by drinking and so reminded them constantly of the need to change their drinking habits. Thirdly, a third were helped by a new and rewarding personal relationship.

Although many people with alcohol problems help themselves, a large number look to other people for help. General practitioners have special opportunities for helping patients with alcohol problems as they are ideally placed to recognize the problem early and intervene. In terms of prevention we should be concentrating on the heavy drinker rather than the alcohol dependant. Most alcohol dependants only present themselves for help in or around their mid-forties when there has often been a 10–20-year history of heavy drinking during which assistance might have prevented the onset of serious difficulties. A general practitioner with an average size list is likely to have 120 heavy drinkers, 36 with alcohol related problems, and six alcohol addicts amongst his/her patients. Because heavy drinkers experience more health problems than average (OPCS 1980) it is likely that they will more often consult their general practitioner.

Effectiveness of treatment

General practitioners are frequently pessimistic about outcomes of efforts to help alcohol dependants and problem drinkers, and this seems to be confirmed by the results of several studies. There is little evidence that minimal forms of treatment are any more effective in modifying alcoholic patterns of drinking than no treatment at all, nor is there much evidence to suggest that the intensity of treatment affects the outcome (Emrick 1975). However, much of the available data about treatment relate only to samples of severely dependent individuals. Outcomes might be more encouraging in the earlier stages of the problem cycle since heavy drinkers are more likely to be able to cut down their drinking than alcohol dependents.

Polich (1980) followed up 758 men who had been admitted to an alcohol treatment unit in the United States for four years. At four year follow up 14 per cent of the sample had died. Of the survivors 28 per cent were abstainers, 18 per cent were non-problem drinkers, and 54 per cent were problem drinkers, a distribution very similar to other studies (Vaillant 1980). The outcome at four years was strongly influenced by the drinking state at 18 months. Those subjects who reported at least one symptom of dependence at 18 months, and those who had only abstained for a short period at 18 months were twice as likely to experience continued symptoms at four years and about three times as likely to die from an alcoholic-related cause. However, those alcoholics who had returned to social drinking at 18 months were no more likely to relapse at four years than those who were long-term abstainers at 18 months (Armor 1980) suggesting that for many social drinking is an acceptable goal for treatment.

Edwards' well-known study compared intensive conventional treatment with simple advice (Edwards *et al.* 1977). One hundred married men were studied and randomly allocated to treatment or advice groups. The treatment group was offered an introduction to Alcoholics Anonymous, and drugs to cover withdrawal; they were seen repeatedly by psychiatrists and social workers; their wives were counselled and if response to outpatient care was poor then the men were offered inpatient care in a specialist unit. After three hour assessments and initial counselling sessions, with their wives, those in the advice group were told that they were alcoholics, that they should aim at complete abstinence and that the responsibility was theirs. They were not seen again at the clinic. After 12 months there was no significant differences between the two groups in terms of drinking behaviour, subjective ratings, or social adjustment. The results of this study might be taken as meaning that a general practitioner can do a great deal to help patients with alcohol problems in a short time and with limited resources. Russell *et al.* (1979) have shown that general practitioners are effective in influencing patients' smoking behaviour and perhaps a similar study with alcohol patients would give equally encouraging results. Although many people with alcohol problems help themselves some, whose problems remit without specialist intervention attribute the change in their drinking habits to advice from their general practitioner.

Awareness of alcohol problems

One of the difficulties of dealing with alcohol problems is recognizing the problem in the first place and to help increase awareness about patients with alcohol problems it is useful to have a check list or at risk register (Table 12.5).

Table 12.5. *Alcohol problem check list*

Accidents work, home, road	**Occupations** catering trade publicans seamen
Alcoholic symptoms smelling of alcohol at consultation morning shakes memory losses withdrawal fits known alcoholic	**Physical symptoms** gastrointestinal upset – pain, vomiting, diarrhoea obesity, especially in men
Blood tests raised MCV particularly above 98 fl raised γ-glutamyl transpeptidase particularly above 50 iu/l	**Psychological symptoms** anxiety attempted suicide depression sexual problems
Family psychological problems in spouse psychological problems in children battering of wife or child	**Social** criminal offences financial problems work problems

Using a similar register, Wilkins (1974) in Manchester noted that during one year 5 per cent of his adult population consulted his practice with one of the at risk characteristics. Of the 546 at risk, 28 per cent were found either to be addicted or have problems associated with alcohol, compared to only 3 per cent of those without any characteristics that were problem drinkers.

Teenagers with drinking problems are seldom seen in surgery but may be known to the police for drinking under age or drinking driving offences. Housewives may take to drink because they feel lonely or unvalued and this may lead to sexual discord and family friction. In the elderly, drinking may be lost amongst the physical deterioration, intellectual failure and social isolation to which they are prone. Professional people may use their status to conceal their drinking and their intelligence to rationalize their trouble. Child abuse and non-accidental injury may be secondary to a drink problem in the parent. Members of the family are often the presenting sign of a drinking problem, but it is easily overlooked.

The physical complaints of heavy drinkers are frequently vague and without obvious cause: loss of appetite, stomach upsets, morning shakes, sweats, backache, memory lapses, and accidents. Symptoms of psychological difficulties include unhappiness, erratic moods, sexual failure, family conflicts, and confusion. Social inadequacy is shown by requests for a sickness certificate, under-achievement, work problems, money shortage, and trouble with the law.

The patient must be asked how much he drinks, when, how often and whether his drinking has ever caused problems. This needs to be done with sympathy and without embarrassment. Consumption is best elicited by taking a recent period and asking the patient in detail about each drinking occasion during that period. He should be asked to recall his leisure activities and his daily routine for each day to jog his memory. The last seven days suffice and it has been shown that in working populations those who claim their last seven days were atypically heavy tend to be reporting trivial differences (Sherlock 1982). If the patient resents such questions, why is this so? The drink may lessen his feelings of isolation and worthlessness and because he sees his problems as the cause and not the result of drinking, he may become aggressive or clamp down if this solution is threatened. The doctor should be direct and specific, challenging any vagueness, wariness, evasion, inconsistencies, bluff, or facile assurances. The patient will not give a true answer until he can be honest with himself. If he will talk the doctor should encourage any sign that he is beginning to examine himself. Progress depends on his confidence in the doctor and on the doctor's sensitivity as to when the patient is ready to accept some insight. When the subject is brought into the open most patients appreciate a frank discussion of the role alcohol plays in their life.

Records are the general practitioner's paper instrument for detecting problem drinkers and accurate records are important, especially in a group practice where the patient may consult with a different partner. Any suspicion of alcohol difficulty should be recorded in the notes.

Although several blood tests may be abnormal in regular drinkers they are not very reliable as screening tests as they are not particularly sensitive and lack power, having too high a false positive rate. Mean red cell volume (MCV) and γ-glutamyl transpeptidase (γ-GT) are the cheapest and most commonly available. Excluding men with other causes of raised values, 50 per cent who admit drinking over 56 units a week have a γ-GT more than 50 iu/l (false-positives 15 per cent) and 23–32 per cent have a MCV of over 98 (false-positives 5 per cent). For clinical purposes the tests have a use in supplementing self-report and in following problem drinkers (Chick *et al.* 1981).

General practitioner's advice

It is surprising how many people will adjust their drinking habits when it is pointed out to them the difficulties that drinking is causing. This is particularly so of those who have developed a medical problem that is instantly made worse by drinking and so reminds them constantly of the need to change their drinking habits. It is necessary to tell people what is a safe level of drinking. The Royal College of Psychiatrists (1979) recommended that the equivalent of four pints of beer for men and three pints for women was the uppermost acceptable daily intake. However, this was designed to stop an individual developing dependence or cirrhosis of the liver and damage may result from consumption of much smaller amounts. A more acceptable level may be the equivalent of two or three pints of beer two or three times a week. It is important to discover what harm the patient thinks results from drinking and whether that harm applies to him. Discussion of alcohol related harm can then be based on the patient's beliefs. Individuals need to be made aware of the health hazards of drinking since heavy drinkers are less aware of the consequences of drinking than light drinkers (OPCS 1980). It should also be pointed out that alcohol is an addictive drug and that anyone could, in given combinations of circumstances, become alcohol dependent.

Attention also needs to be paid to the benefits of reducing drinking rather than to the harm of continuing excessive consumption. One obvious benefit is the financial one. Others include better judgement and performance, safer driving, and less obesity. The benefits on personal characteristics and sexual performance may carry particular weight with some.

Although many people succeed in cutting down their drinking without any help, others do need help and the doctor should be willing to do this. The advice should be offered not only when requested but also whenever the opportunity presents in any consultation, especially if it can be related to the presenting medical problem. Literature is of supplementary value in reinforcing the advice and informing the patient. The Health Education Council has two leaflets: *Good health?* and *Facts about alcohol.*

Treatment

Although the patient has acquired a drinking habit which is damaging his personality, his family and social life and his health, habits are hard to change and the patient may be ambivalent about changing his drinking pattern. This ambivalence can be met by asking the patient to draw up a balance sheet of the good and bad consequences of his continued drinking, prompted by the doctor, and these can be discussed. Armed with such evidence the patient should set a realistic strategy for changing his lifestyle. It is best to aim for specific short-term goals at first, rather than long-term goals and general intentions. This allows the patient to concentrate on the short term and gain positive reinforcement from a sense of achievement. The advice of Alcoholics Anonymous to concentrate on one day at a time is a basic principle of self-control. Under pressure, it may be necessary to focus on one hour at a time. Short-term goals may be a week's abstinence, a night at the pub taking soft drinks or the ability to say no to a drink when offered. The long-term aim for heavy drinkers is to drink less and return to controlled social drinking is a realistic aim for a proportion of alcohol dependants.

For many heavy drinkers, drinking has become their predominant interest and to achieve their desired goal they may have to make major changes in their way of life. The patient will need help to look at impediments to change and alternatives to drinking. Impediments may be, for example, a job where drink is readily available, family stress with which the drinker cannot cope without alcohol, or the occurrence of withdrawal symptoms when he tries to stop drinking. The patient needs to look out for situations and feelings which trigger off drinking and work out new ways of coping with them. Anxiety as a trigger to drinking may be relieved by yoga or other appropriate relaxation training. If craving arises at lunchtime then an alteration of mental state and a change in environment may be achieved by going out for a walk, and going to a coffee bar rather than a pub. When the patient feels the urge to drink he can be taught to imagine the bad consequences of drinking heavily and the pleasant consequences of remaining sober. Many heavy drinkers are particularly influenced by social cues, such as the business lunch, and the problem drinker often reports that he does not have a ready answer when drink is offered. The problem drinker needs to be taught how to say no effectively and advised that to say no is not as difficult as it seems. Some people with drinking problems are unemployed and others are employed in occupations which have a high prevalence of drinking problems and patients may need help in finding new jobs or changing their employment. Sometimes more elaborate help, focused for example on tensions within the family, may be necessary. The more obvious mechanical and naive solutions should not be discounted as these often prove surprisingly effective. To help change their lifestyle patients can be asked to think of activities that they enjoy which do not involve drinking. Alternatives may become clearer if specific attention is paid to past triggers for drinking – for example the pre-match drink may be avoided by meeting at the ground.

The family will need help in supporting the problem drinker. The family may feel confused, bitter, and devalued and will welcome the chance of being understood and participating in the process of recovery.

The goal of intervention will depend on the extent of the patient's drinking problem. If the drinking is excessive but hitherto harm free, the doctor should advise about safe limits for drinking such as two or three pints two or three times a week. Some drinkers with established problems will return to moderate drinking. However, it seems that abstinence remains the preferred goal for those who are over 40, are seriously physically addicted, have evidence of physical damage or have tried controlled drinking without success. For younger people whose problem drinking has been detected at an early stage and who are not seriously addicted or damaged, modified drinking may be a more acceptable and feasible goal.

Whatever the agreed goals it is essential to review the patient's progress, to offer continuing help and support as well as advice on managing difficulties. A diary in which the patient makes a note of any drinks consumed, the time, their quantity, and the occasion, is a useful aid to self-audit. γ-GT, MCV, and blood alcohol can be useful means of monitoring progress and the results and their implications can be discussed with the patient. γ-GT activity returns rapidly to normal with abstention and may be misleading if measured 48 hours after the last drink. A subsequent rise of 50 per cent or more is strong evidence of resumption of heavy drinking. The MCV takes several weeks to return to normal after abstinence. In health alcohol is removed from the blood at a rate of about 15 mg per 100 ml/h. Detectable blood concentrations are present for over eight hours after three pints of beer in normal people. Metabolism is accelerated in heavy drinkers, whereas in patients with liver damage, concentrations may remain high for over 24 hours. Progress should be reviewed regularly over a year. The first six months of progress often give a good impression of longer-term prognosis.

Most patients will drink again whatever the original goal of treatment but this should not be regarded as a loss of all that has been achieved. It should be viewed as an opportunity for the patient to learn more about himself and the problem. Once the relapse has been openly discussed the patient can recognize strategies for preventing a further recurrence. The family often feels particularly threatened and confused by a relapse and will need extra support at this time.

Drugs

Drugs have very little place in the long-term management of alcohol problems. They may be needed to help withdrawal symptoms for someone who is physically dependent on alcohol and this can sometimes be achieved at home if the patient is willing to stay off work for five days and has a reasonably supportive family. An initial starting dose of diazepam 5 mg four times a day, reducing over 5–7 days and then stopping, is one regime. Chlormethiazole starting off at 2–3 capsules four times a day and reducing over 5–7 days is another regime. With chlormethiazole dependence is a danger if treatment is prolonged. The dose prescribed and the rate of reduction should be related to the clinical state of the patient but tranquillizers should not be mixed with alcohol and should not be continued beyond one week. There is no point in changing one drug, alcohol, for another drug, tranquillizer.

Disulfiram (200 mg daily) or citrated calcium carbimide (100 mg daily) can be used to sensitize the body to alcohol, causing flushing, headache, palpitations, nausea, faintness, and collapse when alcohol is taken. The reaction may be severe and fatal and those with established heart disease and those who are suicidal should not take these drugs. They have a small role to play although some patients find them useful.

Referral

The majority of heavy drinkers and patients with alcohol problems can be helped by their general practitioner with support from other members of the primary health care team, including health visitor, social worker, and psychiatric nurse. However, there are going to be some patients whose care the general practitioner wishes or needs to share, particularly those who are severely dependent on alcohol, those who lack a supportive family, those with a severe underlying neurosis or psychosis, and those for whom general practitioner care has previously failed. When referral takes place it is important to maintain a relationship with the patient and to give a further appointment after the initial referral to discuss what took place.

Alcoholics Anonymous provides a very supportive self-help group. It asks members to acknowledge that they are alcoholic and that abstinence is the only way to recovery. Some are deterred by its quasi-religious undertones, but there is no requirement to worship or accept religion. It may be necessary to shop around before finding a group that suits a particular personality. The general practitioner could get to know a few AA members personally and refer his patients to them. Al-anon and Al-alteen provide support for respectively the spouses and teenage children of alcoholics.

Many areas have local councils on alcoholism which are voluntary agencies whose responsibilities include co-ordinating available services and which provide counselling and advice to problem drinkers and their families.

Alcoholism treatment units are usually associated with psychiatric units, have facilities for detoxification and offer a range of approaches for treatment. Some units use a psychoanalytical approach with emphasis on group work whereas other use more of a behaviourist approach; some operate mostly in the psychiatric hospital whereas other run more of their service in the community; some run detoxification and treatment as an integrated service whereas others keep the detoxification period separate from the treatment programme. It may be, therefore, that the service offered will not suit the needs of the individual who is having problems with alcohol and this can create problems for the general practitioner. The patient who admits he has a problem but who does not consider that it is a psychiatric problem or does not like his first experience of group therapy may be helped by a voluntary counselling service if one is operated by the local council on alcoholism. Alternatively, if he has physical complications of alcohol abuse, referral to the liver clinic will be helpful because the medical social worker in the liver clinic is usually experienced in counselling the person with drinking problems.

Hostels are provided by some local authorities and by voluntary bodies. They cater principally but not exclusively for homeless alcoholics and also provide a halfway house for alcoholics discharged from hospital and for habitual drunken offenders discharged from prison.

In summary, the role of the general practitioner in relation to drinking is to:

be aware of drink related problems
offer advice when requested
seek opportunity to offer advice in any consultation
advise on how to cut down or stop drinking
give support to the family
supplement advice with appropriate literature
follow-up attempts to reduce drinking

The advice offered should include:

reference to presenting problem when possible
information about the safe level of drinking
information about the health and personal hazards of excessive drinking
information about the nature and meaning of dependence
emphasis on the benefit of reducing drinking
plan for a short-term goal
ways to cope with the difficulties after reducing drinking
warning of the dangers of relapse
explanation of the need for follow-up.

ALCOHOL AND WORK

Many general practitioners work in occupational health and there are several reasons why a response to alcohol problems at work may be productive. Firstly, most people with alcohol problems are employed and those problems often first become apparent at work. Secondly, certain occupations are known to be associated with an increased prevalence of alcohol problems. Thirdly, the costs to employers of alcohol abuse are considerable. Fourthly, people whose livelihood is at stake are likely to be strongly motivated to overcome their problems.

Programmes at work have three prongs: prevention, case identification, and referral or counselling. Employers and unions must work together and the programme must apply to both blue- and white-collar workers. Programmes need to be based on a written policy which must be made known so that everybody in the company knows that it exists. The booklet, *The problem drinker at work*, produced by the Health and Safety Executive (1981) gives detailed suggestions on what such a policy should include. Preventive measures will include not only education but also policies on drinking in the workplace. The main part of most programmes is the detection of problem drinkers. Important signs to look out for are:

frequent lateness
repeated brief periods of absence
minor accidents on the job
drinking at work
changes of mood
borrowing money
lowering of quality of work
reducing quantity of work
medical certificates for absence including diagnoses like gastro-enteritis, dyspepsia, and nervous debility

One approach at work is for supervisors to report all workers whose performance deteriorates and then for a suitably trained colleague to find out which of them have alcohol problems; some two-thirds probably will. They can then be referred to the Works' doctor who may be in a position to help them.

POLITICS OF ALCOHOL

Since the more alcohol a group consumes the more alcohol-associated damage results, the answer to the prevention of alcohol problems may lie less with individual health workers and more with politicians. There are a number of influences on alcohol consumption.

Price

Figure 12.6 shows the price relative to income per litre of absolute alcohol consumed in the United Kingdom during the period 1949–1979, the percentage consumer spending on alcoholic drink, and litres of alcohol consumed. As the relative price of alcohol has fallen by over 50 per cent, alcohol consumption has increased accordingly.

A report by HM Treasury (1980) suggests that for a 1 per cent rise in its relative price, consumer demand for beer might be expected to fall by about ¼ per cent, for spirits 1½ per cent, and for wine 1 per cent. However, a 1 per cent rise in real incomes might be expected to increase consumer demand for beer by about ¾ per cent, for spirits 2¼ per cent, and wine 2½ per cent. This suggests that over the years consumption of beer has been less sensitive to changes in price and income than wine and spirits and that consumption of alcoholic drinks is less sensitive to rises in prices than to rises in disposable incomes. Figure 12.6 also shows that the percentage of consumer spending on alcoholic drink has increased from 6 per cent in 1960 to just under 8 per cent in 1979.

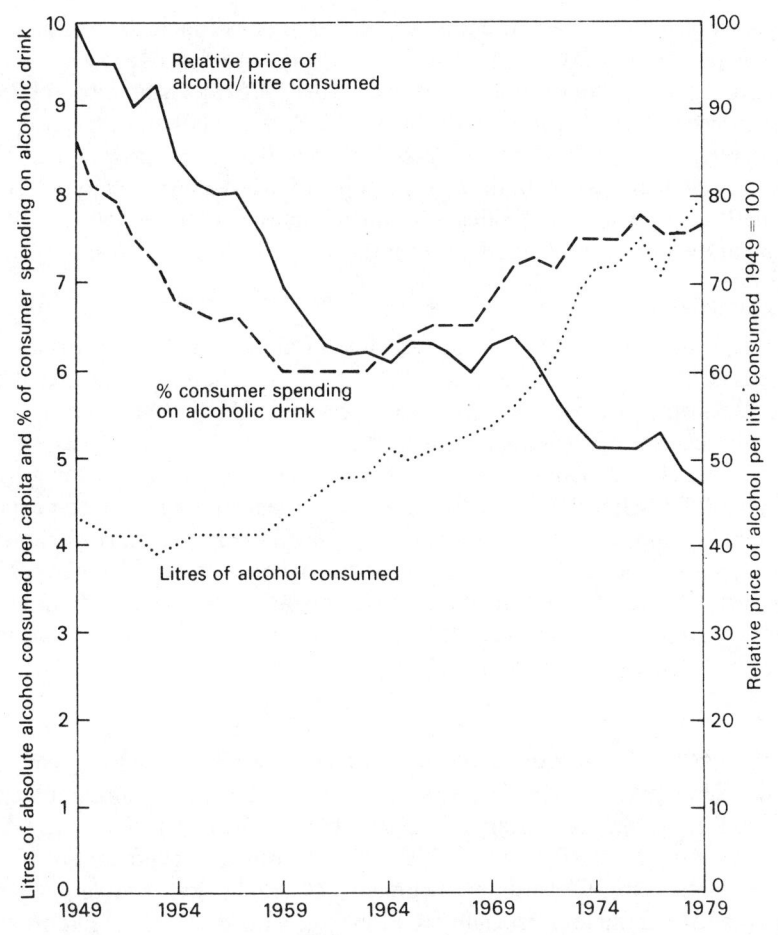

Fig. 12.6. The relative price of alcohol in Britain 1949-1979. (From Office of Health Economics (1981).)

However, there are strong political and economic objections to reducing the demand for alcohol. The excise duties and VAT on alcoholic drinks are estimated to have raised £4000 million in 1980-81, 6 per cent of central government revenue. Production of alcoholic drinks accounts for just over 2 per cent of total UK industrial activity; some 700 000 jobs are dependent on the alcohol industry and total exports of alcoholic drinks in 1980 amounted to £880 million, 1.9 per cent of the value of total exports (DHSS 1981).

Advertising

The drink trade spends about £100 million a year on advertising and the example of vodka which over 20 years has changed from being an almost unknown drink in Britain to one as popular as gin has convinced many people of the power of advertising. British Columbia introduced a total ban on advertising of alcohol in 1972 (Smart and Cutler 1976) and Manitoba applied a ban on beer advertising in 1974 (Ogborne and Smart 1980) and for both cases there were no dramatic changes in alcohol consumption. Interpretation of these results is difficult since in both cases the populations were exposed to the media of the United States and other Canadian States and there was a lack of community and mass media support for the ban.

Licensing laws

Although the total number of outlets to retail or supply alcoholic drinks has increased by 29 per cent between 1945 and 1980, relative to the size of the population the increase has only been 8 per cent (DHSS 1981). Scotland has recently relaxed its licensing laws, extending evening hours on weekdays from 10 p.m. to 11 p.m. from December 1976 and allowing Sunday opening from October 1977. After the later closing there was a reduction in the average speed of drinking and for younger women a slight increase in overall consumption. After Sunday opening there was a 10 per cent increase in overall consumption for men aged 18–45 and this increase was higher for those already drinking heavily. After Sunday opening there was no change in older men's or women's consumption (Knight and Wilson 1980).

Health education

So far, health education about alcohol problems has not succeeded in reducing these problems. In 1976 the Scottish Health Education Unit mounted a national campaign on alcoholism (Plant *et al.* 1979). The campaign used television and press advertising and its main aim was to encourage people with problems to come forward for treatment. Although more people did come forward for treatment, after eight months the general level of public knowledge had not significantly increased and patterns of alcohol consumption had not changed. Evaluations of the Health Education Council campaign in the North East of England have shown no change in drinking behaviour but a small change in attitudes towards drink and drunkenness (Cust 1980).

While a considerable amount may be known about the broad social conditions in which alcohol harm can be minimized, relatively little is known about how attitudes to drinking once formed are changed or the extent to which such attitudinal changes may cause desired behavioural changes. Health education may well be more effectively undertaken at an individual level, emphasizing the importance of general practitioners in relation to their patients.

It has been said that an alcoholic is someone who drinks more than his doctor. Doctors have a mortality from liver cirrhosis three times the national average and there is a lot more that we could do in altering our own drinking behaviour and helping our colleagues with drink-related problems. Doctors' responses to the knowledge of the health risks associated with cigarette smoking sets an important precedent.

REFERENCES

Aitken, P. P. and Leathar, D. S. (1981). *Adults' attitudes towards drinking and smoking among young people in Scotland.* HMSO, London.

Armor, D. J. (1980). The Rand Reports and the analysis of relapse. In *Alcoholism treatment in transition* (ed. G. Edwards and M. Grant) pp. 81–94. Croom Helm, London.

Bruun, K., Edwards, G., Lumio, M., Makela, K., Pan, L., Popham, R. E., Room, R., Schmidt, W., Skog, O-J., Sulkunen, P., and Osterberg, E. (1975). *Alcohol control policies in public health perspective.* Finnish Foundation for Alcohol Studies, Helsinki.

Cartwright, A. K. J., Shaw, S. J., and Spratley, T. A. (1978). Relationships between per capita consumption, drinking patterns and alcohol related problems in a population sample, 1965–1974. *Br. J. Addict.* 73, 237–46.

Central Statistical Office (1981). *Social Trends 12.* HMSO, London.

Chick, J. and Duffy, D. C. (1980). The developmental ordering of symptoms in the alcohol dependence syndrome. In *Aspects of Alcohol and Drug Dependence* (ed. J. S. Madden, R. Walker, and W. H. Kenyon) pp. 54–59. Pitman Medical, Tunbridge Wells.

——, Kreitman, N., and Plant, M. (1981). Mean cell volume and gamma-glutamyl-transpeptidase as markers of drinking in working men. *Lancet* i, 1249–51.

Cust, G. (1980). Health education about alcohol in the Tyne Tees area. In *Aspects of alcohol and drug dependence* (ed. J. S. Madden, R. Walker, and W. H. Kenyon). Pitman Medical, Tunbridge Wells.

Davies, J. and Stacey, N. (1972). *Teenagers and alcohol.* HMSO, London.

Department of the Environment (1976). *Drinking and driving. Report of a Departmental Committee (Blennerhasset).* HMSO, London.

Department of Health and Social Security (1981). *Drinking sensibly.* HMSO, London.

Edwards, G., Orford, J.,Egert S., Guthrie, S., Hawkes, A., Hensman, C., Mitcheson, M., Oppenheimer, E., and Taylor, C. (1977). Alcoholism: a controlled trial of 'treatment' and 'advice'. *J. Stud. Alcohol* 38, 1004–31.

Emrick, C. D. (1975). A Review of psychologically oriented treatments of alcoholism. *J. Stud. Alcohol.* 36, 88–108.

Harlap, S. and Shiono, P. H. (1980). Alcohol, smoking and incidence of spontaneous abortions in the first and second trimester. *Lancet* i, 173–6.

Hawton, K., Fagg, J., Marsack, P. and Wells, P. (1982). Deliberate self-poisoning and self-injury in the Oxford area 1972–1980. *Social Psychiat.* in press.

Health and Safety Executive (1981). *The problem drinker at work.* HMSO, London.

HM Treasury (1980). *Macroeconomic model equation and variable listing.* London.

Jahoda, G. and Cramond, J. (1972). *Children and alcohol.* HMSO, London.

Klatsky, A. L., Friedman, G. D., and Siegelaub, A. B. (1981). Alcohol and mortality. *Ann. intern. Med.* 95, 139–45.

Knight, I. and Wilson, P. (1980). *Scottish licensing laws.* HMSO, London.

Kozarevic, D. J., McGee, D., Vojvodic, N., Racic, Z., Dawber, T., Gordon, T., and Zukel, W. (1980). Frequency of alcohol consumption and morbidity and mortality. *Lancet* i, 613-16.

Observer, and Maxwell, M. A. (1959). A study of absenteeism, accidents and sickness payments in problem drinkers in one industry. *Q. J. Stud. Alcohol* **20**, 302-12.

O'Connor, J. (1978). *The young drinkers*. Tavistock, London.

Ogborne, A. C. and Smart, R. G. (1980). Will restrictions on alcohol advertising reduce alcohol consumption? *Br. J. Addict.* **75**, 293-6.

Office of Health Economics (1981). *Alcohol. Reducing the harm*. London.

OPCS (1979). *Morbidity statistics from general practice 1971-2*. Studies on Medical and Population Subjects No. 36. HMSO, London.

—— (1980). *General Household Survey 1978*. Series GHS No. 8, HMSO, London.

Pequinot, G., Tuyna, A. J., and Berta, J. L. (1978). Ascitic cirrhosis in relation to alcohol consumption. *Int. J. Epidemiol.* **7**, 113-20.

Plant, M. A. (1979). *Drinking careers*. Tavistock, London.

—— (1981). Risk factors in employment. In *Alcohol problems in employment* (ed. B. D. F. Hore and M. A. Plant) pp. 18-34. Croom Helm, London.

——, Peck, D. F., and Stuart, R. (1982). Self-reported drinking habits and alcohol related consequences among a cohort of Scottish teenagers. *Br. J. Addict.* **77**, 75-90.

——, Pirie, F., and Kreitman, N. (1979). Evaluation of the Scottish Health Education Unit's 1976 campaign on alcoholism. *Social Psychiat.* **14**, 11-24.

Polich, J. M. (1980). Patterns of remission in alcoholism. In *Alcoholism treatment in transition* (ed. G. Edwards and M. Grant) pp. 95-112. Croom Helm, London.

Producktschap voor Gedistilleerde Dranken (1981). *Consumption of alcoholic beverages throughout the world*. Shiedam.

Royal College of Psychiatrists (1979). *Alcohol and alcoholism*. Tavistock, London.

Russell, M. A. H., Wilson, C., Taylor, C., and Baker, C. D. (1979). Effect of general practitioners' advice against smoking. *Br. med. J.* ii, 231-5.

Saunders, J. B., Beevers, D. S., and Paton, A. (1981*a*). Alcohol induced hypertension. *Lancet* ii, 653-6.

——, Davis, M., and Williams, R. (1981*b*). Do women develop alcoholic liver disease more readily than men? *Br. med. J.* **282**, 1140-3.

Schmidt, W. (1977). Cirrhosis and alcohol consumption: an epidemiological perspective. In *Alcholism: new knowledge and new responses* (ed. G. Edwards and M. Grant) pp. 15-47. Croom Helm, London.

Shaw, S. (1980). Causes of increasing drinking problems amongst women. In *Camberwell Council on alcoholism. Women and alcohol,* pp. 1-40. Tavistock, London.

Sherlock, S. (ed.) (1982). Alcohol and disease. *Br. med. Bull.* **38**, 3-108.

Smart, R. J. and Cutler, R. E. (1976). The alcohol advertising ban in British Columbia: problems and effects on beverage consumption. *Br. J. Addict.* **71**, 13-21.

Snyder, C. R. (1958). *Alcohol and the Jews*. Rutgers Center of Alcohol Studies, New Jersey.

Spring, J. A. and Buss, D. H. (1977). Three centuries of alcohol in the British diet. *Nature,* Lond. **270**, 567-72.

Vaillant, G. E. (1980). The doctor's dilemma. In *Alcoholism treatment in transition* (ed. G. Edwards and M. Grant) pp. 13-31. Croom Helm, London.

World Health Organization (1980). Problems related to alcohol consumption. Technical Report Series 650. Geneva.

Wilkins, R. H. (1974). *The hidden alcoholic in general practice.* Elek Science, London.

Wilson, P. (1980*a*). Drinking habit in the United Kingdom. *Population Trends* 22, 14–18.

—— (1980*b*). *Drinking in England and Wales* HMSO, London.

13 Mental illness

I. Gordon Lennox

THE NATURE OF THE PROBLEM

Symptoms of mental ill health are surprisingly common in family practice: the major difficulty is in knowing what they mean. General practitioners have long known that psychological symptoms and psychiatric illness present one of the most difficult problems in medical care. Symptoms of psychological distress are common in the population at large and psychiatric illness, despite increased pharmaceutical resources, remains a major problem. Surveys in the community of non-presenting persons (they can hardly be called patients) reveal an undiagnosed and hence untreated population. Those who present to the doctor are mostly dealt with at the GP level and few, some 5%, reach specialist care. In a situation in which 15% of women in Camberwell have clearly defined formal depression (Brown and Harris 1978) the need to look for ways of preventing this problem needs careful consideration and trial.

In the general practice setting Fry (1966) has shown some 12% of all consultation are for emotional disorder, and a general practitioner with a practice of 2500 persons can expect to see 200 patients per annum with emotional disorders (RCGP 1970). Other surveys show that 10–29 per cent of patients can be expected to present with psychiatric disorder each year (Shepherd *et al.* 1966). Goldberg and Blackwell (1970) report a study which allowed a psychiatrist to screen each patient after the GP consultation, albeit with a highly psychiatrically trained and orientated general practitioner. Screening discovered the general practitioner 'missed' one-third of the total cases.

The figures mentioned above are all dependent on definition and in practice this is difficult. The general practitioner is in a particularly difficult situation: he has large numbers of consultations of short duration – not the best setting for psychiatric history taking: he has limited experience of the more serious psychiatric illnesses, seeing them only a few times per annum: he has great experience of drugs and their use, little experience of psychological methods and a healthy scepticism of the finer points of psychoanalytic theory. This leads naturally to an early diagnosis of illness and of early prescription. He works in a disease-orientated model of illness, often regarding 'non-disease' presentation as a soft area requiring low investment, and regarding 'non-medical' treatment as of low value (Table 13.1).

Much effort has gone into accurate operational definitions of psychiatric illness: it is often considered that while this has obvious importance in research,

Table 13.1. *Models of illness*

Medical model	Social model
Affects individual alone, e.g. gene	Affects the family relationships, e.g. marriage
Defined pathological process, e.g. biochemical change	Disturbed functioning in the group, e.g. delinquency
One diagnosis	Multiple factors
Aetiology usually single	Causes usually many
Single treatment, drug	Multiple therapies, usually together

it has less relevance to ordinary practice: in fact, it is in ordinary practice that accurate diagnosis in psychiatry is most important. For example, reactive depression responds much less well to tricyclic antidepressants than endogenous depression: if personality disorders are not recognized the prescription of hypnotics can easily lead to addiction: a missed depression is often a successful suicide.

On the other hand, over-investment in a medical or disease-orientated model of illness can lead to a narrow and unproductive approach to the prevention of mental illness. The central role of the general practitioner as a family doctor enables him to effect continuity of care, often over long periods. His ability to maintain contact by easy access, his opportunity to make a therapeutic relationship, his open door to any complaint in the person or the family, in the body or the mind, enables him to both know the patient and the setting, and enables him, to a degree, to influence both. A narrow choice of disease as the interest of medicine can blind the doctor to the wider aspects of aetiology of mental disorders and close his eyes to the major opportunities that exist to influence his patient prior to the formation of the disease.

Thus the model of psychiatric illness in general practice needs to be broad and if possible inclusive (Fig. 13.2): the idea that depression is a function of depleted brain amines may be true but is a partial truth and often an unhelpful one. Equally the idea that depression is a function of the breakdown of society may be true, but less than helpful. Given that each personality is different one might assume that personality is the interaction of gene and environment, of experiences, good and bad that the individual has gone through. On this person, now established with traits and temperament learnt from experience comes a stress, usually identified as exogenous. This must react with factors within the personality, the aspirations, goals, drives of the individual to produce a reaction. The nature of this reaction is as infinitely variable as there are people, but must be in two types – a coping reaction in which the pressure is absorbed in a functional way or breakdown reaction in which resources within the person prove inadequate or a learnt pattern of dysfunctional behaviour is activated. It is at this point that the patient presents to the doctor wanting help, so called illness behaviour.

210 *Mental illness*

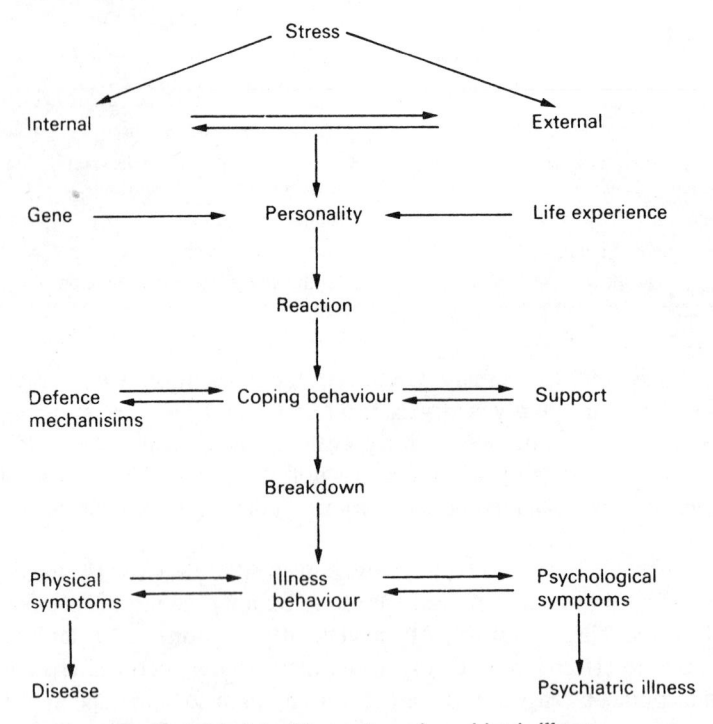

Fig. 13.1. Model of formation of psychiatric illness.

In some presentations, e.g. recurrent endogenous depression, it is perfectly valid to consider the gene as determinative of the reaction: occasionally the illness may be without reactive features, but usually there has been a precipating factor and in all cases the disease occurs within a whole person: social, family, occupational factors must always be taken into consideration both in the analysis of causation and therapy.

A broad social model of disease is as valuable to the family doctor as his pharmacopeia. Within this broad framework there is room to share the patient with other help-giving professionals, each bringing new insights and view points. The hallmark of the mature general practitioner is his network of intra-professional relationships and his skill in maintaining them: the mark of the amateur is the belief that he can do it all by himself, usually with drugs.

The genetic element
Over the past 20 years great effort has been expended on examining the genetic element in psychiatric illness: it has traditionally been held to be high but actual risk rates have only recently been obtained and only now are we able to inform the patient or his relatives of the risk their children run. There is no general awareness of the topic either by doctors or the general public and requests for genetic counselling are rare, except in adoption cases. It is, of course, always

impossible to state what will happen to any one individual no matter what the family background: risk, not certainty, is the coinage of the consultation. Whatever the genetic background, environment plays a most important role even in strongly genetically determined cases.

The first question to determine accurately is the proband's illness: this may be difficult. Without a clear diagnosis made in standard psychiatric terminology no opinion can be made. The use of terms across the Atlantic is particularly fraught. Secondly, the background of the problem must be sought, e.g. if both grandparents were institutionalized schizophrenics and the proband suffers the same condition, then the risks to the offspring must be high. Thirdly, if the illness was severe, occurred early in life, recurred, had few reactive features, then the risk is probably higher.

In general a distinction can be made between the neuroses and the psychoses. The neuroses have a low genetic element: many studies have found none. Yet twin studies have shown increased correlation of neuroticism in the specialized definition. Anxiety as a trait is well established in twin studies: for a good review see Murray and Reveley (1981).

The psychoses have a markedly greater genetic element. Schizophrenia has been carefully studied and split-twin studies of monozygous twins show higher correlation than in dizygous twins. While there is much argument about the mode of inheritance, polygenic or mongenic, most writers agree that genetic influence is strong but modified by environment. In the affective psychoses, bipolar, manic plus depressive disorder, and unipolar, usually depressive illness, the evidence for the gene is high. Manic depressive psychosis is inherited by a single autosomal dominant: bipolar disease has higher penetration than unipolar.

Clearly to prevent these serious disorders genetic counselling has a part to play (Kay 1978).

Factors in childbirth and childhood

The child, the product of its parents' genes, is nurtured by its mother until parturition, a process liable to many problems. Brain damage commonly occurs by asphyxia or trauma which may predispose to later illness. However, the major examined factor has been the effect of the first few days of mother child interaction and its effect on the subsequent relationship. Bonding or attachment (Bowlby 1977) is the term used to describe that close intimate relationship of affection in which mother and child regard each other. Failure of bonding, has been held to produce disorders as various as delinquency, depression, and affectionless psychopathy. The subject is well reviewed by Rutter (1972) and although the basic conclusions of Bowlby's original studies, that the poor quality of care provided for children in institutions could be detrimental is accepted, the further expansions of the theory have been well beyond proof. That every child who has failed to have a satisfactory experience of breast-feeding is doomed for life is clearly untrue (Rutter 1980).

Mental illness

It is generally true that affectionless homes tend to breed delinquency, psychopathy, and, on occasion, emotional dwarfism. Also accepted are age-specific factors in the character of the deprivation. Not so clear is the proposition that there is a distinction between the failure to create a bond leading to psychopathy and the rupture of a bond leading always to distress in the short term but without long-term damage if the bond was firm before and renewed afterwards. Thus the enormous pressure of well-bonded middle-class mothers to attend their children during tonsillectomy has little relation to lasting mental ill health. Rather the mother who lacks any desire to share her child's experience needs help and encouragement to attend. Clearly this is important in cases of family breakdown: the child should go to the bonded parent, be it mother or father: children should be taken into care as infrequently as possible and for as short a time as possible. The danger of staying at home with the risk of nonaccidental injury may be much greater than the risk of ruptured bonding. Unfortunately, much of the work on maternal deprivation has been non-specific: we need to know in much more detail what is lost in bonding failure. Bowlby said in 1951 that 'mother love in infancy and childhood is as important for mental health as are vitamins and proteins for physical health'. We need to know more of the specific effect of each deficiency.

PRIMARY PREVENTION

The theory is attractively simple: define a disease, ascertain its cause, collect the population on which the cause falls, prevent the cause, and prevent the disease. The disease is ended, or to use a word applicable to the almost evangelical attitude that prevention produces, conquered. Mental ill health has, unfortunately, problems in each of these steps. The definition of disease in mental illness is difficult as the range of both symptoms and their severity varies in smooth progression from the normal to the diseased individual. Who is to say when distress at the loss of a loved one ceases to be a normal bereavement reaction and becomes morbid grief or depression? Although each end of the spectrum is clear, the middle ground defies simple definition. Clear categories of disease applied for example to general practitioners' surgeries, fails to classify a considerable proportion of cases: equally there is no psychiatrist who has not wrestled to cram his patients into the Procrustean bed of the glossary. The question 'What is a case?' remains unanswered. If the disease is difficult to define the collection of a population suffering from it becomes difficult, and without that population who can investigate aetiology? Where should the 'cases' be sought – in the hospital bed, or the outpatient department or in the Health Centre or in the community whether they are complaining or not?

Aetiology in mental illness appears to be almost always multifactorial. Single cases of genetic nature acting without the influence of environment, are unusual outside of mental handicap. Taking the affective disorder, depressive type, as an example, the gene may well be important but the timing of the disease seems to be brought about by a combination of vulnerability factors, that is to say past life experience, and current loss events. But people vary and what to one person may be too much, may be weathered by another. Life has its meaning, but not the same to each one, thus the personal, idiosyncratic factor must be allowed for in the aetiology of the illness.

When this complex process has been gone through, far from ending with a clear diagnosis, the formulation is often a mixture of various factors in various strengths. Crystal-clear simplicity in psychiatry is often diagnostic poverty.

Much has been made in recent years of the concept of mental health and the associated process of promoting it. Protagonists seem to contemplate a new state of the human organism when by education, (and often analysis), with conflicts resolved and stresses eliminated, each will become the psychological equivalent of the pentathlete, capable of doing all things well. The unlikeliness of this golden age has failed to prevent the outpouring of mainly dollars in the search. 'Walk In' mental health facilities with free psychotherapy are highly desirable: they meet human need, may well resolve pain, occasionally pick up mental illness at an early stage. But like Marriage Guidance and Samaritans, proof that they prevent disease is hard to come by. Most writers on the topic assume a psychological orientation that understands all mental illness in terms of a developmental theory: while this is far from proven it seems clearer that the presentation of mental illness is often dictated by the family rather than the family being the primary aetiology. While we go mad within the family, does the family drive us mad? Probably not, and to the extent to which it does, it is personal reaction that determines the illness. While not fully proven, some preventive programmes appear to be worthwhile if not for their preventive aspect at least for their orientation to good care. Good fostering, as distinct from bad fostering, the value judgements can only be made in terms of one or other psychodynamic theory, appears to be more humane and, therefore, desirable. The effort put into the prevention of child abuse by helping the abusing family has the appearance of being better social policy than simple sequestration of the child. It is clearly good that voluntary organizations such as Alcoholics Anonymous and Samaritans exist, they deserve wholehearted medical support, but it has proved impossible to show that they alter either mortality or morbidity rates for alcoholism or suicide.

SECONDARY PREVENTION

While primary prevention often seems remote to the family doctor, secondary prevention is the stuff of daily life. Enabling patients to regain normal functioning after illness, the prevention of relapse, reducing the severity of the illness by early diagnosis and the provision of effective treatment where available, especially being careful not to increase illness or disablement by iatrogenic disaster, this is the daily event. Interest must be focused on how and when to intervene to produce the best therapeutic result. The family doctor will always

214 Mental illness

Table 13.2. *Vulnerability factors in depression*

In women (Brown *et al.* 1977; Roy 1978)
1. Parental loss before 17, especially loss of mother before 11
2. Three or more children aged 14 or less at home
3. Poor, non-confiding marital relationship
4. Lack of full or part-time employment

In men (Roy 1981)
1. Parental loss before 17 years of age
2. Poor marriage
3. Unemployment

be aware that some patients are more vulnerable than others: some of these factors are now clear (Table 13.2).

INTERVENTION

When the patient presents to the family doctor there is a repertoire of responses available: no one method excludes another and consideration of the alternative strategies reveals the poverty of the 'diagnosis–automatic prescription' policy.

Consultation

Often the patient orientation in the consultation is one of helplessness. In the face of their anxiety or depression there is a need to find a father-figure who will take over responsibility for the illness. Paradoxically this response tends to occur more often in the minor illness and is often the first clue to a dependent personality. Careful history taking not only establishes both diagnosis and severity of the illness: it also enables a therapeutic alliance to be set up in which the role expectation of both doctor and patient can be defined. Any orientation to self-help and self-sufficiency and a clear limitation of the medical role can be helpful: failure to do this while implying omniscience and infallibility seems doomed to failure.

It is unusual to be able to understand the patient's complaint without help from other members of the family: people live in groups and an insight from some other member of the patient's group is usually essential. It is useless to speed over this phase: rarely unless suicidal risk is paramount does the whole history need to be taken at one interview: an appointment for half an hour tomorrow with the spouse can lead to a completely fresh picture. Often the distress of one day is markedly changed by the next and the necessity for biochemical treatment lost. Equally the immobility of say endogenous depression with psychomotor retardation, unchanged from day to day may become apparent. A second interview, with less pressure, perhaps outside the usual booked appointments, allows time for the patient to relax and reveal the meaning of the illness, without which prevention of recurrence is unlikely. The interval between the interviews can be used for self completion of questionnaires, e.g. the Beck depressive inventory. The result is often surprising, revealing a greater depth of depression than was thought at first sight. At each interview, thought should be given to suicidal risk as suicide is almost the only cause of death in psychiatric illness. The doctor need have no fear that discussion of suicidal feelings will either introduce the ideas into the patient's mind or induce the act. Experience suggests the reverse, most patients are grateful for the chance to discuss these feelings, not often shared with relatives and at least for a while, ventilation of the subject reduces psychic tension. However, in the presence of severe depression denial of suicidal intent by the patient should not be relied on.

History taken, a pause for reflection is worthwhile: has the patient communicated anything else, particularly extra- or non-verbally. Does the patient make the doctor feel anxious, depressed, or psychotic? It is worthwhile asking if the patient is inducing negative feelings in the doctor – does the doctor feel he hates the patient? This occasional event, if recognized, can avoid many excesses of therapy and sometimes keep these patients safe. Physical examination may be rewarding, indeed mandatory in the presence of loss of weight. The doctor's previous experience of the patient may suggest organic aetiology, e.g. a secondary brain tumour; occasionally biochemical investigation or chest X-ray may be indicated.

In psychiatry the diagnosis is made, not in the usual single term of general medicine, but in the formulation. Just as many diagnoses have by the nature of medicine to be provisional, so the formulation should be tentative: it must include all the relevant features.

Mrs Jones, a 39-year old who was widowed a year ago, has felt depressed for four months: she has lost one stone in weight, wakes regularly at 4 a.m. and has clear suicidal ideation. In the past she has had moderate to severe depression that responded to tricyclic antidepressives. She lives alone, is unemployed, and was recently noted to smell of alcohol in a morning surgery.

The formulation is not a single word, it is not concise: but it is a better description of the patient's predicament than the word 'depressed'.

Following the consultation and formulation there begins the process of therapy option.

Crisis intervention

Caplan (1961) defined crisis as a failure of coping with transient situational difficulties. The state often includes a critical role transition, e.g. redundancy at work. Clearly these crises occur around life events.

In the first phase of therapy the therapist accepts the responsibility for the patient, takes over the immediate tasks and removes the patient from the maximal stress. By a problem-solving approach the situation is defined, alternative solutions are assessed, one chosen, and with support, a logical sequence of behavioural steps is gone through to solve the problem. The approach is essentially practical: it can appeal to those who do not work with psychodynamic insights and has been evaluated as effective. The subject has been well reviewed by Bancroft (1979).

An approach that has much in common is the coping model of Lazarus (1966). Few professionals in medicine or social work argue any more about which approach is best: a benign eclecticism appears to rule and elements of each are combined. There is tentative evidence that reference to a regional poisoning treatment centre may reduce the recurrence rate in para-suicide to one-third of those admitted as against those not admitted. Psychiatric help appears to be more effective at the time of crisis and crisis intervention is the optimal technique at this time.

Psychotherapy

The response of most family doctors to the suggestion that the patient needs psychotherapy is negative. It would appear that the treatment is long, lasting years rather than months, takes several hours per week, is private and expensive, and not available on the National Health Service: finally it is the field of the dedicated specialist analyst and his alone. Few stereotypes could be further from the truth: in the last 20 years psychotherapy, stimulated by the changes induced by the rapid development of behaviour therapy, has expanded into numerous fields. Perhaps the major change has been into family and group therapy with the discovery of high effectiveness to low time investment. As the techniques have become defined the family doctor is in an increasingly better position to use them. While training is clearly important, support is even more so and many will find that like M. Jourdain who had been talking prose for 40 years, they have being doing unexamined brief psychotherapy all their professional lives. The interest in the consultation in general practice, a byproduct of the trainee year, has produced literature with distinct parallels to the psychotherapeutic field.

Far from psychotherapy being an alien field, general practitioners have moved easily into it. Teaching in the past has clearly been inadequate and recent teaching is only marginally better. A group of general practitioners presenting problems with a psychodynamically trained leader, would seem the optimal way to learning (Balint 1964). Some patients need specialist help, usually to be obtained via the psychiatrist or the psychologist, but they will always be the minority. The major load of supportive psychotherapy will always be done by the family doctor be it so named or not. The topic is well discussed by Bloch (1979b, Chapter 9). This inexpensive but invaluable handbook deserves a place on each general practitioner's desk.

Psychotherapy—individual

While much informal supportive psychotherapy is possible in the practice setting, and many conditions can be dealth with in this treatment module, some conditions require a more formal approach and a fully trained therapist – medical or lay. The major therapeutic factor in the interaction of therapist and patient is the personality of the therapist: in this sense the therapist uses himself. This is well described by Storr (1979), an excellent outline of the psychotherapeutic process.

Psychotherapy—group

Groups can be found in many settings, from the mental hospital, often under the aegis of a therapeutic community, to the Outpatient Department and the Day Hospital, and out into the general community organized by the social work department, or the family doctor. Given that the basic training and support is available, each of these therapy settings is suitable for group work. It is difficult to deliniate which problem or better which patient is suitable: much depends on the orientation of the group leader/therapist (Bloch 1981).

Family therapy

The family doctor is of all health-care practitioners, ideally placed for this type of therapy. A variety of models exists enabling the therapist to suit his own style. In essence, the central concept is to see the family as the patient, rather than one individual in it. Each member has to accept his or her responsibility for the problem and to bring his or her resources to the solution. The therapist's role is like the conductor of an orchestra – far from deciding how the family will resolve its difficulties, his part is to ensure each gets a fair hearing and to enable the pace of the interaction to proceed with maximal effectiveness. Meetings are traditionally infrequent and most of the change takes place at home and not in the surgery. So gratifying are the results of this form of therapy that some practitioners are now adamant that therapy of the marital duo is essential. Children of any age take the process well: anxiety may be experienced of the 'not in front of the children' type but damage does not seem to occur and it is unlikely that any interaction in the consulting room will be more bitter or violent than round the domestic hearth.

Family therapy in the disabled family

It is becoming increasingly obvious that the family with a physically or mentally handicapped child is greatly disadvantaged: in physical and financial resources and by stigma within the community. Until recently it has been thought sufficient to consider the handicapped member as the problem but viewpoints are now including the whole family: the place of the general practitioner in this type of family therapy is obvious – good examples of this can be found in Gath (1977, 1978).

Marital therapy

A specialized varient of family therapy is marital therapy when the interest is focused on the marital relationship. All doctors become involved in difficult marriages: the problem is to obtain a useful model that enables therapy to be directed at the pair. Dominion (1979a) offers a short chapter and a series of invaluable articles (Dominion 1979b).

Sex therapy

Since the work of Masters and Johnson (1970) the treatment of sexual dysfunction has been revolutionized. Prior to their behavioural technique the analytic approach was largely unfruitful. Now the combination of insightful and behavioural methods is much more successful. 'M & J', as it is always known, is very easy to learn: the best text is Kaplan (1974). Some sexual dysfunctions can be predicted and are thus relatively easy to screen for:

after myocardial infarction;
after female sterilization;
occasionally after termination;
in the late marriage and especially the very late second marriages of widows/widowers.

The presentation of sexual dysfunction may be quite occult so that all persons presenting with vague complaints or even full-blown psychiatric illness must be screened for marital or sexual problems. If these are present and resolvable, the symptoms and illness may clear quickly and completely. It is almost as if the patient presents distress for the family in an unorganized way enabling the physician to choose his favourable mode of therapy: research is needed to see if each therapy is equally curative.

Psychotherapy

While it is quite clear that psychotherapy has much to offer in the prevention and treatment of mental ill health, there are many areas in which research is urgently required. The relative efficacy of treatment regimes, the selection of patients, the training of the therapists, remain unresolved.

Techniques of the psychologist: behavioural modification

There are a series of special techniques usually available from the psychologist that can be more than helpful. Little can be done here except to list them but they illustrate modes of help that family doctors may well feel appropriate to their patient and an approach to the psychologist can well be fruitful: once the doctor has understood the technique he may well want to use it in his own therapeutic repertoire:

social skills training;
cognitive therapy;
biofeedback;
guided mourning;
group exposure for agoraphobia;
desensitization;
flooding.

For a general helpful discussion see Marks (1981) and Gelder (1980); for details of treatment see Wolpe (1973).

All the above treatment and many more are considered behavioural therapy: many of the techniques find a way into a broader psychotherapy as part of each therapist's expertise. Nurse therapists are now being trained.

Meditation

All cultures seem to have techniques of meditation: currently in our culture several models are in the process of development. Undoubtedly some patients find anxiety relaxation by this practice. For a general review see West (1979).

Relaxation

Again an anxiety reduction technique often associated with either meditation or hypnosis. 'Relaxation for Living' is a semi-lay group with branches throughout the United Kingdom – a registered charity.

Hypnosis

Like so many methods of medical intervention, this one has had its historical ups and downs. A growing number of medical practitioners, largely taught and supported by the British Society of Medical and Dental Hypnosis, are finding a definite place in the treatment of anxiety and tension, especially phobic disorder. Research is taking place into its use in hypertension. Most practitioners now combine the technique with the teaching of autohypnotic relaxation that the patient practises at home. The process is greatly accelerated by using imaginal conditioning (Kroger and Fesler 1976). For a general viewpoint see Shaw (1977).

Self-help groups

The support function of self-help groups can be much more valuable than that of the doctor: there is a certain stage in the management of, say, a spina bifida at home, at which a group of parents sharing the same experience will be most supportive. The medical role is to act as a resource to these groups and to point interested parents in their direction.

Alcoholics Anonymous and Cruse (for widows and widowers) are well known; the Phobic Society, less so.

Local groups can often be found of ex-mental hospital patients, who run a semi-social programme with support; they can be highly effective.

'Alternative' therapies

Patients constantly come to their family doctors claiming cure by means of yeast tablets, dianetics, psionic medicine, or rolfing. As none of the above appear in the BNF, practitioners naturally feel lost. Information can be obtained from Hulke (1978).

Consultation with colleagues

Within the primary health care team help can often be obtained by consultation over the problem patient with the health visitor. Few patients object or refuse permission for this intradisciplinary consultation as the health visitor is a well-known and trusted member of the team: she has the capacity to make apparently casual home visit, usually to return with a new viewpoint that is often crucial. Reference to the social work departments is much more difficult: either the patient may be reluctant to see the social worker or the social work department may not have time to accept the client. If the relationship can be set up and if the general practitioner can maintain the intradisciplinary consultation, i.e. if the doctor and the social worker actually meet to share views and create common therapy goals, a very forceful therapy can be gained. Clearly a social work 'attachment' scheme can be of value to the general practitioner in that one member of the area department becomes known and trusted (Paine 1976; Gilchrist *et al.* 1978).

Often, given the goodwill and the resources, the Marriage Guidance Council can be invited to attach a counsellor to the practice. Rarely a psychologist or a community psychiatric nurse can be inveigled into fulfilling a counselling role in the general medical setting (Johnson 1978). The value of these 'attachments' have been well assessed and are now of proven value. Less often discussed is the educational and supportive effect that these workers have on the practice itself. Too few practitioners provide education or support from within by regular case discussion meetings or joint consultations.

The use of consultant colleagues is largely dependent on their attitudes: some welcome a relationship with general practice and revel in support roles that leave the patient within the community: others tend to occupy the ivory towers of either academia or the local mental hospital, and descend only for domiciliary visits. Too often referral means loss to the general practitioner: if the second opinion does not educate both the general practitioner and the consultant much of its value is wasted as it has become a disposal pattern rather than a consultation.

Overriding all other considerations in the making of intraprofessional relationships is the desire to have contacts that enable the family doctor to obtain help at the earliest possible moment. Only so, can prevention be a feasible project. Using the model, intervention at the phase of reaction before breakdown offers hope of avoidance of illness behaviour. However, these interventions depend upon the recognition by primary health care professionals of distress before disease. For the general practitioner to recognize deviation from normal bereavement and grieving from pathological mourning, a clear understanding of the range of normal processes is required, not at present to be found in standard texts.

All workers in the field of mental health are in need of support both to enable them to continue to involve themselves in areas that are personally painful and to learn from the experience. One major use of the psychodynamically trained psychiatrist is to provide the focus for support groups, membership of which should be open to doctors of all descriptions and ages. The more sophisticated and mature of such groups are opening their doors to all local professionals who share a similar role generally described by the broad term psychotherapy (Caplan 1970).

SPECIFIC ISSUES

Bereavement

Since Lindeman's work (1944) after the Coconut Grove Night Club disaster, the hope has been expressed that consultation with the recently bereaved will reduce the incidence of pathological grieving and depression and possibly of suicide. The evaluation of this concept is still in progress but a review by Parkes (1980) examines work professionals, volunteers supported by professionals, and self-help groups. Matching of case and control is particularly important to make comparisons valid. One outcome of such a study showed a greater than 50 per cent reduction in consultation rates. Much of the result was that which could have been given by a supportive family had one existed – thus effort must be best expended where other supports are least.

The intention of work with the recently bereaved is to provide support for normal mourning process, that is the expression of grief including anger and despair, a review of the positive and negative elements in the lost relationship. A practical problem solving approach, a way to decide and solve difficulties rather than collecting them, is indicated, and to make plans for the future. Clearly this is not an easy task and will be painful for the therapist: but need not be time consuming as several short, 15-minute appointments over some six months seem to be sufficient.

The evidence suggests that intervention in the normal bereavement is worthwhile in reducing later psychiatric and physical morbidity. This would tend to imply that early recognition of the pathological bereavement would be even more effective: however, to do this requires some form of supervision and reference to standard patterns of bereavement behaviour. Parkes (1975) offers a splendid overview.

Closely paralleled to the area of bereavement counselling are the problems of the care of the dying and his family. Considerable interest has arisen in recent years in the creation of hospices for terminal care and the psychotherapy of dying, if it may be so called, is just being written (Stedeford 1979, 1981). The care of the relatives is equally important and occasionally the two can most usefullly be conjoined in a family therapy. The greatest care is needed in this area and the backing of the whole primary health care team. Clearly research is needed at an operational level to find out who can do what most usefully: for details of management, see Bloch (1978).

The loss of a child is a particularly painful bereavement: those who read Harman (1981) will not have forgotten it; those who have not, might do so.

Anticipation as a defence against loss

Since Lindemann (1944) wrote about normal grieving process, the idea has been current that 'anticipatory grief' might in some way defend against the subsequent experience of loss. This concept has been extensively used as a *raison d'etre* for psychotherapists in their involvement with many areas but especially in the care of the dying and their relatives (Stededord 1979). For a critical review of the concept see Fulbon and Gottesmann (1980).

Affective disorders

Of all psychiatric illness affective disorder is by far the commonest. The classification is fraught with argument and the following outline will not be universally accepted.

All affective disease divides into two groups:

1. Those with mania, which are called bipolar, whether depression has occurred or not: this is in the belief that depression will occur in due course. Hence the diagnosis of mania, dangerous in itself, is a predictor of a later severe depression. The notes should be marked and a high degree of suspucion exercised.

2. Those with depression alone, which are called unipolar – by far the commonest group.

The major argument now begins to decide between cases within this group. Some believe that there are two distinct groups: the reactive whose depression has been precipitated by a traumatic loss event and the endogenous where the cause is thought to be internal and probably biochemical.

A further discrimination between primary, those acting without another disease and secondary those occurring with a presenting disease, say alcoholism, is important. Secondary disease demands treatment of the cause of the depression, e.g. the alcoholism.

While it is easy to list the features of neurotic/reactive as against psychotic/endogenous depression (Table 13.3) in fact there are many cases in the middle ground. It might be better to refer to mild (neurotic) moderate (mixed) and severe (endogenous) types of depression. However, it is important to realize that suicidal risk exists in all types and always requires careful assessment.

The term masked depression is used to describe, usually an endogenous depression, in which organic features predominates. It is often impossible to get the patient to accept that he is depressed but careful questioning will usually reveal the true affective state. The condition is dangerous because continued somatic investigations, all negative, leads rapidly to loss of confidence and sometimes conflict between patient and physician. Often the patient presents with a smile – so called smiling depression (Shulman 1977). A further feature,

Table 13.3. *Features in depression*

	Neurotic reactive	Psychotic/endogenous
Onset:	often abrupt	usually slow
Complaints:	often fluctuate often markedly variable, can cheer up but relapses quickly, retardation rare, transient	often steady state, little change from day to day or moment to moment
Variation:	no set variation	diurnal variation of mood, worst in mornings
Sleep problems:	can't get off to sleep	early morning waking
Sexual appetite:	normal or reduced	total loss of sexual appetite
Weight:	slight or gaining	loss of weight marked
Treatment:	responds best to psychotherapy	
Tricyclics:	only 20% respond, often feel worse on treatment	responds fairly well to tricyclics 60%
MAOIs:	50% respond	only 10% respond
ECT:	not effective	ECT highly effective.

sometimes used descriptively, is to say that a depression is agitated when anxiety is high and retarded when psychomotor retardation fills the picture.

Reactive depression

Reactive depression is a condition of mood (affect) which is beyond the normal experience and in which gloom, sadness, misery, and unhappiness are out of proportion to the precipitating factor in intensity or duration or both.

Engdogenous depression

Endogenous depression has a severe lowering of affect markedly beyond normal experience, usually without precipitating factors. The depth of depression is marked and usually accompanied by psychomotor retardation in which both mind and body appear to be frozen: thought processes slow down, posture and face become fixed, tears are often uncontrollable, the mind plays and replays a gramophone record of guilt, unworthiness, and self-reproach. Hypochondiacal thoughts are accepted as real and the patient may believe in worms in his head or rot in his gut – a depressive delusional state. Somatic features are usually marked: loss of weight, loss of energy, early morning waking, diurnal variation.

Suicidal ideation is universal and planning often far advanced.

In the diagnostic process, first establish that the depression is primary, i.e. that it is not secondary to organic brain disease or schizophrenia. In the elderly beware of making the diagnosis of dementia without excluding depression.

The assessment of the severity

1. The clinical features.
2. Rating scales. Two types of rating scale are useful in practice, quite apart from their use as a research tool: (i) *Self-rating scales*, e.g. the Beck depressive inventory (Beck *et al.* 1961), and the Zung self-rating depressive scale (Zung 1965). (ii) *Observer rating scales*, e.g. Hamilton depressive rating scale (Hamilton 1960).

Self-rating scales can only be completed by the mild to moderate group: it is almost always possible to make a Hamilton rating. The validity of these scales is well established and correlates well with global scales of severity based on clinical judgement. The value of the scale to the general practitioner, who sees severe depression infrequently, is that it enables him to grasp at once the severity and hence seriousness of the illness: repetition of the test will show changes; again this can be most helpful as a guide to treatment. Remembering that the prevention of suicide is the major task in the treatment of depression, any parameter is to be valued. For a general review see Snaith (1981).

Use of lithium

A highly toxic substance, lithium requires careful monitoring by blood level: it can only be used when patient compliance and supervision are good. Evidence has rapidly accumulated that it is highly effective in preventing recurrence in bipolar affective disorders and currently evidence is appearing of its value in recurrent unipolar. While amitriptyline may be equally effective in unipolar disease, lithium is more useful in bipolar. One unusual side-effect of the tricyclics is worth comment: tricyclics can induce mania while lithium does not, it may this be better to use lithium than amitriptyline in the long-term treatment of both unipolar and bipolar depression.

The patient must be carefully instructed in the side-effects and a handout is obviously valuable; a follow up of the patient who fails to attend for his blood test would appear wise and in view of the very low therapeutic index, the control of the tablets should be rested in a relative in times of mania or depression. Routine checks of renal and thyroid function are mandatory. Beware of using diuretics with lithium unless in hospital with daily lithium levels. The topic is well reviewed by Srinivasan and Hullin (1980) and *Drug and Therapeutic Bulletin* (1981).

Reducing the incidence and severity of suicidal behaviour

It would seem obvious that the first effort must be to identify those at risk: perhaps the easiest to recognize in family practice is the previous overdose patient. The notes should be clearly marked not merely to remind each doctor of the potentiality of recurrence but also to ensure that so far as possible prescriptions are safe and small in quantity.

Secondly, the early recognition of depression is of importance: depression is notoriously recurrent so again a clear note should be made and the recurrence looked for. Treatment, if pharmaceutical, should again be safe and small.

If alcoholism (proven or suspected) is noted then the risk is obviously higher.

Some loss situations tend to be well known to the whole primary health care team: a death at home may leave a widower quite unsupported and almost incapable of caring for himself. There is much to be said for one member of the team staying in touch for the next six months or more. A bereavement register is a useful method of supervision. However, marital break up is much less often known to the practice: the distress experienced at this time may be thought to be unsuitable as a subject for consultation and confidences may well reside in the bar-maid rather than the doctor.

Prevention of suicide

Success in this area will always be difficult to measure: and in view of the relatively low frequency of the event, one per 2500 patients each 3–4 years, much effort must go into relatively little obvious reward. The primary rule must be to have considered the suicidal risk: to do this the patient's notes must be clearly marked: a simple sticker will suffice, no matter how cryptic, see example (Table 13.4).

Table 13.4. *Sticker for case notes*

Risk factors	
History of	
Previous psychiatric disorder	Overdose
Depression	Attempted suicide
Mania	Alcoholism

Once identified, the risk must be assessed and treatment chosen in terms of it. Large doses of toxic drugs, e.g. barbiturates or tricyclic antidepressants are unwise: small quantities to relatives may prevent hoarding. The provision of drugs in plastic bubble packs may be of value but as yet unproven. Highly dangerous drugs such as Distalgesic should be avoided or used in strictly limited circumstances in small quantities. The topic is well reviewed in Office of Health Economics (1981).

Alcohol is a very common accompaniment to any overdose: the sudden asphyxias that occur when dextropopoxyphene is combined with alcohol have been well documented. It appears to be little known how toxic this drug is, 15–20 tablets of Distalgesic plus alcohol being a fatal dose. These deaths largely occur in the community. As there is good evidence that the efficacy of the combination tablet of dextropopoxyphene and paracetamol is the effect of the paracetamol there are good grounds for the total avoidance of the combination (Hawton and Blackstock 1977; Young and Lawson 1980).

Repeaters: recurrent attempters

Repeaters are a very high-risk group: unfortunately, by reason of their other numerous previous attempts they are treated with scant respect. They prove difficult to help as relationships are hard to establish and they demand care, often at unsocial times. The psychopathic nature of the personality disorder produces a feeling of helplessness in all professionals: sometimes only the Samaritans go on listening. Further these patients may actively reject help: any suggestion of aid from another agency is rejected until the helper himself feels persecuted and helpless. There is much to be said for making arrangements within the practice to ensure that this patient is always seen by the same doctor: it would appear that 'divide-and-rule' is the family motto of the personality disordered – a single therapist can avoid some of the traps. Overt hostility is common in this group: they are difficult to get into therapy and fail at follow up.

The assessment of a para-suicide or overdose in the community

The only useful rule is to refer all cases to hospital: failure to do so leaves the responsibility for a potentially fatal situation squarely in the GP's hands. The benefits that accrue from admission lie in the assessment of further risk, rapid psychiatric opinion and the toxicology service of the hospital. Late hepatic necrosis from paracetamol overdose, fatal without treatment, can be predicted and treated at an early stage if blood levels for paracetamol are examined. Despite pressure to minimize the incident, all cases should be admitted. The GP's role lies in the longer term: enter the event in the notes and tag it, e.g. with a sticker: make a plan of supportive therapy over the next few months: examine the social setting, perhaps arrange marital therapy: enquire if a social work approach might be useful – but initially, admit. For a useful review see Hawton and Catalán (1981).

CONCLUSION

Prevention is not so much specific action as an attitude. Opportunistic intervention can occur throughout the doctor's day, often in consultations that would appear to be orientated in a completely different direction. Primary prevention remains largely unproven but highly interesting. Secondary prevention is a stance that underpins the whole general practitioner's role. It must be obvious that we need more information, more research: and that this will need to be carried out within the field of general practice.

REFERENCES

Balint, M. (1964). *The doctor, his patient and the illness.* Pitman, London.
Bancroft, J. (1979). In *An introduction to the psychotherapies* (ed. S. Bloch). Oxford University Press.
Beck, A. T., Ward, C. H., Mendelson, K., Moch, J., and Erbauch, J. (1961). An inventory for measuring depression. *Archs gen. Psychiat.* 4, 53–63.

References 227

Bloch, S. (1978). Psychological management of the dying patient. *Medicine* 3, 1837–41.
—— (1979*a*). Assessment of patients for psychotherapy. *Br. J. Psychiat.* 135, 193–208.
—— (ed.) (1979*b*). *An introduction to the psychotherapies.* Oxford University Press.
—— (1981). Reading about group psychotherapy. *Br. J. Psychiat.* 138, 167–8.
Bowlby, J. (1977). The making and breaking of affectional bonds. *Br. J. Psychiat.* 130, 201–10; *Br. J. Psychiat.* 130, 421–31.
Brown, G. W. and Harris, T. (1978). *Social origins of depression.* Tavistock, London.
—— —— and Copeland, R. (1977). Depression and loss. *Br. J. Psychiat.* 130, 1–18.
Caplan, G. (1961). *An approach to community mental health.* Tavistock, London.
—— (1964). *Principles of preventive psychiatry.* Tavistock, London.
—— (1970). *The theory and practice of mental health consultation.* Tavistock, London.
Dominian, J. (1979*a*). Marital therapy. In *An introduction to the psychotherapies* (ed. S. Bloch). Oxford University Press.
—— (1979*b*). Introduction to marital pathology. *Br. med. J.* ii, 424–5; 478–9; 531–2; 594–6; 654–6; 720–2; 781–3; 854–5; 915–16; 987–9; 1053–4.
Drug and Therapeutics Bulletin (1981). Lithium updated. Editorial. *Drug Therapeut. Bull.* 19 (6), 21–46.
Fry, J. (1966), *Profiles of disease.* Livingstone, London.
—— (1979). *Common diseases.* Redwood Burn, Trowbridge.
Fulton, R. and Gottesman, D. J. (1980). Anticipatory grief: a psycho-social concept reconsidered. *Br. J. Psychiat.* 137, 45–54.
Gath. A. (1977). Impact of an abnormal child upon the parents. *Br. J. Psychiat.* 130, 405–10.
—— (1978). *Down's syndrome and the family: the early years.* Academic Press, London.
Gelder, K. (1980). The behaviour therapies. *Oxford Med. School Gaz.* XXXI, 3.
Gilchrist, L. C., Gough, J. B., Horsfall-Turner, Y. R., Ineson, E. M., Keele, G., Marks, M., and Scott, M. J. (1978). Social work in general practice. *J. R. Coll. Gen. Pract.* 28, 675–86.
Goldberg, D. P. and Blackwell, B. (1970). Psychiatric illness in a general practice – a detailed study using a new method of case identification. *Br. med. J.* ii, 439–43.
Hamilton, M. (1960). A rating scale for depression. *J. Neurol. Neurosurg. Psychiat.* 23, 56–62.
Harman, W. V. (1981). Death of my baby. *Br. med. J.* 282, 35–7.
Hawton, K. and Blackstock, E. (1976). Deliberate self-poisoning: implications for psychotropic drug prescribing in general practice. *J. R. Coll. Gen. Practns* 27, 560–3.
—— and Catalán J. (1981). Psychiatric management of attempted suicide patients. *Br. J. hosp. Med.* 25, 365–76.
——, Gath, D., and Smith, E. (1979). Management of attempted suicide in Oxford. *Br. med. J.* ii, 1040–2.
Hulke, M. (ed.) (1978). *Encyclopedia of alternative medicine and self-help.* Ryder, London.
Johnson, M. (1978). Work of a clinical psychologist in primary care. *J. R. Coll. Gen. Practns* 28, 661–7.
Kaplan, H. S. (1974). *The new sex therapy: active treatment of sexual dysfunction.* Ballière Tindall, London.
Kay, D. W. K. (1978). Assessment of familial risks in the functional psychosis and their application to genetic counselling. *Br. J. Psychiat.* 133, 385–403.
Kroger, W. S. and Fesler, W. D. (1976). *Hypnosis and behaviour modification: imagery and conditioning.* Lippincott, New York.

Lazarus, R. S. (1966). *Psychological stress and the coping process.* McGraw-Hill, New York.

Lindemann, E. (1944). The symptomatology and management of acute grief. *Am. J. Psychiat.* **101**, 141–8.

Marks, I. (1981). Psychiatry and behavioural psychotherapy. *Br. J. Psychiat.* **139**, 74–8.

Masters, W. H. and Johnson, V. E. (1970). *Human sexual inadequacy.* Churchill, London.

Murray, R. M. and Reveley, A. (1981). The genetic contribution to the neuroses. *Br. J. hosp. Med.* **25**, 185–90.

Office of Health Economics (1981). *Suicide and deliberate self-harm.* OHE, London.

Paine, T. F. (1976). Role of part-time social workers in general practice. *J. R. Coll. Gen. Practns* **26**, 695–7.

Parkes, C. M. (1975). *Bereavement: studies in grief in adult life.* Penguin, London.

Parkes, C. M. (1980). Bereavement counselling: does it work? *Br. med. J.* **281**, 3–6.

Roy, A. (1978). Vulnerability factors and depression in women. *Br. J. Psychiat.* **133**, 106–10.

—— (1981). Vulnerability factors and depression in men. *Br. J. Psychiat.* **138**, 75–7.

Royal College of General Practitioners (1970(. Report from General Practice. *Present state and future needs of general practice,* (2nd edn.). RCGP, London.

Rutter, M. (1972). *Maternal deprivation reassessed.* Penguin, Harmondsworth, England.

—— (1980). Long-term effects of early experience. *Devl. Med. Child Neurol.* **22**, 800–15.

Shaw, H. L. (1977). *Hypnosis in practice.* Baillière Tindall, London.

Shepherd, M., Cooper, B., Brown, A. C., and Kalton, G. W. (1966). *Psychiatric illness in general practice.* Oxford University Press.

Shulman, R. (1977). Psychogenic illness with physical manifestations and the other side of the coin. *Lancet* **i**, 524–6.

Snaith, R. P. (1981). Rating scales. *Br. J. Psychiat.* **138**, 512–14.

Srinivasan, D. P. and Hullin, R. P. (1980). Current concepts of lithium therapy. *Br. J. hosp. Med.* **24**, 466–81.

Stedeford, A. (1979). Psychotherapy of the dying patient. *Br. J. Psychol.* **135**, 7–14.

—— (1981). Couples facing death: i Psycho-social aspects. *Br. med. J.* **283**, 1033–6; ii Unsatisfactory communication. *Br. med. J.* **283**, 1098–101.

Storr, A. (1979). *The art of psychotherapy.* Secher and Warburg/Heinmann, London.

West, M. (1979). Meditation. *Br. J. Psychiat.* **135**, 457–67.

Wolpe, J. (1973). *The practice of behaviour therapy.* Pergamon Press, Oxford.

Young, R. J. and Lawson, A. A. H. (1980). Distalgesic poisoning: a cause for concern. *Br. med. J.* **ii**, 1045–7.

Zung, W. W. K. (1965). A self-rating depressive scale. *Archs. gen. Psychiat.* **12**, 63–70.

14 Accident prevention
Muir Gray

ACCIDENT OR 'ACCIDENT'?

The *Shorter Oxford English Dictionary* defines an accident as 'an unforeseen contingency' and it is the unforeseeable, and therefore the unpreventable, aspects of accidents which impress many people. One of the main problems in accident prevention is, therefore, to convince people that accidents are preventable and do not occur because of 'fate' or 'bad luck' but that they have causes and that the causes can often be modified.

When speaking to a group or advising an individual it can be helpful to use the term 'events which are called accidents' to counteract the assumption that accidents cannot be prevented. It would, however, be unnecessarily tedious to use this phrase throughout the chapter so the word 'accident' will be placed within quotation marks to remind the reader of the problems which the connotations of the term 'accident' can create.

The causes of 'accidents' can be grouped into environmental causes and personal causes.

THE CONTRIBUTION OF THE GENERAL PRACTITIONER

Environmental causes are those which result from the design or state of repair of an individual's environment. The condition of the snow on which a mountaineer is climbing, the camber on an acutely angled bend, or the state of repair of a lathe or piece of household apparatus are examples of environmental causes of accidents. The reduction of the risks associated with such factors is the responsibility of engineers, designers, and architects, suitably stimulated by politicians, but the individual general practitioner can play a small but significant part in this process by political action (see p. 86) or, more simply, by writing to the person who is responsible for the risk.

The personal causes of 'accidents' may be divided into two types. Firstly a high proportion of 'accidents' occur because of human error. The person either does not perceive the risk, or does not know how to take avoiding action, or is incapable of taking appropriate action. The perception of risk and the skill to reduce risk can be taught and teaching is primarily the responsibility of health visitors and environmental health officers for home accidents, and of road safety education officers for road traffic accidents. However, the general practitioner can also be an effective educator and can reinforce the message of the health educator.

In addition, the ability of a person to perceive risks, to learn how to reduce them and to take appropriate avoiding action can be impaired by mental and physical disease, and the general practitioner obviously has a contribution to make to accident prevention by ensuring that his patients are as fit as possible.

Secondly, some 'accidents' are direct consequences of disease. In this type of 'accident' disease does not merely increase the individual's liability to commit an error; it actually causes him to lose control. A small proportion of road-traffic accidents, perhaps one or two in every thousand, and a considerable proportion of falls in old age are caused in this way. Some of these diseases cannot be prevented but the general practitioner is able to prevent some by accurate diagnosis and appropriate treatment. Therefore the contribution of the general practitioner to 'accident' prevention has four aspects. He can prevent 'accidents'

(i) By helping his patients keep as fit as possible to reduce the probability that they will fail to perceive risks or be unable to respond to them;

(ii) By careful anticipatory care of those diseases which can directly cause home and road traffic 'accidents';

(iii) By educating patients about risks;

(iv) By trying to educate designers, architects, and politicians.

There are four common types of 'accident':
- Road;
- Home;
- Work;
- Sport and play.

This chapter will concentrate on the first two types because the prevention of accidents at work is more the concern of occupational health physicians than of general practitioners and the prevention of sports injuries is also a specialized subject. Accidents on playgrounds are, of course, sustained by children whose problems are not covered in this book.

HOME 'ACCIDENTS'

People of all ages are injured in the home. Fortunately the contribution of the general practitioner is greatest among the two age groups in which the 'accident' rates are highest – children, whose problems will not be discussed, and elderly people. The general practitioner can influence both the personal, or medical, and the environmental causes of home accidents and he can also educate older patients how to reduce the risks of accidental injury.

Medical factors

The commonest type of home accident in old age is a fall and although it is often difficult to elicit a clear history from old people who have had a fall three common causes of falling can be defined.

(i) Loss of balance;
(ii) Tripping;
(iii) Drop attacks.

The diseases which cause these problems do not solely occur in old age but they are more common in old age and this, combined with the fact that osteoporosis increases with age, means that the type of 'accidents' which require medical attention occur more frequently in older age groups. However, people who suffer from the diseases which cause loss of balance, tripping, and drop attacks are at risk of falling whatever their age.

Loss of balance

The following conditions predispose to loss of balance:

1. Disorders of balance occur in some people as they grow older. If asked to stand upright such a person sways markedly and will respond slowly and ineffectively to a gently push on the sternum.

2. Disorders of the gait can be detected by watching the old person walking. Some old people lean backwards, others lean forwards. Leaning forwards if often associated with a shuffling step, for example in Parkinson's disease, which also increases the risk of tripping. Forward leaning may also result from anxiety: the person who has had one fall leans forward and takes small steps because he thinks this will reduce the risk of a fall whereas it increases the risk of a fall by creating instability.

Full medical assessment and the advice of a physiotherapist is indicated if there is a disorder of gait or balance.

3. Postural hypotension is often caused by antihypertensive drugs. Falls which occur at night when the person has risen from bed should be suspected as being due to postural hypotension. The failure of the person's autonomic nervous system may be aggravated by a decrease in venous return resulting from micturition or coughing. In addition old people are more likely to fall when in darkness because people with disorders of balance rely on visual cues more than the person whose powers of co-ordination and balance are unimpaired.

4. Psychotropic drugs.

Tripping

Any condition which reduces the ability of the person to step normally increases the risk of tripping:

(i) Parkinson's disease;
(ii) osteoarthritis;
(iii) loss of muscle power due to prolonged immobility;
(iv) stroke;
(v) blindness or visual impairment.

Both the ability to lift the foot and the ability to lift the toes should be observed, because foot drop predisposes to tripping.

232 Accident prevention

A full medical assessment is always indicated and the advice of a physiotherapist is also essential. In addition particular attention must be paid to the old person's environment if the old person is at risk of tripping.

Drop attacks

The cause of these is often difficult to determine without special tests such as a 24-hour ECG and a drop attack, or any episode which could be considered as one even though the history is not classical, is an indication for referral to a consultant in geriatric medicine or to a cardiologist.

Environmental factors

Rather than giving a long list of all the hazards which may occur in the home it is easier to advise that the general practitioner who is paying a call to the home of a person who is at greater than average risk of a fall because of physical or mental disability should look for equipment, fittings or furniture which are in disorder or disarray or disrepair. The more disabled a person is the less can he cope with disorder, disrepair, and disarray, with crumpled rugs, or faulty paraffin heaters, or with a stair carpet springing loose from the stair rods. The stair and the kitchen are areas of danger which may not be visited unless the general practitioner is alert to the risk of a patient falling.

The advice of a domiciliary occupational therapist is particularly helpful if hazards are identified in the kitchen, bathroom, on steps or stairs.

All environmental hazards are aggravated by inadequate lighting and several studies have demonstrated the fact that domestic lighting is very often dangerously inadequate, usually for the simple reason that the person is using a bulb which is too weak. If the person is blind or partially sighted the advice of a technical officer for the blind will be valuable in reducing the risk of a home accident. Her job is to help the blind person learn how to cope at home safely. She is usually based in the social services department.

Prevention by education

Having ensured that an old person is as fit as possible the general practitioner should also try to educate the old person how to use her environment safely. This can be difficult. Some old people are unwilling to admit that they are at risk but the old person who refuses to admit that any adaptation of her environment is necessary or that she is at risk of falling may be doing so because the decay of her environment or the deterioration of her condition have been so slow that they are imperceptible to her. She may, however, deny that she is at risk because she is afraid that such an admission will result in pressure being applied on her to go into a home. Furthermore some old people are prepared to admit that they are at risk but maintain that it is 'in God's hands' or adopt a fatalistic attitude which does not involve a religious belief, for example by saying 'what will be, will be' (see p. 76). It is only by changing such beliefs and attitudes that the person who denies that she is at risk can be persuaded to admit that some action is necessary to reduce the risk.

Anyone who points out environmental factors which require to be changed must appreciate that the person at risk may have considerable practical and financial problems to do so. It may be impossible for a disabled elderly person to replace linoleum with a dangerous edge or pay for the rewiring of her house and the general practitioner interested in accident prevention should be prepared to mobilize appropriate help – volunteers for small jobs, the domiciliary occupational therapist for house adaptations for disabled people, and the environmental health officer for major structure problems such as rewiring or rotten floors. Finally the old person should be taught how she can stand up should she fall, how she can call for help if she cannot stand up and how important it is to keep her house warm so that a fall does not result in hypothermia. Relatives and supporters also need education. They may need to have the risks pointed out to them but they are usually well aware of the risks and need advice how to help the old person accept that she is at risk, and therefore accept the necessary changes. They also need advice on how best to help the physiotherapist and finally they may need considerable help to tolerate the fact that the old person is 'at risk' (see p. 258).

ROAD TRAFFIC 'ACCIDENTS'

Pedestrian accidents

Any disorder which slows down the rate at which a person can walk or which impairs his hearing or seeing puts him at increased risk while crossing the road. It would be inappropriate to suggest to such a person that he did not go out, but it is good practice to advise him to remember his disabilities, to wear light clothing if going out in the dusk or dark, and, most important of all, to cross the road at a zebra or pelican crossing or at traffic lights.

A person who is blind or partially sighted can be taught how to walk outside safely by a mobility officer for the blind who can be contacted at the eye hospital or social services department. The job of a mobility officer is to help the person retain or regain his independence, perhaps with the aid of a white stick, by teaching him how to move about inside his house and outside confidently and safely.

Cycling accidents

Cycling is an excellent form of exercise for older people (see p. 174). However, while encouraging an elderly person to take up or continue cycling it is important to emphasize that slower cyclists are at greater risk than those who can accelerate quickly. They should, therefore wear light clothes and reflective bandoliers at night, and dismount to walk across busy junctions. At all ages cyclists are most at risk when turning to the right, and those who are unable to cycle quickly enough to move into the middle of the road or complete the turn across the stream of oncoming traffic quickly or who have poor vision are at high risk.

Motor car and motor cycle accidents

The proportion of road traffic 'accidents' which result from disease is small. Disease is a major cause in only one or two 'accidents' in every thousand. This is very small compared with the major causes of accidents – driver errors, road design and maintenance, and faults in the car or motorcycle (Table 14.1).

Table 14.1. *Causes of road 'accidents'*

Cause	Total percentage contribution
The behaviour of the road user	95
Road conditions	28
Defects in the vehicle	9
Illness	0.1

In 29 per cent of 'accidents' two causes contribute.
In 1 per cent of 'accidents' three causes contribute.

Although the proportion is small it is significant because the reason that it is so small is due to the regulations which control the issue of driving licences to people who are suffering from certain diseases and the care with which the medical profession interprets these regulations.

The legal position

Applicants. The 1974 Road Traffic Act laid down that every applicant for a driving licence is required to declare whether or not he is suffering from any of the four 'prescribed disabilities':
 1. epilepsy;
 2. severe mental subnormality;
 3. liability to sudden attacks of disabling giddiness or fainting;
 4. Inability to meet the prescribed eyesight requirements, that is to read in good daylight, with the aid of corrective lenses if worn, a registration mark fixed to a motor vehicle, the letters of which are 3½ inches high, at a distance of 75 feet or 3⅛ inches high at 67 feet.

In addition the person is asked to inform the Licensing Centre if he suffers from any other disability likely to cause the driving of a vehicle by him to be a source of danger to the public. An example of this type of disability is a 'limb disability', namely the absence, deformity, loss, or weakness of one or more limbs or parts of limbs.

Such disabilities are termed 'relevant disabilities'. The applicant is also required to state whether or not he is suffering from a disability or condition which may deteriorate to such a degree that it may become a 'relevant disability'. Such disabilities are called 'prospective disabilities'.

If the prescribed or relevant disability is being satisfactorily controlled the applicant will be granted a licence for one, two, or three years. A fixed-term licence is also granted to people who have prospective disability. If, however, the disability is not being satisfactorily controlled or if the person has a limb disability the application will be refused or the licence may be restricted to take the disability into account, for example by laying the onus on the person with the limb disability to make any necessary adaptations to ensure safe driving.

Licence holders. The person who holds a driving licence is required by law to notify the Licensing Centre if:

1. he develops a relevant or prospective disability;
2. a disability becomes worse.

Disabilities which are expected to last for less than three months are excluded from this rule.

The general practitioner's position. A doctor is not under any legal obligation to tell his patient that he is suffering from a relevant or prospective disability. However, a leader in the *British Medical Journal* stated that it 'should be regarded as good medical practice' to tell a driver that he is suffering from a relevant disability and that he should notify the Licensing Centre. However, the British Medical Association booklet on Medical Ethics states that 'rarely, the public interest may persuade the doctor that his duty to the community may override his duty to maintain his patient's confidence'. If a doctor is worried about whether or not to inform the Driver and Vehicle Licensing Centre he can discuss the dilemma with an adviser from his Defence Society.

With prospective disabilities the position is different and the Government has accepted that a doctor may not wish to tell his patient that his condition is one in which progressive deterioration occurs or may occur.

For his own protection the general practitioner who informs a patient that he is suffering from a relevant disability should record this fact in the patient's notes so that he cannot be said to have failed to do so if the patient decides that he would rather not inform the Licensing Centre and then causes an 'accident'. Doctors are not under any legal obligation to inform the Licensing Centre if a patient is suffering from a relevant disability, indeed it would be a breach of confidence to do so. However, the Licensing Centre may require the applicant or licence holder who has stated that he is suffering from a relevant or prospective disability to authorise his general practitioner to release information to the Centre. If this information is insufficient for the Licensing Centre to reach a decision on his fitness to drive it can require the licence holder to have a medical examination by a doctor nominated by the Centre.

The general practitioner who wishes advice can phone the Medical Advisory Branch of the Driver and Vehicle Licensing Centre at Swansea (0792 42731). However, many problems can be solved by consulting the booklet called

Medical Aspects of Fitness to Drive which is published by the Medical Commission on Accident Prevention. It is very clearly written and is both brief and comprehensive.

Relevant disabilities

Most of the booklet is devoted to a discussion of those diseases which commonly cause relevant disabilities and the authors give guidelines which the general practitioner can use as a basis for advising patients.

Cardiac conditions

The person who has suffered a myocardial infarction should be advised not to drive within the two months following clinical recovery.

Angina pectoris which is easily provoked by the physical effort of driving or by the annoyance caused by other road users is a cause for concern and patients who have this type of angina should be advised not to drive. The person who has had coronary artery bypass surgery is not held to be suffering from a relevant disability but if he continues to have angina which is provoked by driving he should be advised not to drive. Coronary artery bypass surgery is classified as a prospective disability and if the patient is free from angina he will be issued with a fixed-term licence for one, two, or three years.

People who are hypertensive can drive provided that their treatment is not causing vertigo, faintness, or postural hypotension but a 'Till 70' will not be given. However, every driver who is being treated for hypertension should be warned of the dangers of fatigue. This applies particularly to elderly drivers who are receiving treatment for hypertension.

The diagnosis of an arrhythmia or of aortic valvular disease is not relevant to the patient's ability to drive unless the disease is causing syncopal attacks, or transient ischaemic attacks, which may occur after heart valve replacement but the patient should notify the DVLC. The regulations state that 'liability to sudden attacks of fainting or giddiness' is a relevant disability. Complete heart block is a common cause of this type of disability and the licensing centre will not issue a licence unless a pacemaker has been inserted and the person agrees to have regular medical reviews. The licence issued will only be a fixed-term licence, usually for three years. Drug treatment of heart block is regarded as insufficiently reliable for a licence to be granted.

If in doubt about the advice to give the most appropriate step is usually to refer the patient for the opinion of a cardiologist because an accurate diagnosis is fundamentally important.

Diabetes

All patients with diabetes should notify the Licensing Centre because diabetes is regarded as a prospective disability. However, people with insulin-dependent diabetes will not necessarily be barred from driving provided that they do not suffer from complications such as neuropathy, peripheral vascular disease, or visual impairment.

If the person with diabetes continues to drive, as the great majority do, the general practitioner should warn him about the dangers of hypoglycaemia. He should be told to ask himself 'am I liable to have a hypoglycaemic attack' every time he inserts his ignition key. He should also be told to carry at least ten lumps of sugar within easy reach for those occasions when the risk of hypoglycaemia is greatest, for example when a meal has been missed, or when he has had to push the car or change a tyre. Some sufferers from diabetes receive virtually no warning of a hypoglycaemic attack and they are obviously at special risk. So high is the risk associated with hypoglycaemic attacks which come on without warning that the patient will probably not be granted a licence.

Young people may have to be advised to give up driving for the first few months after the onset of the disease if it is proving difficult to achieve stabilization or to decide on a dose which will not produce hypoglycaemia.

Neurological conditions

Epilepsy is a prescribed disability and specific rules have been laid down by the Licensing Centre.

The young person applying for his first licence will probably be granted a licence if the Licensing Centre is satisfied that he has been free from any epileptic attacks while awake for at least three years prior to the date from which the licence is to be valid. If the applicant has had epileptic attacks while asleep during this three-year period he will not be disqualified provided that the attacks have occurred only when he was asleep. The fact that the young person has not had attacks because he has been having effective treatment is immaterial; it is only the occurrence of attacks which is taken into account.

The development of epilepsy by someone who holds a normal drinving licence presents the general practitioner with a different type of problem. The occurrence of a single fit is not sufficient evidence for the label of 'epilepsy' to be applied but the patient should stop driving for one year from the time of the fit. If he has no further fits during that year his licence will probably be returned to him but if another fit occurs he will be considered to have epilepsy and will lose his licence for three years.

It is essential to warn the patient on treatment that anticonvulsant drugs and alcohol interact and that he should never drink any alcohol before driving. Although the rules set out in this section appear simple they are only generalizations and their interpretation in particular cases is often very difficult. If a general practitioner is in any doubt he should refer the patient to a consultant neurologist.

Other neurological diseases can cause disabilities which impair the ability to drive safely.

Transient ischaemic attacks can cause 'disabling giddiness or fainting' and patients should not drive for a period of 12 months. If no other attacks occur during that year a licence for a limited period may be offered.

In Ménière's disease the licence will be revoked until he has had a six-month period free from symptoms. Then a limited period licence will be offered.

A stroke which results in 'limb disability' will not necessarily result in loss of the licence but a limited period licence may be issued. If limb function is impaired the licence will require the driver to make necessary adaptations to his car.

Parkinson's disease can cause impairment in motor skills.

Multiple sclerosis can cause both motor and sensory defects which should be notified to the DVLC.

The advice given to a patient is determined not only by the diagnosis but also by other factors but the diagnosis is of fundamental importance and referral to a consultant neurologist is often very helpful. The consultant will be able to give a more accurate prognosis for both 'prospective disabilities', that is conditions in which deterioration usually occurs, and he is also very useful in assessing the risk of driving in conditions in which recovery is taking place. When a patient who is recovering wishes to begin driving again it is often appropriate to arrange a special driving test in which the person's need for a specially adapted car will be assessed in addition to his ability to drive.

Psychiatric disorders

As in many branches of medicine assessment is most difficult when the person is suffering from mental disorder. In a florid psychosis with hallucinations the person's inability to drive is self-evident but the decision can be very difficult if the person is not so severely disturbed or has a personality disorder.

The advice of a consultant psychiatrist or the Medical Advisory Branch of the Licensing Centre is often necessary, particularly in cases in which the patient believes that he is fit to drive and is not prepared to accept or follow the doctor's advice.

Of all the psychiatric illnesses alcoholism is the most important because it has the greatest relevance to driving and because it is commonly denied by those who are affected. It is common for people who admit to having problems with alcohol to have had at least one serious 'accident' in the preceding two years and there is no doubt that those who are dependent on alcohol are much more commonly involved in 'accidents' than the average drinker. It often happens, therefore, that a person who is dependent on alcohol will have lost his licence before he is prepared to admit his dependence.

However, it is also common for people to refuse to admit their dependence or accept referral to a specialist clinic while they still have a valid licence and this presents general practitioners with a difficult decision. Often the person who is dependent on alcohol is also dependent on his car for his job. If the general practitioner suspects that the person will continue to drink he should advise him to inform the Licensing Centre of his problem, although many people will not follow this advice, and this is the type of case in which the doctor may have to consult his Defence Society to discuss whether or not the Licensing Authority should be informed of the patient's condition.

Visual disorders

Any disease which impairs visual acuity to a degree at which the person is unable to pass the visual test – certain visual-field defects, diplopia, and defects in night vision – are relevant disabilities and render the affected person unsafe to drive. However, even the person who can pass the visual test may still be dangerous if allowed to drive. For example, diplopia and complete homonymous hemianopia are bars to driving and a partial homonymous hemianopia may lead to disqualification. In Britain a right-sided hemianopia is more dangerous, particularly if the right lower quandrant is affected; in countries in which they drive on the right, left-sided field defects are of course the more dangerous. If there is thought to be a field defect and the field defect may only be significant at night, full assessment by an ophthalmologist is always necessary. Eye diseases which are prospective disabilities. They would be notified to the Licensing Centre and kept under regular review.

In all cases of visual disorder the assessment of an ophthalmologist to establish the diagnosis will be helpful and the Medical Advisory Branch of the Licensing Centre can be contacted if there is any doubt or difficulty about the advice which should be given.

Aging

The driving licence automatically becomes invalid on the driver's seventieth birthday except in those cases in which a person has been granted a three-year licence some time during the three years prior to the person's seventieth birthday. Such a licence will be allowed to run its full course. On the expiry of the licence the older driver has to make a specific health declaration when he applies for a new licence which has to be renewed every three years.

There is, of course, no good reason why the age of 70 was chosen and not any other age. The choice of 70 was arbitrary but reflects the fact that the incidence of disabling disease rises quickly after that age. People aged over 70 are more likely to have one or more relevant disabilities and when advising an older patient about his fitness to drive the same criteria and principles are used as for drivers of any age. However, the rule has been set not only because the incidence of disabling disease increases with age but also because other changes that may be regarded as the consequences of normal aging take place and these changes increase the risk of 'accidents'.

The 'accident' rate does not increase greatly in old age, partly because old people are more cautious and have more experience than younger drivers. There is, however, one type of accident in which the rate is greatly increased – accidents at junctions when one driver is coming out from a minor road to turn to his left or right. Older drivers are more likely to pull out from the minor road into the path of an oncoming car or motorcycle. They react more slowly and less appropriately than younger drivers do.

The reason for this is not that sensory or motor defects develop as people age. While it is true that some people develop diseases which impair their sensory or motor powers the effect of the aging process is primarily on the central nervous pathways concerned with data processing. It is because of this failure of central nervous pathways that older drivers respond more slowly and less appropriately to oncoming traffic or emergencies even though they are not suffering from any specific disease or disability, and it is for this reason also that older drivers are more easily distracted by conversation or a car radio.

The implication of this is that the older a driver is the more likely will it be that a disability will be a relevant disability. However, it is sometimes necessary to discuss cases with the DLVC in which the person has suffered a degree of intellectual deterioration that leads the doctor to suspect that he would not be able to act safely in a crisis, even though he were unable to diagnose a specific disability.

Drugs and medicines

The drug which most commonly causes road traffic accidents is of course ethanol but other drugs cause accidents. Psychotropic drugs are the class most likely to cause an accident, partly because of their pharmacological effects but also because abuse of psychotropic drugs and abuse of alcohol not infrequently co-exist. However, other drugs such as antihistamines, vasodilators, anticholinergic and cholinergic drugs, anticonvulsants, oral hypoglycaemic agents, and cardiac glycosides can affect driving. Distalgesic indomethacin, and phenylbutazone can also impair driving ability. General anaesthetics also impair the ability to drive and patients should be instructed not to drive in the 48 hours following a general anaesthetic.

The general practitioner who wishes to warn his patients about the risks which prescribed drugs have on driving faces a number of difficulties. Firstly because explicit warnings about driving are not always to be found in the information on adverse reactions and interactions which is provided by the drug company. A second difficulty is that some drugs which can be bought over the counter impair driving skills, for example many cold cures contain stimulant substances and many travel sickness preparations contain antihistamines. In addition many proprietary analgesics contain caffeine which can also impair driving ability.

It is impossible for a general practitioner to be aware of all the side-effects and interactions of every drug he prescribes but it is essential that he remembers the effects of those drugs which most commonly have an influence on an individual's ability to drive and to warn the patient that significant effects often occur during the first ten days of treatment.

Types of drugs which most often impair the ability to drive
Barbiturates and other hypnotics.
Tranquillizers, both major and minor.
Tricyclic and monoamine oxidase inhibiting antidepressants.
Stimulants.
Narcotics.
Antihistamines.

In addition to the advice usually given when prescribing these drugs patients who drive should also be told:
1. not to drink *any* alcohol or take other drugs before driving;
2. not to drive if feeling unwell;
3. not to drive if very tired.

This advice is particularly important for elderly people and for those who have to drive in the course of their work. Particular care should be taken when prescribing any drug for someone who drives every day because he will often have to drive when feeling unwell or tired and he may be under considerable pressure to drink alcohol while working.

HGV and PSV licences

To drive a heavy goods vehicle (HGV) or a public service vehicle (PSV) requires special licences which are governed by much more stringent medical regulations, for example the law states that anyone who has had an epileptic attack since the age of three cannot hold a PSV or HGV licence. The decisions often have difficult social implications because loss or refusal of a licence means the loss of a job. The general practitioner who has to advise one of his patients who drives, or wishes to drive, a heavy goods or public services vehicle should read the booklet on *Medical Aspects of Fitness to Drive* because each of the chapters in it has a section clarifying the criteria as they apply to applicants for, or holders of, PSV or HGV licences. In addition the doctors working in the Medical Advisory Branch of the Licensing Centre can be consulted and are very experienced not only in giving an opinion on the relationship between disease and driving ability but also in advising general practitioners faced with ethical dilemmas and decisions which will have serious social consequences.

Prevention by education

It is not easy to influence the behaviour of road users by education for a number of reasons. Firstly, the image of safe driving is unattractive to many drivers who are more likely to equate 'fast' driving with 'good' driving. Secondly, education is difficult because the risks are low. This may seem surprising considering the large numbers of people killed and injured on the road but a serious 'accident' happens only once every several million trips. Furthermore driving creates anxiety and a considerable proportion of drivers use magical techniques to control their anxiety and these magical techniques, such as fatalistic beliefs or a St Christopher's medal, impair the ability to think logically about the risks they run (see p. 77).

Nevertheless it is possible for a general practitioner to educate his patients about road safety in the following ways.

1. By advising vulnerable patients to wear seat belts; elderly people or those with cervical spondylitis should be advised to wear a seat belt and to use a head rest. In addition the parents of small children should be advised that their children will be more amenable to seat belts if they see their parents putting on a seat belt every trip. In addition parents need sensible advice on the most appropriate types of restraint.

2. By participating in, or initiating, local campaigns on the prevention of road traffic 'accidents'.

Prevention by legislation

There is no doubt that legislation can prevent deaths and injuries on the road and general practitioners can press for legislative changes and press for the implementation of that which exists. If, for example, a Member of Parliament were to introduce a Private Member's Bill advocating the abolition of the law requiring motorcyclists to wear crash helmets letters from general practitioners to the Members for their constituencies would have influence (see p. 87). Similarly if a general practitioner learns that the roads in his rural practice are to receive less salt because of constraints on local authority expenditure he should inform his local councillors of his concern.

15 The prevention of disability and handicap

Muir Gray

The Office of Population Censuses and Surveys conducted an important and influential survey of the problems of handicapped people in Great Britain which was published in 1971 (Harris 1971). The author, Amelia Harris, emphasized the different meanings of the terms 'disability' and 'handicap', which many people still use as synonyms. She used disability for the effects of disease, for example restricted hip movement, whereas the handicap was the social consequence of the disability; in the case of restricted hip movement the handicap may be inability to climb stairs to reach the toilet (Wood 1981). Tertiary prevention is the prevention of disability by accurate diagnosis and appropriate treatment. This chapter discusses that part which the general practitioner can play in the prevention of handicap.

The many different handicaps which may result from disabling diseases may be summarized under three main headings.

1. Immobility (see p. 243).
2. Educational and employment difficulties which may result in poverty (see p. 247).
3. Difficulties with self-care (see p. 250).

The probability that someone will be handicapped by a disabling disease is obviously related to the degree of disability, but three other factors are always important.

1. The design of the environment in which the person lives.
2. The strength of the person's motivation which is influenced by many factors, notably his personality before the onset of disability, his reaction to the disabling disease and the attitude of other people (Blaxter 1976).
3. His income.

It is these social factors which influence the degree of dependence of the handicapped person.

HANDICAP AND DEPENDENCE

A person who is handicapped in any way is either deprived by being unable to perform a certain task or he becomes dependent on others to do it for him. It is always important to consider the needs of people who are dependent as well as the needs of those who are deprived because the person who depends on someone else to perform a task which would be regarded as normal for someone of his age and background may feel humiliated and inadequate. It is also essential to take into account the needs of those on whom the disabled person is dependent. Their primary need may be for relief but this should not be assumed automatically. Some people receive considerable rewards from helping a handicapped person and in some cases the rewards may be so great that they are reluctant to see the handicapped person regain his independence.

The disabled person may also benefit from his dependence. A housebound disabled person may depend upon the home help, nursing auxiliary, and the person who delivers meals on wheels not only for the service they perform but for their company. If he appreciates that independence in the tasks which they perform will increase his isolation his motivation may be affected. The disabled person is not usually aware of this process but it is insufficient simply to expose and discuss it. Steps have to be taken to reduce the person's isolation and to reduce his dependence on those who perform tasks as the main means of alleviating his isolation. When planning an approach to a handicapped person's problems it is often essential to try to re-establish the social contacts which disability has interrupted, for example regular visits to the pub or to church, as a means of improving his morale and his motivation. The most important way of achieving this is usually to increase the person's mobility.

It is, therefore, essential to consider the emotional consequences of being handicapped.

Emotional consequences of handicap

No-one is completely independent but disabled people are more dependent than those who are not, and dependence is often depressing and sometimes humiliating.

Although depression is a cause for concern the handicapped person who is not depressed is sometimes also a cause for concern because it may be that she has become hopelessly resigned to her problems and the person who has gone past the stage of depression is less likely to comply with any measures suggested by her doctor.

Anxiety is also common because the life of a severely handicapped person contains many uncertainties, for example uncertainty about one's ability to continue living at home, and the uncertainties are magnified if the disabled person lives alone and has no-one to reassure her.

Rejection and alienation are feelings experienced by some handicapped people. Discriminated against in the job market and ostracized socially on some occasions they feel that they are outsiders, treated as second-class citizens as the result of having a disease for which they are not responsible. The manifestations of these feelings may be a constructive type of anger, channelled into a determination to improve their own lot and the lot of other disabled people but it may be expressed as bitterness, with hostility towards those who offer to

Immobility 245

help. Even those who have not experienced rejection may become angry because of the feelings of humiliation which can result from dependence.

A person who becomes handicapped should be offered opportunity to discuss her reactions to prevent feelings of depression and alienation. If, however, the person is not forthcoming about her feelings her general practitioner may have to try to lead that discussion in this direction if he is of the opinion that her adjustment to her disability and handicap is not as satisfactory as it could be because she has unresolved conflicts about the change in herself and in her situation imposed by the disability (Stevenson 1981; Topliss 1978).

Practical implications

Four questions cover the more important psychological issues when assessing a handicapped person.
 1. How has the person adapted to his handicap?
 2. Has he or others noticed any change in his personality or mood since becoming handicapped?
 3. What does he feel about being dependent on others?
 4. What do other people feel about his dependence on them?

Comprehensive assessment

Important though it is to consider the factors affecting the person's motivation there are many other factors which have to be considered when making a comprehensive assessment with the intention of preventing handicap. These can be set out as an algorithm (Fig. 15.1).

IMMOBILITY

The most important contribution of the general practitioner is of course the effective management of the disease which is immobilizing the person, namely accurate diagnosis, appropriate therapy, and careful education of the person to ensure compliance, the first three steps in the algorithm.

Physiotherapy

The second important contribution which the general practitioner can make is the appropriate use of the skills of a physiotherapist who is trained to treat the secondary effects of disease.
 Muscle weakness resulting from immobility.
 Joint stiffness resulting from immobility.
 Loss of confidence.

In some parts of the country it is impossible for a general practitioner to consult a physiotherapist without referral to a consultant but if the general practitioner is satisfied that he has answered the first three questions satisfactorily there is little need for the opinion of another doctor.

246 *The prevention of disability and handicap*

```
┌─────────────────────────────┐   No    ┌─────────────────────────────┐
│ 1. Have I diagnosed all the │────────▶│ Review clinical data        │
│    relevant diseases        │         │ Consider referral for       │
│    accurately?              │         │ consultant opinion.         │
└─────────────────────────────┘         └─────────────────────────────┘
              │ Yes
              ▼
┌─────────────────────────────┐   No    ┌─────────────────────────────┐
│ 2. Have I prescribed the    │────────▶│ Review therapy, consider    │
│    most appropriate         │         │ referral for consultant     │
│    treatment?               │         │ opinion.                    │
└─────────────────────────────┘         └─────────────────────────────┘
              │ Yes
              ▼
┌─────────────────────────────┐   No    ┌─────────────────────────────┐
│ 3. Is the person taking the │────────▶│ Re-educate the patient,     │
│    treatment correctly?     │         │ simplify treatment regime   │
│                             │         │ if possible                 │
└─────────────────────────────┘         └─────────────────────────────┘
              │ Yes
              ▼
┌─────────────────────────────┐   No    ┌─────────────────────────────┐
│ 4. Could the person's       │────────▶│ Review social aspects of    │
│    motivation be stronger?  │         │ disability in discussion    │
│                             │         │ with relatives and any      │
│                             │         │ other professionals who     │
│                             │         │ are involved.               │
└─────────────────────────────┘         └─────────────────────────────┘
              │ No
              ▼
┌─────────────────────────────┐   No    ┌─────────────────────────────┐
│ 5. Are the secondary        │────────▶│ As for the advice of a      │
│    effects of disease       │         │ physiotherapist             │
│    (muscle wasting, joint   │         │                             │
│    stiffness, and loss of   │         │                             │
│    confidence) significant  │         │                             │
│    problems?                │         │                             │
└─────────────────────────────┘         └─────────────────────────────┘
              │ No
              ▼
┌─────────────────────────────┐   Yes
│ 6. Is it possible to teach  │────────▶┐
│    the person how to        │         │
│    overcome her disability  │         │
│    without the use of aids  │         │
│    or appliances?           │         │
└─────────────────────────────┘         │
              │ No                      │
              ▼                         ▼
┌─────────────────────────────┐   Yes  ╱─────────────╲
│ 7. Could she be independent │───────▶│ Ask for the  │
│    with the provision of    │        │ advice of a  │
│    an aid?                  │        │ domiciliary  │
└─────────────────────────────┘        │ occupational │
              │ No                     │ therapist.   │
              ▼                        ╲─────────────╱
┌─────────────────────────────┐   Yes     ▲
│ 8. Could she be independent │───────────┘
│    if her dwelling were     │
│    adapted, for example     │
│    the installation of a    │
│    downstairs toilet?       │
└─────────────────────────────┘
```

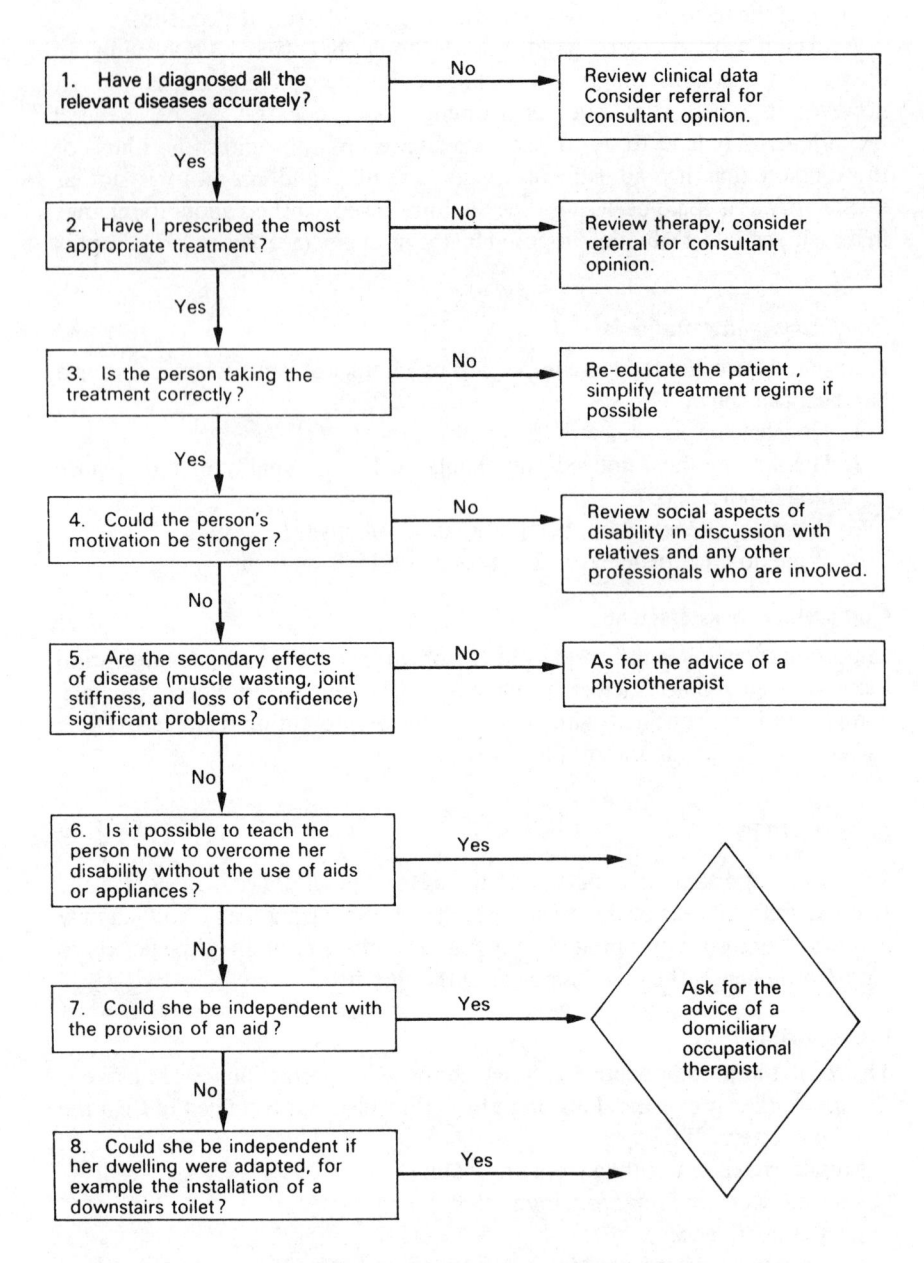

Fig. 15.1. The handicap algorithm.

Effective intervention by a physiotherapist requires the general practitioner to offer her:

1. Adequate information about diagnosis, therapy, the person's personality, and relevant social factors, such as isolation.

2. The opportunity to pay a home visit with the doctor, district nurse, or health visitor.

3. Support, by reinforcing her advice to the patient and his family. Physiotherapists try to educate the disabled person how he can make the best use of his residual abilities and try to restore his confidence, for many disabled people underestimate both their abilities and their potential for improvement. She also tries to educate the disabled person's supporters. In both cases her educational efforts need frequent reinforcement.

Walking aids

Three types of walking frames are in common use.

1. The walking stick.

2. The quadrapod stick – the tripod stick is unstable and in my opinion should not be recommended.

3. The walking frame, for example the Zimmer frame.

Many people prescribe a stick for themselves and use it on the correct side but assessment by a physiotherapist or occupational therapist is often helpful because the provision of a walking aid converts a biped into a triped or a quintaped animal with permanent effects on that person's gait. The easiest approach for a general practitioner who does not consider hospital referral indicated but has no access to a physiotherapist is to ask the advice of the domiciliary occupational therapist.

If mobility within the home is the main problem an adaptation of the dwelling may be more appropriate.

Home adaptations

Mobility problems within the home can be prevented by fixing a handrail along a corridor or up the stairs, or by attaching a short grabrail where there is one or two steps, or by the provision of a stairlift. The advice of the domiciliary occupational therapist will be helpful and patients should be discouraged from buying a stairlift, or from undertaking any structural adaptations, until they have discussed it with her.

Wheelchairs

If the disabled person is only going to use a wheelchair for the occasional trip out of the house, the general practitioner can recommend its use and suggest that the person or her family try to borrow one from a local voluntary society, such as The Red Cross. If, however, the patient wants the wheelchair for everyday use about her home the decision is much more difficult because of the complications which will follow if a person takes to a wheelchair unnecessarily.

It is almost always useful to have a second opinion in such cases and referral to a wheelchair assessment clinic is the appropriate means of achieving this.

Mobility allowance

Poverty is a common cause of immobility outside the home but the Mobility Allowance can prevent this. It was introduced for people who are:

Unable to walk using artificial limbs or other aids;
likely to remain so for at least a year;
able to make use of the allowance;
under pension age.

Although the Department of Health and Social Security (DHSS) often arranges for a medical examination by one of their doctors supporting evidence from the person's general practitioner is helpful. Application can be made by the disabled person or a relative using the form attached to the explanatory leaflet 'Mobility Allowance – Leaflet NI 211' with the general practitioner providing a covering letter.

War pensioners should consult 'War Pensioners – help with personal transport – Leaflet 211 A'.

If a severely disabled person wishes to purchase a specially adapted car he may be eligible for financial help from the Motability scheme. The domiciliary occupational therapist will be able to provide information about this scheme.

Public transport

Holidays and trips away from home prevent the disabled person from becoming depressed and isolated and should be encouraged. Full details of holidays and public transport opportunities are contained in the *Directory for the Disabled* (Darnborough and Kinrade 1977) but the following points offer helpful general guidelines to the disabled person.

1. It is possible to hire a car specially adapted for disabled people.

2. Wheelchairs are available at most main railway stations for moving people between car or taxi and train. In addition special wheelchairs for use inside carriages are available and some of the most modern carriages have seats near a toilet which can be removed to provide space for a wheelchair.

3. Travel by plane is possible for someone in a wheelchair but it helps if notice is given to the airport before the trip is made.

Coping with isolation

If the person is isolated at home by his immobility it is important to try to reduce the degree of isolation. This can be done in three ways.

1. Trips out of the home.
2. Visitors into the home.
3. Stimulation in the home through radio, television, books, and newspapers.

EDUCATION, EMPLOYMENT, AND INCOME PROBLEMS

These three problems are closely inter-related because the person who has difficulty in fulfilling her educational potential because of disability is at a disadvantage in the job market and will be more likely to suffer from unemployment or to work in a job with a low income. It is true that some employers are prejudiced against disabled people and that some workplaces are unsuitable but the employment problems of very disabled people result from the fact that they are less well qualified than those who are not disabled.

Education

The education of disabled schoolchildren leaves much to be desired but at least all schoolchildren are assessed and offered an education. The difficulties increase when the young person leaves school, for in some parts of the country the arrangements for disabled school leavers are inadequate. The first steps in helping the disabled school leaver should, of course, be taken long before the end of his school career and the Careers Officer of the education careers service is the most important person in this respect. Usually she will rely on the school doctor for medical advice but she may wish to consult the young person's general practitioner.

When trying to assess the most appropriate type of further education or employment when giving advice of this sort it is necessary to be careful. It is easy to underestimate a disabled person's ability and to overestimate the influence which the person's disability will have on his ability to attend an institution or to work, particularly if the doctor is uncertain about the exact nature of the work for which the person is being considered. In my opinion it is better to err on the side of optimism than to be over-cautious even though the young person is exposed to the possibility of failure and disappointment. Further education is often necessary for disabled people, as it is for those who are not disabled. It is necessary both for the school leaver and for the person who becomes so disabled in adult life that he or she requires re-training. Education at home, through the medium of the Open University, is one option but it is probably better to aim for attendance at a college, polytechnic, or university in the first instance because the disabled students will receive the benefits of forming friendships with other people in addition to acquiring qualifications; in general integration is better than segregation. The National Bureau of Handicapped Students (City of London Polytechnic), Old Castle Street, London E1 7NT, telephone 01 283 1030) and the Association for Disabled Professionals (73 Pound Road, Banstead, Surrey, telephone Burgh Heath 52366) give advice about the availability of special facilities at colleges and polytechnics and the Open University at Milton Keynes has a counsellor with special responsibilities for disabled students.

Employment

The disablement resettlement officer (the DRO) is the key person in the search for suitable employment. Working from a Job Centre or Employment Office the DRO has to be aware of all the employment opportunities for disabled people and able to advise on the types of the special training which may be required. He has also, of course, to be able to assess the skills and limitations of the disabled person who consults him and to try to place the individual in an appropriate job.

The disabled person may be advised to register under the Disabled Persons (Employment) Act and obtain the 'Green card', a procedure which is completely separate from registration with the Social Services, or Social Work, department under the Chronically Sick and Disabled Persons Act. To be eligible a medical certificate has to be issued stating that the person suffers from a disability that is likely to last for at least 12 months. Holding a green card helps the person find employment as part of the 'quota' of disabled people which large firms are legally required to employ. There are, however, disadvantages to registration because the person may be refused employment or be offered a job which is below his capabilities, for example a carpark attendant or lift operator, if it is known that he holds a green card. However, the DRO is usually able to anticipate and preclude such problems.

The DRO may advise the person to attend an employment rehabilitation centre for retraining and vocational guidance, or he may advise the person to make contact with Professional and Executive Recruitment (PER) which is a Government employment service for managers and technicians and for professional and scientific staff.

The object of this system of vocational guidance and retraining is to allow the disabled person to be able to work in the same type of job as people who are not disabled but it is sometimes necessary for the person to do 'sheltered work' which is specially geared to disabled people, in a Remploy factory for example. Once more the DRO is the main source of advice but there are some useful organizations, for example the Association of Disabled Professionals and Home Opportunities for Professional Employment (Oakwood Further Education Centre, High Street, Kelvedon, Essex). The *Directory for the Disabled* gives a very useful guide to employment opportunities.

Poverty

The income tax deducted from any income being earned by a disabled person, or by a member of his household, should be carefully checked to ensure that the person being taxed is receiving all the allowances for which they are eligible. There is, for example, a dependent relative allowance for the taxpayer who supports a disabled relative and a daughter's services allowance for those who have to rely on the help of a daughter who lives in the same dwelling.

Many disabled people have to depend on social security either in addition to, or in lieu of, income from a job and although the social security system is extremely complicated there are a few simple points which summarize the types of benefit available and the criteria by which eligibility is decided. The reference numbers for the Department of Health and Social Security leaflets are included as it is useful to have at least one copy of each leaflet in the health centre or surgery for reference and it is also useful to have at least one on display.

Invalidity benefit (leaflet NI 16A) is paid to people who have been receiving Sickness Benefit for six months. There are additions for a wife, or any economically dependent adult, and for each child. Men under the age of 60 and women under the age of 55 receive an additional allowance called the Invalidity Allowance, which is also described in Leaflet NI 16A. The Invalidity Benefit is a National Insurance benefit, that is it is only paid to people who have paid enough contributions. Some disabled people have not been able to pay sufficient contributions to qualify and a benefit was introduced for such people. This is the Non-Contributory Invalidity Pension which is for people of working age who have not been able to work for at least six months but who are ineligible for invalidity benefit because they have not paid sufficient National Insurance contributions. Married women can also claim the non-contributory Invalidity Pension provided that they are unable to do normal household work. There are two leaflets about this benefit – leaflet NI 210 for single women and for men and leaflet NI 214 for married women.

Industrial Disablement Benefit is paid to people who have been disabled either by an accident at work, or by a prescribed industrial disease, or by industrial deafness or pneumoconiosis or byssinosis. It can be paid in addition to invalidity or unemployment benefit and consists of a basic allowance which can be supplemented by additional allowances such as the special hardship allowance. Leaflet NI 6, Industrial Disablement Benefit, gives a summary of the criteria and advice on how to apply.

A War Disablement Pension is payable to anyone who is disabled as a result of service in the armed forces. The disabled person should write to the Controller, Central Office (War Pensions), DHSS, Norcross, Blackpool, FX5 3TA.

The Attendance Allowance (leaflet NI 20J) is payable to any disabled person who has needed 'a lot of looking after', in the Department's terms, for at least six months. There are two rates. A higher rate is paid to those who need attendance both night and day, and a lower rate to those whose needs are for attendance during either the day or night. The Invalid Care Allowance (leaflet NI 212) is payable to men and single women of working ages who are unable to work because they have to stay at home to look after a severely disabled relative who is receiving the Attendance Allowance. The advantage of this benefit is not only financial. Even more important, especially for single daughters, is the fact that the recipient is awarded a National Insurance stamp as though she were in paid employment.

In addition to those benefits which are specially for disabled people, people may be eligible for help with their rates because of low income. Application should be made to the Town Hall but a rate or rent rebate officer is usually available to pay a home visit if the person cannot reach the office or has difficulty in writing or phoning.

There are two other financial benefits for low income households. Family Income Supplement (FIS), Leaflet FIS I, for people in fulltime work and Supplementary Benefit (Leaflet SB1) for people who are not working. If the disabled person is in doubt whether or not she is eligible she should apply, although she may need some encouragement to do so.

SELF-CARE PROBLEMS

A disabled person who has become dependent has experienced a series of failures and becomes increasingly pessimistic about his ability to succeed and more dependent on other people for emotional support as well as for practical help. When trying to prevent an increase in dependence it is therefore important to start by setting goals which can be reached so that the disabled person sees that she can succeed; it is more effective to set specific goals such as 'I'm sure that we can teach you how to cook toast and scrambled eggs again', rather than general aims such as 'I'm sure that we can help you become completely independent again'.

The basic functions in which independence is important can be summarized in the following checklist.
- Getting out of and in to bed
- Dressing and undressing
- Reaching the toilet in time
- Washing all over
- Getting enough to eat and drink
- Doing light housework and gardening

Each of these tasks can be analysed in more detail and this is very helpful in identifying the specific problems. If, for example, there is concern about whether or not the disabled person is getting enough to eat it is helpful to determine whether this results from a practical difficulty with shopping or with food preparation, or with cooking or with eating. Having identified the specific problem and problems the next step is to review the management of the disabling disease, and to consider whether there are any relevant psychological factors; for example, a person may have been referred because it is felt by here relatives that she is not getting enough to eat and drink, when the problem is not disability but depression.

The person's disability can be quickly reviewed using the approach summarized in Fig. 15.1 (p. 244).
- Have all the relevant diseases been diagnosed?
- Is the patient complying?
- Are there any relevant social and psychological factors?
- Would physiotherapy help reduce the secondary effects of disease?
- Could the domiciliary occupational therapist prevent handicap?

Self-care problems

Once confident that the person's disability is reduced to its lowest level, an attempt can then be made to overcome her handicap either by teaching her a new way to perform the task which is becoming difficult, or be giving her an aid, or by adapting her house, and the advice of a domiciliary occupational therapist is very useful in the prevention of handicap and dependence.

Getting out of and into bed

If the person is finding difficulty it is often possible to teach him how to get out of bed, and into it, by using another technique. People in wheelchairs are always taught how to transfer from chair to bed, but if the person's disability has increased since a physiotherapist taught him how to transfer it will be useful to seek the advice of a physiotherapist again. It may be helpful to teach the person to transfer from his bed to a chair and then to get up. Sometimes a small handrail on the wall beside the bed head helps the person to stand up but a 'monkey-pole' may be necessary.

It may be necessary to alter the height of the bed. Some beds are too low for the person to get out of, others are too high to get into, and care must therefore be taken to ensure that the advice given to solve one problem does not create another. Sometimes a new bed is necessary, for example when the person's bed has a deep hollow in the middle which traps him.

Dressing and undressing

The advice of an occupational or physiotherapist is particularly useful in this area. Often it is possible to teach someone how to dress and undress independently even though they are severely disabled. Sometimes it is necessary to provide a dressing aid, such as a stick with a rubber tip, with which the person can lift a jacket or cardigan round his paralysed side or an aid which helps him put on his socks. The Red Cross publish a useful catalogue of aids for disabled people but the occupational therapist is the best source of advice for aids and for special clothing.

It is possible to adapt ordinary clothing, for example by replacing buttons with Velcro fastenings. It is also possible to buy specially designed clothing which is easier to manage, for example by having a Velcro flap in the front of a pair of trousers rather than a fly, and the advice and assistance of an occupational therapist is useful if special clothing is being considered. She will, however, often be able to preclude the need for special clothing by advising the person to buy those types of ordinary clothing which are more suitable, for example to buy a wrap-around skirt rather than one which has to be pulled on.

Washing all over

Many disabled people develop their own method of washing all over without using the bath. For example by using a towelling mitten or a sponge on a stick the person who cannot use his bath unaided may be able to wash all over. However, it is often possible to help someone who says that he is unable or

254 *The prevention of disability and handicap*

afraid to get into his bath to learn how to use it safely while alone by the provision of aids, such as a rail on the wall beside the bath or a bath board.

The advice of an occupational therapist is always helpful with bathing problems and if a bath board or seat does not give independence she will consider whether a shower would allow the person to regain independence or whether the person has to accept that he needs help with bathing. If help is needed the contribution which a hoist can make to the wellbeing of the helper – spouse, relative, or district nurse – should be considered.

Reaching the toilet in time

Incontinence is particularly distressing both for the disabled person and his supporters and its prevention is of great importance. In some cases it is due to disease of the genito-urinary system or of the nervous system in which cases its prevention depends upon the effective management of the causal disease. In other people, however, it results solely from the disabled person's inability to reach the toilet in time and in other instances, following a stroke for example, both factors are present for both nervous control and mobility are impaired.

The steps by which a disabled person can be helped to reach the toilet in time can best be summarized in an algorithm (Fig. 15.2).

Getting enough to eat and drink

The need to identify the specific cause of the problem and the means by which it can be alleviated have already been emphasized. Often the most important factor is either depression or the loss of motivation which results from isolation and nutritional problems should always be regarded as a symptom of some other problem as well as being a problem in their own right. One type of problem which may be presented as a nutritional problem is over-anxiety on the part of relatives. Because there are such fixed cultural beliefs about eating three meals a day relatives sometimes become very alarmed if a disabled person is not eating in a way which is conventionally acceptable. Furthermore, expressions of anxiety about a person's eating may be expressive of much more generalized anxieties about his condition and his circumstances.

In some cases nutritional problems that are the anxiety of the disabled person's supporters, can be prevented by persuading them that three cooked meals are not necessary and that most nutritional needs can be met with well-filled sandwiches and a flask within reach.

Doing light housework and gardening

Disabled people often find their own solution to this problem but the occupational therapist can help by the provision of special housebound gadgets or by the adaptation of the person's kitchen, for example by changing the height of the sink so that the disabled person can use it while in her wheelchair. Independence in light housework is of great importance to many women and this may be underestimated by a male doctor. Dependence on others for

Self-care problems 255

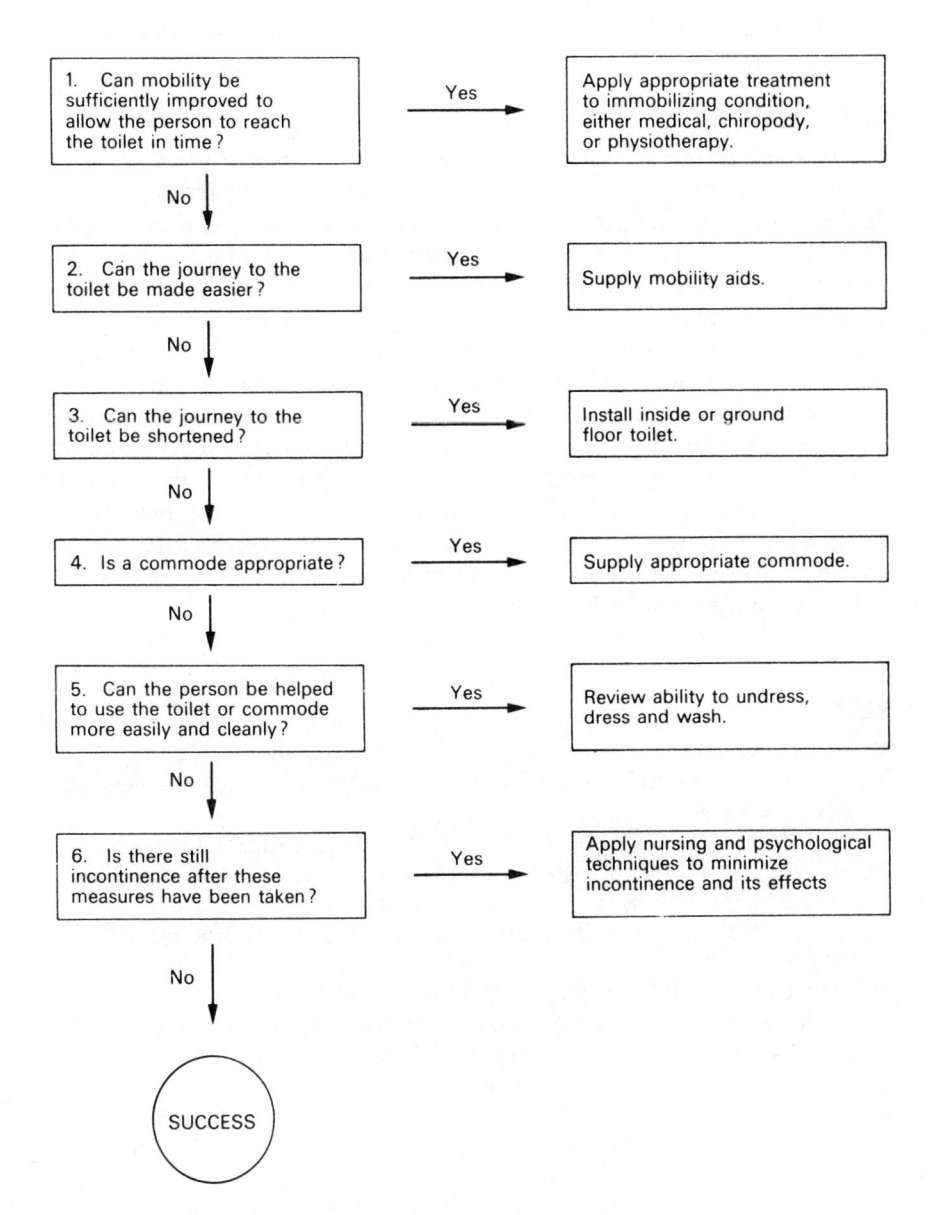

```
┌─────────────────────────┐
│ 1. Can mobility be      │      Yes      ┌──────────────────────────────┐
│ sufficiently improved to│──────────────▶│ Apply appropriate treatment  │
│ allow the person to reach│              │ to immobilizing condition,   │
│ the toilet in time?     │               │ either medical, chiropody,   │
└─────────────────────────┘               │ or physiotherapy.            │
        │ No                              └──────────────────────────────┘
        ▼
┌─────────────────────────┐      Yes      ┌──────────────────────────────┐
│ 2. Can the journey to the│─────────────▶│ Supply mobility aids.        │
│ toilet be made easier?  │               └──────────────────────────────┘
└─────────────────────────┘
        │ No
        ▼
┌─────────────────────────┐      Yes      ┌──────────────────────────────┐
│ 3. Can the journey to the│─────────────▶│ Install inside or ground     │
│ toilet be shortened?    │               │ floor toilet.                │
└─────────────────────────┘               └──────────────────────────────┘
        │ No
        ▼
┌─────────────────────────┐      Yes      ┌──────────────────────────────┐
│ 4. Is a commode appropriate?│─────────▶│ Supply appropriate commode.   │
└─────────────────────────┘               └──────────────────────────────┘
        │ No
        ▼
┌─────────────────────────┐      Yes      ┌──────────────────────────────┐
│ 5. Can the person be helped│───────────▶│ Review ability to undress,   │
│ to use the toilet or commode│             │ dress and wash.             │
│ more easily and cleanly?  │              └──────────────────────────────┘
└─────────────────────────┘
        │ No
        ▼
┌─────────────────────────┐      Yes      ┌──────────────────────────────┐
│ 6. Is there still       │──────────────▶│ Apply nursing and psychological│
│ incontinence after these│               │ techniques to minimize        │
│ measures have been taken?│              │ incontinence and its effects  │
└─────────────────────────┘               └──────────────────────────────┘
        │ No
        ▼
     ( SUCCESS )
```

Fig. 15.2. Algorithm showing steps by which a disabled person can be helped to reach the toilet in time.

housework may result in feelings of inadequacy and depression and the corollary of this is that a decline in the standard of housekeeping may be a sign of depression.

Other care

The disabled person may still be unable to care for himself after all these measures have been taken and help from other people will be required. Most disabled people receive help from their families but it is often as important to offer help in the form of home help or district nursing to a family as it is to offer it to an isolated disabled person to prevent family strains and family breakdown. In some parts of the country Crossroads schemes operate with home care assistants providing both personal and domestic help, but in most areas the home help and district nursing service must be approached individually. Volunteers are also extremely helpful in performing jobs about the home but relatives, volunteers and other untrained helpers require careful and specific advice about which tasks they should perform for the disabled person and which he should perform for himself. Most untrained people err on the side of over-protection and do too much for the person and proper education of the helper is an important means of preventing an increase in dependence and the degree of handicap.

REFERENCES

Blaxter, M. (1976). *The meaning of disability.* Heinemann, London.

Darnborough, A. and Kinrade, D. (1977). *Directory for the disabled.* Woodhead-Faulkner, London.

Harris, A. (1971). *Handicapped and impaired in Great Britain.* HMSO, London.

Stevenson, O. (1981). The frail elderly – a social worker's perspective. In *Health care of the elderly* (ed. T. Arie) pp. 158–75. Croom Helm, London.

Topliss, E. (1978). The disabled. In *The social context of health care,* pp. 122–51. Martin Robertson.

Wood, P. H. N. (1981). The language of disablement. *Int. Rehab. Med.* 2, 86–92.

World Health Organization (1980). *International classification of impairments, disabilities and handicaps.* WHO, Geneva.

16 Prevention in old age

Muir Gray

SETTING OBJECTIVES

One way of describing the objective of preventive medicine is to state that its goal is to maintain the *status quo,* to offer the 30-year-old man the prospect that he still will be as healthy when he is 50 years old. When working with older people, for example those in their eighties, this goal is inappropriate because some decline in the person's physical ability is inevitable and it would be inappropriate to suggest to an 80-year-old man that he could still be fit when he is 100. However, because an elderly persons actual ability is almost always less than his potential ability it is often possible to set a similar goal and to state to an 80-year-old person that he could be as fit when he is 85 as he is at 80, alternatively he could be told that he could be fitter than he is currently (Fig. 16.1).

The objective of intervention may therefore be defined as being to slow down the rate of decline in ability but the means by which this is achieved is not by influencing the aging process but by helping the old person function at the level of ability which is nearer his potential ability.

Before setting any goal, whether therapeutic or preventive, it is essential to appreciate the beliefs of elderly people about their ability and potential and

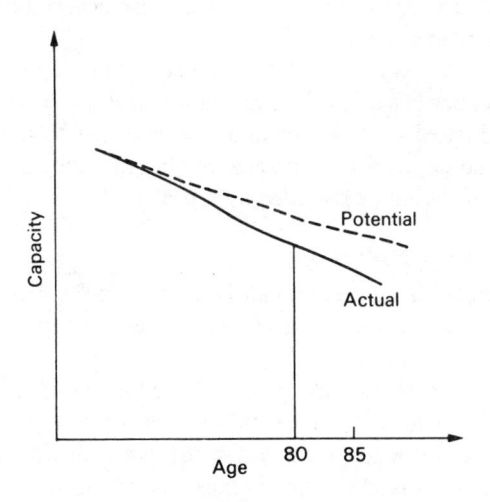

Fig. 16.1.

their attitudes towards their problems, because many of them do not believe that there is any potential for improvement in their present condition nor that their rate of deterioration can be decelerated.

BELIEFS AND ATTITUDES

Health beliefs of older people

Many elderly people take a very pessimistic attitude towards physical or mental symptoms with the result that they are less likely to seek help for symptoms. They are also less easy to persuade that they could be healthier and are less likely to comply with advice than are young people. This pessimism is a consequence of the belief that all the symptoms which occur in old age are the result of the aging process and are not the consequences of treatable pathological processes. 'What else can you expect at my age?' is a common statement and reflects this belief. Regrettably, this belief has sometimes been reinforced by a doctor who said 'What else can you expect at your age?' before he has even examined the person. This is an ageist statement.

The acceptance of disability or discomfort which results from such an aging prejudice is further reinforced in some elderly people by the belief that the reason why they are afflicted is 'God's Will'. Not infrequently this type of religious explanation of the person's suffering, which may of course be a source of comfort to the afflicted elder, is overlooked but it is very important to recognize it and seek the assistance of a priest if it is decided to challenge it (Gray and Wilcock 1981).

Although these beliefs are the cause of the old person's acceptance of her problems and unwillingness to seek help a fatalistic belief may also be the person's means of coping with problems which are believed to be intractable, that is it may be a magical belief.

They may only be ways of adapting to her disability and any attempt to challenge or dispel her beliefs poses a difficult ethical problem. It is justifiable to make her dissatisfied with her lot and to expose her to the risk of failure, disappointment and depression by persuading her that the condition which she previously accepted should be regarded as 'a problem'?

Attitudes towards social problems

Many elderly people also accept social circumstances which younger people would find intolerable. However, this is not the result of their health beliefs, it is the consequences of their biography.

Most people in their eighties and nineties have known such hardship in their youth that difficulties which seem tremendous to prosperous young professionals are often of little consequence to the old people who are affected: to men who had to use their socks soaked in urine because the administration miscalculated the number of gas masks needed, the lack of an inside toilet or the presence of rats in the kitchen are minor problems. Not only are their standards often lower, their expectations may also be much lower than those of younger people because their generation has been disappointed so often, for example by the promise that it was a 'War to end all wars' which would provide 'Homes fit for Heroes'. In addition they are less demanding than younger people because they have a more limited view of their rights, having been brought up in a culture in which landlords and employers had very much more power than their present day equivalents (Blythe 1979).

Finally, it is essential to remember that some old people will be very suspicious of unsolicited offers of 'help'. Most welcome a doctor who takes the initiative but some will believe that the doctor is in league with relatives or neighbours who wish to persuade them to enter a home. The response to professional intervention by someone who holds this belief may be an angry and hostile one, in which case the old person may be labelled as being 'difficult' or 'aggressive'. Alternatively the main impression may be one of suspicion, in which case the elder may be diagnosed as being 'paranoid'. Some old people may say that 'I'm all right' not because they accept their disabilities and difficulties but because they wish to hide them; refusing to reveal their problems because they are afraid that they will be institutionalized if they admit that they are failing to cope.

It should also be said that some elderly people do not ask for help because they 'don't like to trouble the doctor'.

Practical implications

1. Elderly people have to be educated that their physical, mental, and social problems may be preventable and treatable. Every possible opportunity should be taken to present to older people an optimistic and hopeful view of the future and particular emphasis should be given to the distinction between aging and disease and to the need to refer problems.

2. Attempts to alleviate the problems of an old person who accepts them and does not appear too bothered by them undoubtedly pose an ethical dilemma for the doctor, but, in my opinion, the majority of doctors err on the side of caution and should challenge the mistaken beliefs of old people more strongly.

3. The doctor should be prepared to initiate contact with his elderly patients partly because of their attitudes and beliefs and partly because they have more difficulty in communicating with or reaching the surgery than younger patients (Williamson *et al.* 1964; Hannay 1979). The most appropriate means of initiating and maintaining contact depend upon the resources of the practice. Alternative approaches are:

(i) regular home visits by a doctor;
(ii) regular home visits by a health visitor or district nurse;
(iii) attendance at a clinic held at the surgery or health centre.

An age/sex register is essential for an effective programme of prevention (Tulloch and Moore 1979; Williamson 1981; Wilcock *et al.* 1982). It allows the doctor to be sure that the whole population is covered and allows him to select vulnerable subgroups within his practice population. One method of selecting the vulnerable group is by age and to concentrate on those over 75 or over 85, depending upon how much time the doctor can devote to preventive work. This approach is necessary if the doctor knows very little about the whole group but the doctor can select the people who would benefit from an approach initiated by the doctor more specifically by identifying those with one or more of the following characteristics:

(i) being housebound;
(ii) not having a telephone;
(iii) having recently lost their spouse;
(iv) having dementia;
(v) having severely impaired communication because of speech, hearing, or visual problems;
(vi) being depressed.

4. Care must be taken to minimize fear. An explicit statement by the doctor such as 'I'm interested in helping you live on in your own home as long as possible' is often helpful and should always be said but it may take two or three visits before the elderly person begins to trust the doctor if she has not seen him before. Where possible the support of a trusted person, either a professional such as a nurse who has visited regularly for some months or a relative, should be enlisted.

ATTITUDES OF OTHER PEOPLE

Indifference and hostility

It is commonly said and widely believed that British people do not care for their elders as much as they do in 'primitive' cultures or in our own past. This is not the case. There is no evidence to suggest that the society today is less caring or more hostile than it was in the past (Isaacs 1971; Moroney 1976). People are probably less willing to help their elderly neighbours than they were but the reason for this is probably due as much to their belief that the statutory service for which they pay large amounts in rates and taxes should care for elderly people. Some people are even hostile towards professionals whom they see in secure, superannuated jobs paid for by their rates and taxes while they are in jobs threatened by redundancy or run small businesses at risk of bankruptcy. This resentment towards the health and social services may only be expressed as a vehement demand that 'something should be done about Mrs S' who is herself unconcerned by her circumstances.

Guilt

If a person knows that she could help an elderly neighbour, relative, or friend but does not do so, she will probably feel guilty even though she is able to find good reasons why she should not help, for example 'because the social services should help'. She may become extremely anxious about the old person and try to persuade her that she should enter an institution 'to be looked after'. She may also phone the old person's doctor, the social services department, her councillor, and the local press frequently demanding that 'someone should do something'.

It would be wrong to ascribe all the motives of relatives, friends, and neighbours who behave in this way to guilt, some people who are more anxious than appears to be reasonable may be anxious because they underestimate the old person's ability to appreciate that she is at risk.

Underestimation and ageism

The ageist attitude is a prejudice. The person who is ageist believes that all elderly people are of declining intelligence, unable to change or learn, and in a 'second childhood'. Not only do they assume that physical symptoms are due to aging but they believe that any mental or behavioural change is due to dementia and that it is useless to attempt to help an old person solve her problems by any means other than by 'taking care of her' that is doing things for her either in her home or in an institution.

Practical implications

1. Referrals by persons other than the elder are biased by these attitudes. Guilt and resentment towards professionals lead to the over-referral of elderly people who may be in no need of help whereas agism results in the under-referral of treatable problems. These factors strengthen the argument for a style of practice in which the initiative should be taken by the doctor.

2. Ageist underestimations of the intelligence and educability of elderly people may result in reluctance on the part of relatives, friends, and neighbours to participate in rehabilitation. They may believe that the only feasible approach to elderly people is a 'caring' approach and equate caring with doing things for the elder rather helping her to learn to do things for herself. It is as necessary to educate the supporters as it is to educate the elder.

3. People who are guilty about an elderly person will also prefer to do things for her, to 'care for her' rather than encourage her to do things for herself. Guilt may arise from many sources, for example from the feelings of anger towards an elderly parent which co-exist with the feelings of love in a single daughter. The doctor should try to reveal these feelings and relieve the guilt if it is a problem.

TERTIARY PREVENTION

There is scope for tertiary prevention in both acute and chronic disease.

Tertiary prevention in acute conditions

Tertiary prevention is achieved by the accurate diagnosis and appropriate treatment of a disease at an early stage in its evolution. Early detection cannot be achieved by routine visiting or by contacts initiated by professionals. It requires the prompt referral of problems by elderly people themselves and by their relatives, neighbours, friends, and professional helpers. To encourage early referral requires the education of these people that the problems of old age are neither inevitable nor incurable and the doctor should use every opportunity to change the attitudes described in the preceding sections of this chapter.

Tertiary prevention in chronic conditions (Wilcock *et al.* 1982)

Chronic diseases

There are two principal means of tertiary prevention of chronic diseases – surveillance and physiotherapy.

The surveillance of people with chronic conditions by making regular contacts with them allows the doctor to monitor the progress of the disease and the compliance of the patient with his therapeutic advice. The elderly person suffering from a chronic disease or her supporters may fail to report a deterioration not only because they assume any change for the worse to be due to aging but also because it is more difficult for patients or people who see them daily to notice.

This type of surveillance is aimed at the primary effects of the disease but it is essential to try to prevent the secondary effects of disease – muscle wasting, joint stiffness, and loss of confidence – which result from the immobility. To prevent these secondary effects the contribution of a physiotherapist is very helpful after the doctor is satisfied that he has answered the following questions:

1. Have all the relevant diseases been diagnosed accurately?
2. Is the treatment appropriate for each condition?
3. Is the old person taking the treatment as prescribed?

If the answer to these is in the affirmative a home visit by a physiotherapist should be arranged if it is the doctor's opinion that the person is becoming immobilized or demoralized as a consequence of disease. Unfortunately, hospital assessment by a physiotherapist is often the only service on which the general practitioner can call but every effort should be made to develop a domiciliary physiotherapy service to prevent unnecessary disability.

Chronic symptoms

The tertiary prevention of disease is important but it is always necessary to complement the surveillance and treatment of disease by a symptom orientated approach because there are five common symptoms which can cause great distress to the old person and her supporters.

Instability; falling or fear of falling
Immobility

Incontinence or fear of incontinence
Pain
Anxiety and depression.

It is necessary to consider these separately from disease because they may be overlooked and because it is often necessary to try to alleviate each of these symptoms although the causal disease is either obscure or incurable. If, for example, an old person is still incontinent after all possible pathological causes have been diagnosed and are being treated, the doctor has to try to alleviate the problems which the incontinence causes the old person or her supporters.

Chronic handicaps

It is often necessary to treat symptoms in old age even though the underlying disease, is unkown or intractable, as indeed it is in many other aspects of general practice. When working with older patients it is also necessary to consider the functional consequences of disease and for the general practitioner to ensure that steps are being taken to alleviate any which may be present. In older people the most important functional consequence of disease is a handicap in one or more of the activities of daily living.

Getting out of bed
Dressing
Washing all over
Getting to the toilet in time
Getting enough to eat and drink
Doing light housework
Undressing
Getting to bed.

The approach to problems with these functions is the same as it is with younger people (see p. 241).

Remember also that disability may interfere with an elderly couple's ability to enjoy sexual intercourse. This is a severe problem for older couples particularly for those who believe that sexual activity is somewhat improper in old age and are ashamed to admit their difficulties to their doctor as they will have to reveal that they are still interested in sex.

The prevention of iatrogenic disorders

Perhaps the most important aspect of tertiary prevention is the prevention of iatrogenic diseases. The two common causes of iatrogenic disorders are drug side-effects and poor compliance, and often the two are combined for the person who does not take his drugs as the doctor intended is at higher risk of suffering side-effects from the drugs. This is obviously an immense subject but it is possible to summarize the means by which iatrogenic disorders may be prevented by means of a small number of maxims.

Prescribe as few drugs as possible.
Prescribe each drug in as small a dose as possible.

Take special care that drugs will not interact with one another.
Take a careful drug history to identify possible sensitivities.
Take time to educate the elderly person about his drugs (Knox 1980).
Ensure that there is adequate surveillance of elderly people on repeat prescriptions (Tulloch 1981).

Chronic social problems

No doctor has the time to tackle all the social problems of his elderly patients but the general practitioner can make an important contribution to their solution for three reasons. Firstly because he may be the only professional in contact with the elderly person, secondly he may be the person who is most trusted and respected by the elder, and thirdly he should be interested in social problems for his own well-being and that of his partners. In the type of crisis which arises at the weekend or over a public holiday it is frequently the social circumstances which prove more worrying and difficult to improve than the person's medical condition.

A doctor can take four steps which may help an elderly person with a social problem. He can

1. Recognize the presence of a social problem.
2. Inform the elder of the help which is available.
3. Ensure that she can make contact with the appropriate source of help if she has difficulty in communicating.
4. Be prepared to discuss her attitudes towards the help which is available if she refuses to consider seeking help, for example because she considers social security to be 'charity'.

It is usually possible to take these steps during the course of a home visit without unduly increasing the length of time the visit takes.

No doctor can carry all the information about the full range of services available for elderly people and he will often have to refer the old person to another professional, a health visitor or social worker, or to the Citizens Advice Bureau or the local Age Concern Office for detailed information and advice.

Social problem checklist (Gray and Mackenzie 1979)

1. Is the old person at risk of hypothermia because she is not heating her house properly? (Fox *et al.* 1973) If the answer is yes, what is the cause?
    (a) poverty;
    (b) old or inefficient heating apparatus;
    (c) inadequate insulation;
    (d) fear of fuel bills.
2. Is the old person's housing causing her anxiety or depression or creating practical difficulties for herself or her helpers?
3. Is the old person worrying excessively about debt or the cost of living or is she buying inadequate amounts of food or fuel or clothes because of her income problems?

PREVENTION OF MENTAL DISORDER

The many causes of mental disorder can be classified under five headings and the general practitioner can do much to prevent mental or behavioural problems, if he can prevent or alleviate any of these factors
  Physical disease
  Family pressures
  Social pressures
  Isolation
  Sensory deprivation.

Physical disease

If an old person develops a mental or behavioural disorder it should be assumed that is the consequence of physical disease until this possibility has been excluded. The only means by which the doctor can do this is by the education of old people, and of their relatives, friends, neighbours, and professional supporters, that a change in an old person's mental state or in her behaviour is an indication for referral to her general practitioner. Too often it is assumed that any such change is due to 'her age'. It may even be assumed that the old person is 'dementing' if he or she is very elderly, because some people use 'aging' and 'dementing' as synonyms.

Particular emphasis has to be given to this point when the elderly person has definitely been diagnosed as suffering from dementia. Too often physical disease remains undiagnosed and untreated in people with dementia because those who are helping them assume that any change or deterioration is a result of their dementia. Once someone has been labelled as 'a dement' or 'a psycho-geriatric' by her relatives other problems are created. They may not disagree with her if she makes a mistake because they believe that someone with dementia is unable to learn or appreciate an error. This can increase the person's confusion. Similarly, they may not correct her when her behaviour is upsetting and thus she is therefore not the subject of the normal sanctions on which we all depend to regulate our behaviour within acceptable limits. Some allowance must, of course, be made for a person who has dementia but most people make too many allowances and supporters have to be educated about this and helped to decide how to respond to her mistakes and lapses in memory.

Family pressures

The effect of the resentment towards an old person with dementia who is sharing a house with her family, or the effects of moving an old person from one child to another can increase her confusion and can make her depressed, as can many other family pressures.

All the measures described in the section on the prevention of family breakdown are equally appropriate for mental disorder as for physical disorders. The offer of regular assured periods of relief are particularly helpful.

Social pressures

Social pressures can cause:
- Anxiety
- Depression
- Delusions and hallucinations
- Intellectual deterioration and a loss of spirit.

The individual doctor can do little to change the structure of society but he can reduce the adverse influence of some of its aspects by:

1. Trying to minimize the old person's social problems, for these are a common cause of anxiety and depression.

2. Trying to reduce the old person's isolation, because the emotional effect of social problems such as fear of crime, or worry about debt or a feeling of uselessness and almost always greater if the affected person has no-one with whom to discuss them and no-one to be reassured by.

3. Trying to make each elderly person feel that he respects him or her as an individual. One of the most distressing aspects of disability and dependence is that the dependent person may feel useless. Some elderly people have little social life other than with the professionals who come to help them. The number of people who come to visit them as a person decreases and the number who come to visit them 'as a client', to sort out some problem, increases. In an existential sense this can be very destructive and can result in depression, apathy, and depersonalization. Those who have been religious may be helped if links can be reestablished with their church but professionals can also help. One of the most important benefits of regular home visiting is that it allows a personal relationship to develop to complement the professional relationship. Home helps and district nurses become friends with the elderly people they visit and this friendship can be very strengthening and sustaining. Even though his visits may be much less frequent than those of the nurse or home help a general practitioner can help strengthen the nature of the individual to continue coping if a personal relationship can develop.

In my opinion this is certainly an effective type of intervention. Whether or not it is sufficiently efficient, as measured against all the other possible ways of using his time, is up to the individual doctor to decide.

Isolation

Isolation can cause:

Loneliness, although not all isolated old people are lonely; neither are all lonely people isolated.

Disorientation in time and space, delusions, memory impairment: research conducted into brainwashing has demonstrated that many young people display these symptoms after 48 hours isolation. Many elderly people are alone for 70 hours every weekend from noon on Friday until nine on Monday, with significant sensory deprivation as well.

Depression and anxiety.

Nutritional problems: lunch clubs are more effective than meals on wheels for most people.

Dependence.

Some people prefer to be isolated and that is their right. But if a person was previously gregarious and now says that she prefers to stay at home the possibility of some underlying problem should be considered. For example fear that she will be incontinent, shame about her clothes and appearance, or a phobia about leaving home. Other people become isolated because their mobility is impaired but being housebound does not necessarily mean that a person will become isolated, their personality is also important. An old person who is rewarding to visit, who does not dwell on her own problems, who is not bitter, who is moved by the plight of other people less fortunate than herself and who shows an interest in the doings of her friends and relatives and neighbours – is less likely to become isolated than the old person who is self-centred, bitter, and critical of those who come to visit. If such characteristics are new depression should be suspected but they are often characteristics which the individual has had all her life. The prevention of isolation is of great importance in the prevention of mental disorder and the following measures should be tried:

1. The reduction of disability to its lowest possible degree.
2. The organization of as many trips out of the person's home as possible.
3. The facilitation of as many visits to the old person at home as possible.
4. The stimulation of the old person in her home by encouraging her to take an interest in newspapers, the radio, and television and by arranging for a library volunteer to bring her books. Some old people benefit greatly from a pet such as a kitten or a budgie.
5. The provision of a telephone. This is very dificult to arrange in most parts of the country but funds may be able to be raised from local or national charities.
6. Discussion with the old person about the benefits of a move to sheltered housing. In general, elderly people should be encouraged to stay in the dwelling in which they live but it is sometimes preferable to encourage a move to a dwelling with security, elderly neighbours nearby, and the services of a warden. Isolation is rarely a sufficient reason for admission to an old people's home to be indicated but it is often an important contributory factor.

Sensory deprivation

Sensory deprivation can cause a number of problems:

Depression and anxiety.

Delusions and hallucinations; deafness is associated with paranoid delusions.

Disorientation in time and space and intellectual deterioration; research on brainwashing has revealed the effect of sensory deprivation as a means of confusing an individual. Disorientation in time and space and memory disorder may all result from sensory deprivation.

By trying to minimize visual impairment (Disabled Living Foundation 1979), hearing impairment (Herbert and Humphrey 1980), and the communication difficulties which may follow a stroke, the doctor can prevent some of the mental consequences of sensory deprivation.

SECONDARY PREVENTION – SCREENING

The identification of chronic diseases which were not previously diagnosed or social problems which had previously been unknown to any professional is sometimes referred to as 'screening' but I prefer to use the term screening in a narrower, I believe its proper, sense. By screening I mean the detection of a disorder by a sensitive, specific test at an earlier stage in its natural history than the stage at which it would have been diagnosed, namely the symptomatic stage. I will therefore include only those procedures which I believe to meet the criteria cited in the chapter on screening (see p. 96).

A large number of articles have been written on screening in old age and the writers have suggested many procedures which have not been validated against the standard criteria but which have been included in screening programmes. Some of the procedures which have been proposed are listed below.

1. Measurement of blood pressure (see p. 101).
2. Tonometry.
3. Rectal examination.
4. Faecal occult blood test.
5. Vaginal examination.
6. Breast palpation.
7. Haemoglobin estimation.
8. White blood cell count.
9. Erythrocyte sedimentation rate.
10. Mental status questionnaires.

In my opinion there is insufficient evidence to justify the use of the above procedures but there is some scope for screening in old age, although the procedures discussed in this section have not been formally validated using the criteria previously cited (see p. 96).

Cervical cytology

In theory, cervical cytology is still relevant in older age groups. In practice, however, it often proves so difficult to perform satisfactory examination and obtain a smear that it would be inappropriate to attempt the procedure with every old person. If a pelvic examination is being carried out as a result of self-referral for some symptom then a smear should be taken but this screening procedure is of little practical significance for women over the age of 65.

Visual screening

Many elderly people accept visual impairment as being due to the aging process when it is often due to some correctable disorder. The objective of visual screening is to detect disease and visual impairment. The former is best detected by examination of the fundi the latter by the old person's report of a decrease in acuity.

If glaucoma is suspected as a result of the elderly person's account of her visual symptoms or after examination of the fundi she should be referred to an ophthalmologist. If the presence of macular degeneration or cataracts is suspected it is, however, appropriate to refer the person to an optician for examination and refraction initially, unless she has had a recent examination by an optician.

If the old person reports a decrease in visual acuity without any sign of disease she should be referred to an optician for refraction. He acts as a second screen and may detect a disease which the doctor has missed but in most cases accurate refraction is all that is required.

If there is neither any sign of disease nor any report of recent impairment the person should be encouraged to consult an optician if it is more than two years since her vision was last tested. Elderly people should be encouraged to have a biennal refraction because their prescription may require modification due to presbyopia. If the person is unable to say whether or not her vision has deteriorated, for example because of dysphasia or dementia, refraction should be recommended if more than two years have passed since their visual acuity was last tested.

Remember that inadequate lighting is one of the commonest correctable causes of visual impairment (Gilkes 1979).

Auditory screening

To be precise only the detection of glaucoma can be classified as a screening procedure because the other measures described in the previous section are more accurately described as the detection of unreported problems. It could also be argued that an enquiry about the elder's ability to hear and the detection of any impairment are also more appropriately described as being the detection of unreported problems rather than as a screening procedure. The objective of the enquiry is not the treatment of a disease at an early curable stage because otosclerosis is rarely treatable and therefore, is not a screening procedure. However, I include it in the screening section of this chapter because I believe that the early detection and treatment of the effects of the disease is more effective than waiting until the person has become completely deaf. The earlier a person is helped to adjust to a loss of hearing the better will he adjust whether the measure suggested is advice on communication and on how one should ask others to communicate, or tuition in lip reading or a hearing aid.

If the person reports that conversation is becoming difficult, or that it has become more difficult to hear the telephone ringing, auroscopic examination is indicated with referral to a specialist if wax is not the cause of the impairment.

Foot problems

The detection of foot problems could also be considered as being the recognition of unmet need rather then as a screening procedure but it is probable that the correct treatment of minor foot disorders can prevent the development of more serious deformity and disability.

Malnutrition

Obesity is the commonest type of malnutrition in old age. It is easily detected by observation but it is often very difficult to decide on the appropriate response. Obesity undoubtedly causes a number of problems for an elderly person but it is often difficult to achieve a decrease in weight. The old person may believe that her weight is due to her 'glands' or her inactivity, or to her 'age' and be very resistant to suggestions that she could lose weight. Furthermore eating and drinking may be one of the main pleasures left to her. This gives the doctor two difficult decisions, should he inform the elder that her weight is a problem and, if decides to do so, how hard should he try to persuade her to lose weight.

In general the doctor should try to help the elder lose weight, even though he may have to upset her to do so, if he thinks that the obesity is causing symptoms. The approach to obesity in old age is similar to that used for younger people (see p. 153).

Fibre deficiency is also common among older people and it is appropriate to recommend an increase in fibre intake at all ages. If constipation worries the old person advice on fibre is obviously indicated but even if the old person is not worried about her bowel habits the advice is also indicated. There is no definite evidence that an increase in the intake of fibre at the age of 70, or older, reduces the risk of complications from diverticular disease in people who have no symptoms of the disease but the improvement in symptoms of older people who have complications suggests that prevention is possible. The old person must be cautioned not to increase the intake too quickly or explosive and uncomfortable bowel movements may be the consequence.

Vitamin and mineral deficiencies are uncommon (Department of Health and Social Security 1972, 1980). They should be suspected if the old person's food intake has decreased but the best approach to the detection of such deficiencies is to concentrate on those who have some problem which is likely to lead to a reduction in intake; that is people with one or more of the following characteristics:

Isolation.
Depression.
Recent bereavement, particularly in men.
Severe dental or oral problems with difficulty in chewing and swallowing.
Being dependent on social security.
Being handicapped in food preparation or eating.
Severe dementia.

Secondary prevention—screening

The obvious steps to take when considering how best to help an old person who is considered to be at risk of developing a nutritional deficiency is to arrange for her to have meals on wheels. However, before doing so it is appropriate to try to determine why she is at risk and what alternative measures could be taken to help her provide for herself. The following questions are useful.

Is shopping difficult?
Is food preparation difficult?
Is cooking difficult?
Is eating difficult?
Is it a problem of motivation to perform any of those tasks?

Only after these questions have been answered and one is satisfied that it is impossible for the old person to cook for herself should meals on wheels be arranged; although they offer another benefit for isolated elderly people and her supporters – regular visits.

Primary prevention—a pre-retirement checklist

A general practitioner can undertake health education during the course of a consultation which was initiated by a patient seeking help with a problem but he must be careful not to create new anxieties before he has allayed the anxiety which was the original reason for the consultation. He may also be given an opportunity for health education by being asked to address an old people's club or pre-retirement course. When speaking to a group a different approach is required because the speaker rarely knows all the members of the group and must take even greater care not to raise fears which he cannot allay.

In both situations the same subjects should be covered.

Diet
Exercise
Smoking
Accidents
Mental health
Beliefs and attitudes

Diet

The two most common preventable problems are obesity and fibre deficiency. Obesity is common in the older age groups and the preventive approach has two objectives. One is to try to help the old person from becoming heavier, whatever his weight; the second is to help those who are obese to lose weight.

The person in the pre-retirement class can be told to weigh himself during his last week at work and then to make a routine of weighing himself at the same time every week. If there are weight increases on two successive weeks the person should review his diet and his exercise habits and try to take in less energy than he expends for the next four weeks. It is usually necessary to explain energy balance and the energy content of different foods to older people. Many are aware of the energy content of fat and refined carbohydrate but think that bread and potatoes are very fattening foods believing that the avoidance of these two foods constitutes 'a diet'.

Those who wish to lose weight also need this information. In addition they need help to decide whether or not they need to lose weight and they need to be given good reasons for making the effort to do so. To give guidance on whether or not an old person needs to lose weight it is easier to recommend that he looks in the mirror and decides for himself whether or not he has surplus weight to lose than to give advice on 'average' or 'ideal' weight. The motivation to lose weight can be provided if the old person is told that he can reduce the risk of a number of diseases if he does so but an appeal to the person's vanity should not be omitted solely because he or she is old.

Not only are many old people ignorant about the energy content of food, they know very little about fibre content and this topic and the benefits of fibre should also be included in health education.

Exercise (see p. 162)

Almost every old person would benefit from increasing the amount of exercise taken. This applies as much to the chairbound 90-year old as to the person who is retiring early at 60. Cycling and swimming are the best forms of exercise for people who have arthritis (see p. 168) but any type of exercise which is enjoyed is beneficial. An old person may safely increase the amount of exercise he takes without consulting a doctor provided that he does not suffer from heart or lung disease or any other chronic disease and provided that he increases the work load gradually (Fentem and Bassey 1978).

Smoking

Although an old person who stops smoking cannot expect a dramatic increase in his life expectation his health will improve. A chronic cough will clear up, the sense of taste and smell will improve and the elderly cigarette smoker will cope better with acute chest infections if he manages to stop smoking.

Because the benefits of smoking cessation are less than for younger smokers the approach to the older smoker should be less forceful. For example, it is appropriate to say to a group of men at a pre-retirement class that each smoker should note the amount he smokes during his week at work and should take care that he never smokes any more than this during the remainder of his life. The elderly smoker should, or course, not just be encouraged to ensure that his intake does not increase. He should be advised to stop and an appeal to the example he sets to his grandchildren may stimulate him to try. Many elderly people find it inconceivable that they will be able to change the habit of 30 or 40 years and for this reason it may be useful to ask a smoker not to increase his intake for the three months after retirement to demonstrate his ability to control his smoking before encouraging him to stop completely.

Accidents

Elderly people should also be advised to take care on the roads, whether as pedestrian, cyclist, or drivers or passengers. The need to wear a seat belt should be emphasized although this exhortation may be ignored by the person who has driven for 40 years and 'never needed a seat belt yet'. Advice on the benefits of a headrest to prevent whiplash injuries may be adopted more readily because the elderly person will usually have evidence of the changes which are taking place in his spinal column and in this context the need for seat belts may be accepted if the dangers of low speed collisions in traffic jams are emphasized.

Advice on home safety should also be given (see p. 228).

Mental health

Finally it is important to reassure the old person about mental illness because many are very afraid of dementia. Elderly people should be advised to stay active and involved as much as possible, and to try to remember at all times that any physical or mental change which takes place should not be assumed to be a consequence of aging. It is important for an old person to remember his past and to forget his age.

REFERENCES

Blythe, R. (1979). *The view in winter: reflections on old age.* Allan Lane, London.

Department of Health and Social Security (1972). A nutritional survey of the elderly at home. Report on Health and Social Subjects, No. 3. London.

—— (1980). A nutritional survey of the elderly at home. Report on Health and Social Subjects. No. 16. London.

Disabled Living Foundation (1979). *The elderly person with failing vision.*

Fentem, P. H. and Bassey, J. (1978). *The case for exercise.* The Sports Council.

This is an excellent brief summary of the benefits of exercise with all the main references cited. A more detailed, and therefore much longer, review of the subject is *Physical activity and ageing*, by R. J. Shephard, Croom Helm (1981).

Fox, R. H., Woodward, P. M., Exton-Smith, A. N., Green, M. F., Dennison, D. V., and Wicks, M. M. (1973). *Br. med. J.* i, 200–6.

The full report of this study is *Old and cold* by Malcolm Wicks (Heinemann, 1978). In addition *The elderly at home* by Audrey Hunt (HMSO, 1978) gives very useful information about the types of heating used by elderly people.

Gilkes, M. J. (1979). Eyes run on light. *Br. med. J.* i, 1681–3.

Gray, J. A. M. and Mackenzie, H. (1979). *Take care of your elderly relative.* Allen and Unwin, Beaconsfield.

This is a relative's handbook summarizing all the main benefits and services available for relatives who are caring for an elderly parent.

—— and Wilcock, G. (1981). *Our elders,* pp. 26–60. Oxford University Press.

Hannay, D. R. (1979). *The symptom iceberg. A study of community health.* Routledge and Kegan Paul, London.

Herbert, K. G. and Humphrey, C. (1980). Hearing impairment and mental state in the elderly living at home. *Br. med. J.* **ii**, 903–5.

Isaacs, B. (1971). Geriatric patients: do their patients care? *Br. med. J.* **iii**, 282–6.

Knox, J. D. E. (1980). Prescribing for the elderly in general practice. A review of current literature. Supplement I. *J. R. Coll. Gen. Practns* **30**.

See also the article 'Improving drug compliance in general practice' by J. M. Graham and D. A. Supree, *J. R. Coll. Gen. Practns* **29**, 399–404 (1979).

Moroney, R. M. (1976). *The family and the State.* Longman, London.

This short book makes stimulating and encouraging reading reviewing the trends in family care for elderly and mentally handicapped people.

Tulloch, A. J. (1981). Repeat prescribing for elderly patients. *Br. med. J.* **282**, 1672–5.

—— and Moore, V. (1979). A randomized controlled trial of geriatric screening and surveillance in general practice. *J. R. Coll. Gen. Practns* **29**, 733–42.

For a more detailed analysis of screening see Williamson (1981) and for other descriptions of practical approaches to screening see pages 91–115 in *The care of the elderly in the community* by Idris Williams (Croom Helm, 1979), and the paper on 'Assessment of the elderly in general practice' by J. H. Barber and J. B. Wallis, *J. R. Coll. Gen. Practns* **26**, 106–14 (1976).

Wilcock, G. K., Gray, J. A. M., and Pritchard, P. M. M. (1982). *Geriatric medicine in general practice.* Oxford University Press.

Williamson, J. (1981). Screening surveillance and case finding. In *Health care of the elderly* (ed. T. Arie) pp. 194–214. Croom Helm, London.

——, Stokoe, I. H., Gray, S., Fisher, M., Smith, A., McGhee, A., and Stephenson, E. (1969). Old people at home: their unreported needs. *Lancet* **i**, 1117–20.

17 The future of preventive medicine in general practice

Godfrey Fowler and Muir Gray

INTRODUCTION

In the past hundred years medicine has been subject to a therapeutic explosion. As was outlined in Chapter 1, the important developments in medical care in the nineteenth century were based on the preventive approach; opportunities for effective therapeutic intervention were limited. By contrast the present century has seen a vast and escalating development in pharmacological and other treatments with the comparative neglect of prevention. However, it now seems clear that the law of diminishing returns is operating in relation to medical treatment and that the pendulum is swinging again towards prevention.

Acknowledgement of the greater potential for prevention rather than cure in the large proportion of ill health which is now behaviourally determined is an important factor in this change. Recent official statements have highlighted the need for a greater emphasis on prevention (DHSS 1976, 1981).

But a generation of doctors whose education and training have been orientated towards pharmacological magic cannot easily forsake the magician's wand for the teacher's skills. Nor do the demand-orientated nature of medical services and the concern with instant remedy rather than future health facilitate such a change. Moreover, on a practical level such demands and concerns may be so overwhelming that there is little inclination, time, or energy for the additional work involved in prevention.

As has been argued, if preventive medicine is to be practised effectively this must be at the primary care level for many reasons, chief of which is the access which this alone provides to the population concerned, particularly those most at risk, and because it is the identification and management of this group which is most urgent and most important. But its achievement in general practice depends on the incorporation of preventive medicine into existing patterns of work – the union of prevention with cure and care.

But the general practitioner is dependent on many factors which he cannot influence or control. For example, it is difficult to persuade people who are living in conditions of deprivation and uncertainty and who see no prospect of a stable and prosperous future, to review and then try to influence their future health, and factors such as economic stability, the levels of unemployment and the feelings of alienation experienced by those who are deprived materially or socially, all influence the social and cultural context in which the general practitioner works and tries to practise preventive medicine. But the general practitioner will have an important part to play in preventive medicine whatever the state of the economy.

BENEFITS OF GENERAL PRACTICE

As has been pointed out, general practice has considerable advantages as a medium for prevention.

Frequency of contact

The general practitioner sees at least two-thirds of his patients every year and more than 90 per cent at least once every five years. Increasingly important as social mobility increases individuals who move register with a new general practitioner soon after their move, so that the Practice list is the most accurate and up to date Register which is accessible to doctors and health workers.

Trust

In spite of an increase in complaints about general practice, the general practitioner is still the most trusted source of advice for many people; a study of all sources of health advice found that 'of all the many and varied sources of health information available to the adult population, it is the GP who is most trusted and whose advice has most impact' (McCron and Budd 1979). However, this trust is not conferred on general practitioners automatically; it grows as the relationship develops between the doctor and his patients, both individual patients and the population he serves as a whole because the reputation which the doctor has in his community influences individuals who are consulting him for the first time. Because the doctor–patient relationship is so difficult to measure and quantify, the evidence of its effects does not, in our opinion, reflect its importance. However, the studies which have been conducted on the effect of the doctor–patient relationship suggest what many general practitioners will have observed for themselves, that the quality of the relationship is of fundamental importance in achieving compliance (Pendleton *et al.* 1983).

Furthermore, the evidence gathered by Ann Cartwright and Robert Anderson in their study *General practice revisited* showed that home visits were particularly important in establishing the type of relationship in which preventive medicine could be most effectively given. They reported that 'the number of home visits patients had received in the last year was clearly related to their satisfaction with their care, to their views of their relationship with their doctor as being friendly rather than businesslike, to their assessment of whether or not they would consult their doctor about a personal problem that worried them, and to whether they found their doctor an easy person to talk to'

(Cartwright and Anderson 1981). In preventive medicine therefore home visiting has an important part to play.

Liaison with other professionals

Undoubtedly the term Team has been loosely and often inaccurately used, but the opportunity of working with health visitors and district nurses and of developing a closer relationship with social and voluntary services offers tremendous scope for prevention; but it does require a concerted effort and the full involvement of everyone who works with the general practitioner. The importance of the receptionist and practice manager is only beginning to be recognized but there are encouraging signs that real team work is developing (Pritchard 1982).

THE NEEDS OF GENERAL PRACTITIONERS

To improve their effectiveness general practitioners have three main needs: better information, more effective approach, and more time.

Better information

Not only is more information about risk factors needed but this type of information must be presented in ways which the general practitioner can use easily and effectively. Furthermore it must be complemented by information about beliefs and attitudes about disease and risk which prevail in his community, together with information on the approaches which have been most effective in achieving change. To do this requires epidemiologists and social scientists to be prepared to translate their findings into conclusions which will be more useful to those who meet the public than they are at present. National organizations such as the Health Education Council and the Scottish Health Education Group and the various special interest groups such as Action on Smoking and Health or locally community physicians and health education officers, can act as translators, but this does not reduce the need for closer links and greater interchange between research workers and the practitioners of preventive medicine.

A more effective approach

The increasing number of studies on drug compliance demonstrates how ineffective doctors are as educators and this is also true in preventive medicine. In part, effectiveness can be improved by improving the doctor–patient relationship and by observing a few simple rules of communication. As has been discussed in Chapter 4 it would be simplistic to consider the transfer of information as implying education and behaviour change. Amongst the factors influencing compliance are the individual's health beliefs including their perceived personal vulnerability, their perception of the seriousness of the disease and the 'costs' and 'benefits' of the advice. Readiness to accept and act on advice, particularly about lifestyles, may also depend on certain cues such as personal feelings, the influence of family and friends, magazine articles, television programmes, and so on. As has been discussed, satisfaction with the doctor giving the advice and particularly with the consultation in which it is given are also important influences. Doctors must avoid moralizing, being judgmental, imposing their own values, and inducing feelings of blame or guilt. The task is not easy!

Patients too need to help to bring about this shift in the direction of medical care. Their expectations must be of receiving advice rather than medication and there is evidence of a shift in this direction (Cartwright and Anderson 1981).

More time

Preventive medicine may save resources in the long term, but it requires a considerable commitment in the short term and more time needs to be devoted to prevention than is the case at present. One way to give more time to doctors would be to increase their numbers and thus decrease the average list size. Although this could increase the time available for prevention, other options can also be defined and these include:

More effective patient education about the management of self-limiting disease. There is evidence that the consultation rate for acute self-limiting conditions which have probably declined in Britain during the 1970s can be further reduced by appropriate education (Morrell *et al.* 1980).

The management of psychosocial problems by a practice counsellor (Anderson and Hasler 1979) or attached social worker or clinical psychologist.

The performance of tasks such as measurement of blood pressure by other workers who have been suitably trained. The scope for this is limited until we know how effective other workers such as the health visitor or practice nurse are in patient education and how they see their contribution to it, but there is evidence to suggest that they can be equally effective if there is sufficient time for a good relationship between the health worker and the patient to develop (Marsh 1977).

The referral of patients with chronic musculoskeletal problems to a physiotherapist or yoga teacher.

What is required therefore is a reduction in demand on medical time coupled with a reorientation of the work of the doctor and all the other members of the team from a pattern of work which is dominated by patient demand (Tudor Hart's 'medical shopkeeping') to one in which a proportion of the initiatives are those taken by members of the primary health care team.

RESOURCES WITHIN THE TEAM

How well the primary care team actually functions as a team is a matter for debate and research, but there is no doubt that doctors and community nurses and health visitors have worked more closely together since practice attachment was introduced in the 1960s. This, helped and supported by receptionists and, more recently, practice managers, has improved the effectiveness and efficiency of primary care. There is however scope for further development.

The nurse

The main possible contribution of the district (community) nurse to prevention is with older people; the main constraint is again time.

The new style of training introduced in 1981 lays much more emphasis on the social aspects of disease and on patients education than the previous pattern of training which is much more limited both in time and scope. In theory the trained nurse will be able to delegate more of the routine 'general care' tasks to the nursing auxilliary, leaving here time to concentrate on the more difficult nursing tasks and to take on some of the type of work done by the health visitor at present, for example giving advice on prevention either to individual old people or to groups such as old people's clubs. In practice, however, the nurse's ability to develop her work in this way will depend on the amount of resources made available to community nursing. The increase in the number of very elderly will require an increase in the number of district nurses and nursing auxilliaries merely to be able to provide the same type and level of service as they do at present. To take on new tasks will require more resources.

Although community nurses employed by Health Authorities may also work in practice treatment rooms, an increasing number of nurses are directly employed by general practitioners as practice nurses to do such work. While the major role of such 'treatment room sisters' may be seen as the performance of treatment tasks, these team members have an increasingly important function in relation to prevention. Not only may they, like the doctor, offer health education and preventive activities on an opportunistic basis, but they may also play a vital role in programmes for the detection and monitoring of hypertension, in cervical cytology, as well as in their more traditional prophylactic immunization role.

The health visitor

The health visitor is the one member of the team whose training is specifically geared to health education and preventive medicine. She (or more rarely he) is an independent professional who identifies people in need on her own personal initiative as well as acting on referrals from general practitioners, social services, voluntary organizations or members of the community. Her training sharpens her capacity to detect early deviation from the norm and knowledge of the helping organizations enables her to work out a programme of help for the individual when required. Her knowledge of health education means that she can select the method most likely to be successful in any particular instance.

Understanding and appreciation by the general practitioner of the health visitor's role and skills will increase her development and contribution within the primary health care team as well as benefiting the community which both members serve. The interaction between the two is therefore important. It is essential that the fundamental differences between the function of the health visitor and the general practitioner are understood by both parties. The health visitor must, in the majority of cases, make her own decision about whether to offer services, many of her calls being made to clients who may not have asked for a visit. The general practitioner, on the other hand, sees mainly members of the community who have made a request for advice and help usually by coming to the surgery or health centre. It is probably the less practical nursing skills and the emphasis on primary preventive work which is less easy to evaluate and in which to see tangible results which has contributed to the finding that, despite 18 years of general practice attachment of health visitors, many general practitioners are so ignorant of the possibilities of involvement with community nursing staff, let alone the potential of health visitors. Debate continues about the benefit and disadvantages of such attachments. The advantages of knowing the 'at risk' people in a defined geographical neighbourhood must be weighed against the benefits of improved communications between the two professionals which attachment facilitates.

The quality of health visiting is affected by the philosophy and priorities of Health Authorities, some restricting development and others encouraging professional growth. The skills of the health visitor can be used in any situation and although she has to date concentrated here work on the mother and baby and on the care of the elderly, current health problems require a shift of emphasis towards her responsibilities for health education. Suggestions such as health visitors assuming some of the responsibility for health education for middle aged adults in the practice need to be discussed with all members of primary health care teams. If advantage is to be taken of the fact that more than 90 per cent of the population is in contact with general practice at least once every five years, then greater flexibility in the working roles of nurses, health visitors and doctors are needed to accomodate the responsibility for prevention. No other worker at present combines the knowledge and skills which the health visitor gains from her nursing background and post-nursing training and in this she has a unique contribution to make to her colleagues and the public whom she serves.

The receptionist and practice manager

These two team members, sometimes clearly distinguished, sometimes embodied in one person, have a great contribution to make to prevention. But they can only do this if they are drawn fully into the planning of preventive services.

The practice manager can help in the re-orientation of the practice from response only to demands to a position in which it initiates preventive services. In particular she will be responsible for the development and maintenance of a record system which can be used as a basis for prevention. The receptionist is more directly concerned in the delivery of preventive services; in checking the notes when a patient makes an appointment to identify the preventive measures which are needed; in prompting whichever professionals are responsible for performing the test or giving advice; and in booking their follow-up appointment if that should be necessary. There is no reason why the receptionist should not be trained to perform some of the tests, checking the weight or height, or measuring blood pressure for example, for she, like the practice manager, is a health worker, not simply an administrator.

Patient groups

Finally it is important to remember that patients themselves have considerable resources and their participation in prevention can be of assistance to the professionals in the team. Practice patient participation groups may suggest more effective ways of practising prevention than are apparent to health professionals. Patient clubs and groups can help by organizing discussion and support over diet, smoking, alcohol, handicaps, marital stress, and bereavement. Practice classes and groups such as ante-natal classes, post-natal support groups, relaxation and yoga classes, all have a valuable role.

COMMUNITY MEDICINE

The key role that Community Medicine has to play in the promotion of preventive medicine in general practice has been referred to in Chapter 2. Community Medicine has been accused by Acheson of having 'a bird's eye view of medicine that seems all strategy and no combat'. It might equally be said that general practice has a myopic view of medicine which is all combat and no strategy. The scope for co-operation between the two is therefore substantial. Traditionally the role of the medical officer of health in relation to preventive medicine was substantial. This function can best be performed in his successor by the facilitation of preventive medicine in general practice. Practice attachment of Health Authority staff such as nurses and health visitors is one aspect of this. Support for local Health Education Units and encouragement of stronger links with the medical care system should also be pursued. But the main role of Community Medicine in preventive medicine in general practice is that of 'facilitator' – initiating, assisting, and co-ordinating such work in primary care teams.

MEDICAL EDUCATION

But changes in the attitudes and behaviour of doctors are the most important requirements for a shift towards the practice of preventive medicine in primary care. Medical education must play an important part in bringing such changes about by demonstrating that it is no longer sufficient for the doctor to concern himself solely with newly presenting or continuing clinical problems.

Basic medical education remains almost entirely hospital based. Because of this undue emphasis on pathology, advanced disease, and acute, even crisis medical care. The heroics of salvage are what medical care is seen to be about. The causes of ill health and the importance of environmental, occupational, social, and interpersonal influences on health receive little attention. Prevention is seen as unexciting – and impracticable anyway. Compared with the drama of the coronary care unit the prevention of myocardial infarction in middle age by stopping a man in his twenties smoking, is very dull and unglamorous.

But increasing emphasis on using general practice as an environment for medical student teaching, provides opportunities to demonstrate the scope and practice of preventive medicine. Basic medical education has remained under the dominant influence of diagnostic and therapeutic hospital wizards, whose magic has been enhanced by the acquisition of yet more sophisticated tools and skills. Technological advances have encouraged the neglect of the counselling, advisory and educational roles of the doctor. The development in recent years of general practice teaching of medical students provides an opportunity to remedy this, to complement and balance hospital-based, disease-orientated teaching of technologically intensive medical care with that of the less technically sophisticated patient orientated family care in the community.

Increasing awareness of the importance of human behaviour as a major determinant of illness in modern society, especially well illustrated by smoking related diseases, demands that greater emphasis be placed in medical education on learning the skills of patient communication and education. Even in hospital, diagnosis in the majority of cases is established on the basis of history alone, investigations making a significant contribution in less than 10 per cent of cases (Hampton *et al.* 1975). Above all attitudes must change so that preventive medicine is no longer seen as the poor relation of exciting, acute hospital medical care.

General Practice vocational training must become more concerned with health education and with the desirability and feasibility of health promotion through behaviour change. Co-operation with other members of the practice team, with colleagues in Community Medicine, with Health Education Units and with organizations like the Health Education Council, should be encouraged and facilitated. Training programmes should include opportunities to explore with such colleagues the avenues for co-operative effort and should demonstrate the availability and use of relevant teaching aids and other resources.

Continuing education for general practitioners must likewise place greater emphasis on health promotion not – as at present – be largely confined to updating knowledge about disease. As with vocational training it should include opportunities to explore with other health care professionals ways and means of achieving better preventive care. The potential for preventive medicine in general practice needs to be demonstrated to general practitioners and evidence of its effectiveness used to dispel feelings of impotence. Such evidence is now forthcoming (Russell *et al.* 1979; Morrell *et al.* 1980).

At all educational levels the major change required is the attitudinal one – the recognition of health promotion as a respectable medical activity, inseparable from the accepted ones of curing and caring.

THE COMMITMENT OF GENERAL PRACTICE

General practitioners are independent contractors and it is this independence that is attractive to doctors who choose it as a career and that allows for the type of service offered by general practitioners to evolve and adapt to the particular needs of the community they serve. In this world of independent contractors, the Royal College of General Practitioners has a difficult but, we believe, important part to play, for its efforts to encourage the evolution of general practice have been met with indifference in some quarters and with outright hostility in others.

One of the important functions of the College is to collect the views of general practitioners about what could be done to offer a more effective and efficient service to the community and, in 1981/2, it published five reports on health and prevention in primary care which are documents of considerable significance not only for general practitioners but for the Health Service as a whole (RCGP 1981/82). The central theme which emerged was that general practitioners could practise effective preventive medicine, but that to do so they would not only need more resources but also a different approach which took into account the needs of the whole community of patients they served without detracting from the quality of the key element of general practice, the commitment of the general practitioner to the needs of the individual who has trusted him with their health care.

REFERENCES

Anderson, S. and Hasler, J. C. (1979: Counselling in general practice. *J. R. Coll. Gen. Practrs* 29, 352.

Cartwright, A. (1967). *Patients and their doctors. A study of general practice.* Routledge and Kegan Paul, London.

—— and Anderson, R. (1981). *General practice revisited. A second study of patients and their doctors.* Tavistock Publications, London.

Department of Health and Social Security (1976). *Prevention and health: everybody's business. A reassessment of public and personal health.* HMSO, London.

—— (1981). *Care in action. A handbook of policies and priorities for health and personal social services in England.* HMSO, London.

Hampton, J. R., Harrison, M. J. G., Mitchell, J. R. A., Pritchard, J. S., and Seymour, S. (1975). Relative contributions of history taking, physical examination and laboratory investigation to diagnosis and management of medical outpatients. *Br. med. J.* ii, 486–9.

McCron, R. and Budd, J. (1979). Communication and health education: a preliminary study. Unpublished document prepared for the Health Education Council, University of Leicester Centre for Mass Communication Research, October 1979. Chapter 8.

Marsh, G. (1977). 'Curing' minor illness in general practice. *Br. med. J.* **ii**, 1267.

Morrell, D. C., Avery, A. J., and Watkins, C. J. (1980). Management of minor illness. *Br. med. J.* **280**, 769.

Pendleton, D., Tate, P., Havelock, P., and Schofield, T. (1983). *The consultation: an approach to learning and teaching.* Oxford University Press.

Pritchard, P. M. M. (1982). *Manual of primary health care: its nature and organization,* 2nd edn. Oxford University Press.

Russell, M. A. H., Wilson, C., Taylor, C., and Baker, C. D. Effect of general practitioners' advice against smoking. *Br. med. J.* **ii**, 231.

Stott, N. C. H. and Davis, R. H. (1979). The exceptional potential of each primary care consultation. *J. R. Coll. Gen. Practs* **29**, 201.

Index

accident prevention 229–42
  and alcohol 181
airways obstruction, effects of exercise 166
alcohol 180–207
anticipatory care 21
arthritis, effects of exercise 168
ASH (Action on Smoking and Health) 87
asthma 14, 166

back pain, effects of exercise 168
bereavement 221
breast cancer 110–12
bronchitis 14, 136

cancer 8–14
  alcohol and 182
  cervical 107–10
  lung 133
case-finding 21, 94
cervical cytology 107–10
childhood
  screening in 99, 137
  smoking 138
circulatory system, effects of alcohol 182
communication skills 63
community medicine 281
compliance 59
computer 41
consultation 28, 62
coronary heart disease 5, 9–11, 105, 134–6, 149–52
  and exercise 164–5
cost-benefit analysis 70, 117
cycling accidents 233

dental caries 155
depression 221–5
diabetes 106, 112–13
  effects of exercise 167
  and driving 236
diet 149–59
  and cancer 11
dietary fibre 156–9
disability, prevention of 243–56
diverticular disease 154

environmental health officer 124
ethical problems 57, 95
exercise 160–78
  hazards of 169–73
  in old age 272

fitness to drive 235

glaucoma 113–14

handicap, prevention of 243–56
health beliefs 60
  of older people 258
health education 56–85
Health Education Council 125
health education officers 125
health visitors 279
  and home safety 124
high blood pressure 99, 165, 183
  effects of exercise 166
home accidents 230–3

iceberg of morbidity 23
ischaemic heart disease 5, 9–11, 105, 134–6
  and diet 149–52
  and exercise 164–5

lipids 151
lung cancer 133

medical education 281
Members of Parliament 86–93, 125
mental handicap 16
mental illness 16, 208–28
  in old age 268
multiphasic screening 114

nurses in prevention 279–80
nutrition 149–59
  alcohol 181
  in old age 270
obesity 153
  exercise in 167
old age 257–74
  home accidents 230
  exercise in 162
  road traffic accidents 233, 239
osteoporosis 167

passive smoking 139
patient education 56–85
peripheral vascular disease 165
politics of prevention 86–93
practice manager 280
pregnancy, screening in 98
primary prevention 20
psychotherapy 216

receptionist 280
records 33–55
risk factors 20, 105
road traffic accidents 124, 233–42
Royal College of General Practitioners 125

schizophrenia 16
Scottish Health Education Group 125
screening 20, 94–116, 268–71
secondary prevention 20
sickness absence 17–19

smoking 133–48
  in old age 272
stroke 7
suicide 184, 225

team, primary care 278
tertiary prevention 21

voluntary groups 124

women's health problems 136